NGHAM

NEUROPLASTICITY AND REHABILITATION

Neuroplasticity and Rehabilitation

Edited by

Sarah A. Raskin

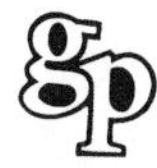

THE GUILFORD PRESS
New York London

A Division of Guilford Publications, Inc.
72 Spring Street, New York, NY 10012
www.guilford.com

Printed in the United States of America

This book is printed on acid-free paper.

Last digit is print number: 9 8 7 6 5 4 3 2 1

The authors have checked with sources believed to be reliable in their efforts to provide information that is complete and generally in accord with the standards of practice that are accepted at the time of publication. However, in view of the possibility of human error or changes in behavioral, mental health, or medical sciences, neither the authors, nor the editor and publisher, nor any other party who has been involved in the preparation or publication of this work warrants that the information contained herein is in every respect accurate or complete, and they are not responsible for any errors or omissions or the results obtained from the use of such information. Readers are encouraged to confirm the information contained in this book with other sources.

Library of Congress Cataloging-in-Publication Data is available from the Publisher

ISBN 978-1-60918-137-6

About the Editor

Sarah A. Raskin, PhD, is a board certified clinical neuropsychologist and Professor of Psychology and Neuroscience at Trinity College in Hartford, Connecticut. Dr. Raskin has published numerous articles investigating neuropsychological functions and cognitive rehabilitation for people with a variety of disorders, including brain injury and Parkinson's disease. She has a particular interest in assessment and treatment of prospective memory. She has served on the Board of Directors of the Brain Injury Association of Connecticut and facilitated a brain injury support group for 15 years. Dr. Raskin is coauthor, with Catherine A. Mateer, of *Neuropsychological Management of Mild Traumatic Brain Injury* and creator of the Memory for Intentions Test, a standardized clinical measure of prospective memory. In addition, she is currently funded for work investigating the cognitive and neurophysiological effects of alcohol use in college students.

Contributors

C. Scott Bickel, PT, PhD, Department of Physical Therapy, School of Health Professions, University of Alabama at Birmingham, Birmingham, Alabama

Scott Bury, PhD, Landon Center on Aging, University of Kansas Medical Center, Kansas City, Kansas

Jan Cioe, PhD, Department of Psychology, University of British Columbia, Kelowna, British Columbia, Canada

Jennifer A. Engle, PhD, Department of Psychology, Sunny Hill Health Centre for Children, Vancouver, British Columbia, Canada

John C. Freeland, PhD, Brain Injury Rehabilitation Trust, York, North Yorkshire, United Kingdom

Julianne T. Garbarino, Department of Psychology, Trinity College, Hartford, Connecticut

Leslie J. Gonzalez Rothi, PhD, CCC-SLP, Brain Rehabilitation Research Center, Malcolm Randall Department of Veterans Affairs Medical Center, Gainesville, Florida

Theresa A. Jones, PhD, Department of Psychology and Neuroscience Institute, University of Texas at Austin, Austin, Texas

Kimberly A. Kerns, PhD, Department of Psychology, University of Victoria, Victoria, British Columbia, Canada

Bryan Kolb, PhD, Canadian Centre for Behavioural Neuroscience, University of Lethbridge, Lethbridge, Alberta, Canada

Susan A. Leon, PhD, CCC-SLP, Department of Neurology, University of Florida, Gainesville, Florida

Rema A. Lillie, MSc, Department of Psychology, University of Victoria, Victoria, British Columbia, Canada

Lynn M. Maher, PhD, CCC-SLP, Department of Communication Sciences and Disorders, University of Houston, Houston, Texas

Catherine A. Mateer, PhD, Department of Psychology, University of Victoria, Victoria, British Columbia, Canada

Ginger N. Mills, Neuroscience Program, Trinity College, Hartford, Connecticut

David M. Morris, PT, MS, PhD, Department of Physical Therapy, School of Health Professions, University of Alabama at Birmingham, Birmingham, Alabama

Randolph J. Nudo, PhD, Landon Center on Aging, University of Kansas Medical Center, Kansas City, Kansas

Redmond G. O'Connell, PhD, School of Psychology and Trinity College Institute of Neuroscience, Trinity College Dublin, Dublin, Ireland

Laurie Ehlhardt Powell, PhD, Teaching Research Institute–Eugene, Western Oregon University, Eugene, Oregon

Sarah A. Raskin, PhD, Department of Psychology and Neuroscience Program, Trinity College, Hartford, Connecticut

Ian H. Robertson, PhD, School of Psychology and Trinity College Institute of Neuroscience, Trinity College Dublin, Dublin, Ireland

Bennett A. Shaywitz, MD, Departments of Pediatrics and Neurology; Yale Center for Dyslexia, Creativity, and Other Learning Attributes; and Yale Center for the Study of Learning, Reading, and Attention, Yale University School of Medicine, New Haven, Connecticut

Sally E. Shaywitz, MD, Departments of Pediatrics and Neurology; Yale Center for Dyslexia, Creativity, and Other Learning Attributes; and Yale Center for the Study of Learning, Reading, and Attention, Yale University School of Medicine, New Haven, Connecticut

McKay Moore Sohlberg, PhD, Department of Communication Disorders and Sciences, University of Oregon, Eugene, Oregon

Yaakov Stern, PhD, Cognitive Neuroscience Division of the Taub Institute, and Departments of Neurology and Psychiatry, Columbia University College of Physicians and Surgeons, New York, New York

Preston Williams, MA, Canadian Centre for Behavioural Neuroscience, University of Lethbridge, Lethbridge, Alberta, Canada

Acknowledgments

I would like to thank all of the individuals who contributed to this volume in countless ways—principally by sharing stories of the impact of their cognitive deficits in daily life, and by volunteering to be research participants in the numerous studies cited throughout this book.

I would also like to thank all of the contributors to this volume. In some ways, the task put before them required them to reinterpret their data from a new perspective. Each of the authors has done tremendous and thoughtful work in trying to translate basic research in plasticity into clinical practice. I am grateful not only for their insights, but for their patience in waiting for all of the chapters to be completed.

At Trinity College, both Holly Brunette and Ann St. Amand have been a tremendous help with the completion of this book. Michael Smith and Carol Buckheit have been instrumental as well. Many Trinity College students have also helped with different aspects of this book, including Amanda Waxman, Elizabeth Gromisch, Ferrinne Spector, Margaret Moult, Elan Jones, Tamara Nicol Medina, Brian Harel, Andrew Castiglione, Deniz Vatansever, Nora Murphy, Carrie Edwards, Hanna Ghaleb, Jacqueline Maye, Navneet Kaur, Christina Palmese, Suzanne Fallon, Kristina Depeau, Miriam Zichlin, Jessica Hansen, and Alexandra Rogers. I would also like to thank all of my colleagues in the Department of Psychology and the Neuroscience Program. Some aspects of this book were supported by funding from the Trinity College Faculty Research Committee. Ideas found in this book were influenced by conversations over the years with Allen Raskin and Wayne Gordon.

Rochelle Serwator at The Guilford Press has been a helpful, encouraging, enthusiastic, and, most of all, patient editor. I thank her not only for her unflagging support, but for all of her editorial insights, suggestions, and comments.

I thank my husband, Brian Waddell, for his constant advice, support, and love, not to mention editorial assistance. I thank Emma and Julian for being exactly who they are.

SARAH A. RASKIN

Contents

NEUROPLASTICITY AND REHABILITATION

CHAPTER 1

Introduction

Current Approaches to Rehabilitation

SARAH A. RASKIN

Perhaps the greatest finding in neuroscience in the past decade is that adult cortical representations are not fixed. Indeed, not only is there the possibility of cortical map plasticity and cortical synaptic plasticity, but is also appears that these mechanisms are responsible for learning. Research is only beginning to reveal the mechanisms that lead to plastic changes in the adult brain. However, recent literature on experience-dependent changes, including ones that are practice-dependent, can be used to inform future studies in motor and cognitive rehabilitation. For example, repeated use of a particular cognitive process during training should strengthen connections in the underlying neural circuitry and consequently should produce an increase in cognitive capacity. The aim for both cognitive and motor rehabilitation is that benefits should generalize to any unpracticed task that recruits the same underlying function; thus the ultimate goal is to produce improvements that are transferable beyond a controlled laboratory setting and can alleviate functional impairments in everyday activities. Toward this end, some rehabilitation researchers are beginning to use findings in plasticity to inform their research, and to use neuroimaging techniques to measure brain changes related to treatment.

Rehabilitation is generally thought of as comprising one of two types of interventions. The first type consists of interventions that target change at the level of behavior (i.e., *behavioral approaches*); the second consists of those that target change at the level of restitution (i.e., *restorative approaches*). Behavioral approaches are thought to involve compensating for a function that has been lost, whereas restorative/restitution approaches aim to improve the lost function itself. In more recent years, a third category has been added: therapies targeting metacognition or self-regulation.

Teaching the use of external compensatory aids to prompt people to complete planned tasks at target times is an example of a behavioral intervention. Such interventions may also include teaching a new behavior or substitute skill (e.g., teaching persons with memory loss to make lists for shopping; teaching persons with hemiplegia to tie their shoes with their less affected arm exclusively) and/or an encouraging increase in time, effort, or both (e.g., more studying). An injured person may also adapt to a new situation by changing self-expectations, selecting new tasks, or relaxing the criteria for success. Whether people are taught to use a compensation or develop it on their own, they are active participants in its application.

Direct restitutive interventions use procedures that aim to improve or restore some underlying ability or cognitive capacity. Examples of restorative, impairment-based interventions include direct attention training (a drill-oriented therapy with hierarchical exercises designed to decrease attention deficits) and the administration of functional activities with the more affected arm to attempt to reestablish pathways affected by hemiplegia.

An example of a metacognitive approach is training people in the use of strategies or systems that facilitate self-monitoring during task completion. All three types of approaches—behavioral, restorative, and metacognitive—are useful as appropriate, and are generally used in combination.

Given these categories, it has been assumed that direct interventions are those most likely to lead to plastic changes in the brain. However, it should be remembered that brain changes can also be considered to be compensations or recovery. A *compensation* occurs when a noninjured brain region takes over the function of the injured region. True *recovery* involves improvement in function in an injured area. Thus, throughout this book, chapter authors discuss a wide variety of brain changes that have been measured and try to map these changes onto potential rehabilitation techniques, be they compensatory (behavioral), direct (restorative), or metacognitive.

In Chapter 2 of this volume, Kolb, Cioe, and Williams provide a basic overview of the mechanisms that underlie both cortical map plasticity and cortical synaptic plasticity. These authors have identified critical principles of plasticity that can be used to inform rehabilitation approaches. The first is that changes in the brain can be shown at many levels, including cellular, synaptic, systems, and *in vivo* levels. The second is that the brain can be altered by a wide range of experiences, and that experience-dependent changes can be long-lasting. The third is that training studies must be aware of the specific systems being targeted by the training and of how these systems react to experience such as the training procedures. The fourth is that experience-dependent changes interact. In addition, of course, some plastic changes reflect compensation while others reflect recovery, and the treatment must specifically be designed with one or the other in mind. In other words, in some cases the plasticity involves an intact cortical region's taking on the tasks once mediated by the damaged region. In other cases, it is now suggested, damaged regions can actually recover and resume previous functions.

The rest of the chapters in Part I of this book focus on experience-based cortical reorganization. First, Jones (Chapter 3) discusses changes observed in nonhuman animal models, particularly rodent models. She provides an important discussion of reactive synaptogenesis and neurogenesis, making the points that not all such connections are functional, and that functional connections take time to develop. She lays out the considerable evidence from her work and that of others for a lesion–behavior interaction, such that lesion-induced degeneration followed by training leads to the formation of new synapses and dendrites only in the cortex contralateral to the behaving limb. She also reviews the literature on enriched environments, demonstrating that these environments promote the capacity for future learning and may lead to behavioral compensation. Thus environmental stimulation may affect the degree of plasticity after brain damage. Furthermore, Jones raises important findings about the benefits and limits of both exercise and forced use before and after brain injury. One of her most important points is that brain damage may place the brain in a particularly dynamic state, where greater plasticity may be possible.

In Chapter 4, Nudo and Bury focus on the current evidence for motor and sensory reorganization in primates, including the plasticity of cortical maps in mature animals. They begin with a comprehensive discussion of dynamic changes in the receptotopic organization of cerebral cortex in response to injury, which they suggest is due to unmasking at multiple levels of the somatosensory system. They provide evidence that this process involves two phases. The first is unmasking due to the disinhibition of tonically suppressed inputs mediated by gamma-aminobutyric acid, subtype a (GABAa). The second, longer phase is dendritic sprouting, perhaps mediated by *N*-methyl-D-aspartate (NMDA). Thus, they provide a theoretical basis for both early and late plasticity following injury. They also raise the importance of context-dependent reinforcement, which certainly has ramifications for human treatment approaches. Another direct human analogy is provided in the comparison of postinjury repetitive motor tasks in nonhuman animals and focal dystonia in humans, including evidence for disorganized primary somatosensory cortex (S1) maps in musicians with dystonia. This finding has led to a theoretically based treatment with splinting to reestablish independent digit sensation and movement. This chapter then turns to the important work of Nudo and others on the dynamic nature of motor maps in a series of seminal studies on motor skill learning and changes in cortical representation. Their exciting work using intracortical microstimulation suggests that compensatory mechanisms utilize unaffected cortical regions. One valuable lesson from their work is the importance of lesion size. That is, after a larger lesion, reorganization of adjacent regions may not be sufficient; therefore, reorganization may need to take place elsewhere in the cortex. They also document not just reorganization but novel postinjury connections formed through intracortical sprouting.

As this volume moves toward creating theoretical constructs to apply findings in neuroplasticity to the postinjury rehabilitation of humans, one of the important concepts to integrate is that of *cognitive reserve*. In Chapter 5, Stern not only reviews the considerable literature supporting the idea of cognitive reserve, but also explores possible explanatory mechanisms. This model has been used to explain why two people with similar lesion sizes may have widely different functional impairments. Cognitive reserve tends to be related to levels of intelligence, education, and occupational attainment. Thus, Stern points out, not only is brain reserve malleable by experience over a lifetime; these same lifetime experiences contribute to cognitive reserve and can affect recovery after brain damage. Cognitive reserve allows an individual with greater brain pathology to demonstrate symptoms and functional abilities equivalent to those of persons with a much lower degree of pathology. In a series of studies, Stern has demonstrated the possibility that individuals with greater cognitive reserve may be recruiting different network of brain regions to perform a cognitively demanding task—a form of neural compensation.

Chapter 6 is intended to provide a transition between the more theoretical experimental studies and those that are more clinical and applied. With my colleagues Mills and Garbarino, I look specifically in this chapter at practice-related changes in humans and research findings in humans, to suggest specific types of neuroplastic changes in response to experience in daily life. In particular, we note that the plasticity of motor and sensory systems may be different from that of cognitive functions. Training on sensory or motor tasks is most likely to result in an expanded cortical representation of the specific skills or processes required to perform the training tasks. In contrast, high-order cognitive tasks recruit a distributed network of regions whose activation is not determined by the specific sensory or motor requirements of the task. Consequently, increased efficiency of this network may be best achieved by increasing connectivity between regions and enhancing neural efficiency within regions.

Part II of the volume then turns to therapeutic approaches that take advantage of these findings. It begins with therapeutic approaches to motor functions. One area of treatment that has shown considerable promise is constraint-induced (CI) therapy. In Chapter 7, Morris and Bickel describe CI therapy, which is a prescribed, integrated, and systematic therapy designed to induce a patient to use a more impaired upper extremity many hours a day for several weeks (depending on the severity of the initial deficit). Some of the important elements are that the therapy requires repetitive, task-oriented training for a significant period of time (several hours a day for 10–15 consecutive weekdays). The use of a generalization procedure to transfer gains made in the research laboratory or clinical setting to the patient's real-world environment is essential. Finally, the hallmark of this therapy is constraining the patient to use the more impaired upper extremity during waking hours over the course of treatment, sometimes by restraining the less impaired upper extremity in a mitt or cuff.

Morris and Bickel also review locomotor training (LT), which is an approach to gait rehabilitation that provides truncal support while giving manual sensory signals on a moving treadmill. Participants are supported in a harness over a treadmill. The theoretical basis for LT is that the spinal cord has the capacity to integrate the afferent input and respond with an appropriate motor output through a network of spinal interneurons. In one study, the amount of body weight support required was reduced from 40% to 0% over a period of weeks. Thus findings from both CI therapy and LT demonstrate that both of these treatments lead to functional generalization in daily life. In the case of CI therapy, these changes are related to plasticity in neural systems. In particular, these authors describe evidence for an expansion of cortical representation of the affected limb, altered cortical activation with movement, altered cortical excitation, and altered cerebral blood flow.

Part II then turns to approaches to rehabilitating cognitive functions. Chapters 8 and 9 deal with treatment of cognitive deficits in children. Chapter 8 focuses on developmental dyslexia, and Chapter 9 focuses on acquired attention deficits in children after brain injury. In Chapter 8, Shaywitz and Shaywitz ground their discussion of treatment in the well-supported theory of dyslexia as a phonological disorder. In a series of studies using functional magnetic resonance imaging (fMRI), these authors demonstrate differences in activation between children with and without dyslexia in areas of activation when the children are required to read words and pseudowords, pointing particularly to a dysfunction in left-hemisphere posterior regions. Moreover, they have been able to show compensatory changes in older children with dyslexia as compared to younger children with dyslexia, suggesting experience-dependent changes in brain regions used for reading.

Engle and Kerns focus in Chapter 9 on children with acquired brain injury, those with attention-deficit/hyperactivity disorder (ADHD), and those with cancer affecting the central nervous system (CNS). One of the main approaches described in this chapter is the process approach to attention training, including the Pay Attention! materials designed by Kerns and her colleagues. These materials are theoretically grounded in a clinical model of attention and demonstrate the need to focus rehabilitation efforts on the specific aspect of attention that is deficient (e.g., sustained, divided, alternating). These materials are also hierarchically based, allowing for greater cognitive demand as an individual becomes proficient at each level.

In the chapter on rehabilitation of language deficits (Chapter 10), Leon, Maher, and Gonzalez Rothi describe an exciting novel application of the principles of CI therapy to language functions. Constraint-induced language therapy (CILT) is designed to eliminate the potential learned non-use of speech in individuals with aphasia. CILT incorporates the principles of repetition, intensity, salience, and specificity of treatment. The idea of constraint in this case is the limiting of the person's responses to speech by using visual barriers that prevent any communication through gestures, drawings, facial expressions, or other alternatives to speech. The therapy is hierarchically organized so that at first only a single word is required, then full sentences, and so on. Results have suggested that improvements are generalized to daily life. In one study, CILT was demonstrated to be superior to Promoting Aphasics' Communicative Effectiveness (PACE) therapy.

The next two chapters focus on two different aspects of executive functioning. In Chapter 11, O'Connell and Robertson review the literature on targeted training of executive attention and working memory, including studies that have included people with brain injury and children with ADHD, in addition to studies of age-related cognitive decline. They review studies that have used imaging techniques to try to measure reorganization of cortical networks. They also discuss their own successful work using strategy training and self-instructional techniques to improve sustained attention.

In Chapter 12, Lillie and Mateer review more metacognitive executive functions, such as error monitoring, problem solving, and multitasking. These authors give solid practical suggestions for treatment, but do so within a context of caution due to a lack of current data. They point out several important considerations for remediating executive functions, including the multiprocess nature of most executive tasks and the need to improve overall cortical tone before executive deficits can be addressed.

In the final chapter on cognitive training (Chapter 13), Sohlberg and Ehlhardt Powell review the literature on instructional practice and make important connections to brain plasticity and remediation. These principles from direct instruction are useful across all cognitive domains, but are particularly important to learning and memory. Some specific aspects of learning and memory approaches that are discussed in this chapter are errorless learning and distributed practice-spaced retrieval. In particular, a treatment protocol developed by these authors and their colleagues called TEACH-M is described and reviewed.

In the final chapter of this volume (Chapter 14), Freeland discusses pharmacological therapies that have been designed to improve cognitive or motor functioning. Many of these can be used in conjunction with nonpharmacological therapies to enhance recovery. Freeland makes the point that in most studies neuroplasticity is not directly measured, but inferred, and he urges researchers to begin examining neuroplastic changes as a theoretical guideline for creating new therapies.

Perhaps one of the most important factors in any rehabilitation approach is the need for generalization (Raskin & Gordon, 1992). One of the first authors to specify an approach to generalization was Gordon (1987), who suggested that the first level of generalization is that gains from rehabilitation hold true in the same setting with the same materials on separate occasions. The second is that improvement on the training tasks is also observed on a similar but not identical set of tasks. The third level of generalization is that the functions gained in training are shown to transfer to functions in day-to-day living. How does generalization occur?

Elsewhere, we (Sohlberg & Raskin, 1996) have suggested a set of generalization principles or strategies that can be broadly adapted to both research and clinical practice. These principles, drawn primarily from the applied behavioral literature (Stokes & Baer, 1977) and from the cognitive psychology literature on transfer or training (Anderson, 1996), are as follows: (1) Actively plan for and program generalization from the beginning of the treatment process; (2) identify reinforcements in the natural environment; (3) program stimuli common to both the training environment and the real world; (4) use sufficient examples when conducting therapy; and (5) select a method for measuring generalization.

These methods are thought to promote generalization through known learning and transfer of training paradigms. The process by which generalization occurs, of course, varies according to the treatment approach. Behavioral (compensation) techniques affect generalization by bypassing defective cognitive or motor functions and allowing a person to apply strategies in a large number of settings. Restorative approaches are thought to actually change the affected functions, thereby allowing the process to be more effective in any setting. However, the keys in any case seem to be to plan for generalization from the start and to have a measure of efficacy in place. In a meta-analysis of 39 papers on cognitive rehabilitation, Geusgens, Winkens, van Heugten, Jolles, and van den Heuvel (2007) concluded that a large number of studies make claims for transfer of training, but that relatively few actually evaluate whether transfer has occurred.

Some of the most exciting new work in the field of rehabilitation is based on models of cortical plasticity. Robertson and Murre (1999) have argued that the extent and nature of neural recovery following targeted intervention will depend largely on the severity of the injury. Thus, in the case of a large lesion, there may not be sufficient residual connectivity with which to reestablish a fully functioning network. In these cases, then, treatment should be targeted at the compensatory recruitment of alternative brain regions or the use of compensatory strategies.

In a similar vein, there is some evidence to suggest that patients with brain injury require training tailored to their specific level of functioning. For example, an analysis of individual differences in a study of the Attention Process Training (APT) program (Sohlberg, McLaughlin, Pavese, Heidrich, & Posner, 2000) indicated differences in treatment efficacy, depending on a patient's initial vigilance level. Only individuals who had poor vigilance levels showed improvements in basic attentional skills after APT, and only individuals with better vigilance levels showed improvement on more demanding attentional or working memory tasks. Further work is required to establish predictors of training efficacy, and future studies should delineate specific patient profiles in order to determine who is likely to benefit.

Research in rehabilitation is increasingly being required to follow evidence-based guidelines, as it has been noted many times that such research tends to be limited by the heterogeneity of subjects, methods, and outcome measures. Although randomized controlled studies are assumed to provide the best evidence of efficacy, it is also accepted that in clinical practice it may be necessary to combine standard treatment protocols and individualized treatments (Cicerone et al., 2000).

As the field of neuroscience provides more evidence for the specific kinds of practice and experience-dependent learning that lead to the most effective cortical plasticity, it should also be possible to target rehabilitation efforts to maximize these potential changes.

REFERENCES

Anderson, J. (1996). ACT: A simple theory of complex cognition. *American Psychologist, 51*, 355–365.

Cicerone, K., Dahlberg, C., Kalmer, K., Langenbahn, D. M., Malec, J. F., Bergquist, T. F., et al. (2000). Evidence-based cognitive rehabilitation: Recommendations for clinical practice. *Archives of Physical Medicine and Rehabilitation, 81*, 1596–1615.

Geusgens, C. A., Winkens, I., van Heugten, C. M., Jolles, J., & van den Heuvel, W. J. (2007). Occurrence and measurement of transfer in cognitive rehabilitation: A critical review. *Journal of Rehabilitation Medicine, 39*(6), 425–439.

Gordon, W. (1987). Methodological considerations in cognitive remediation. In M. Meier, A. Benton, & L. Diller (Eds.), *Neuropsychological rehabilitation*. New York: Guilford Press.

Raskin, S. A., & Gordon, W. (1992). The impact of different approaches to remediation on generalization. *NeuroRehabilitation, 2*, 38–45.

Robertson, I. H., & Murre, J. J. (1999). Rehabilitation of brain damage: Brain plasticity and principles of guided recovery. *Psychological Bulletin, 125*(5), 544–575.

Sohlberg, M. M., McLaughlin, K. A., Pavese, A., Heidrich, A., & Posner, M. I. (2000). Evaluation of attention process training and brain injury education in persons with acquired brain injury. *Journal of Clinical and Experimental Neuropsychology, 22*(5), 656–676.

Sohlberg, M. M., & Raskin, S. A. (1996). Principles of generalization applied to attention and memory interventions. *Journal of Head Trauma Rehabilitation, 11*(2), 65–78.

Stokes, T., & Baer, D. (1977). An implicit technology of generalization. *Journal of Applied Behavioral Analysis, 10*, 349–367.

PART I

Reorganization in the Central Nervous System

CHAPTER 2

Neuronal Organization and Change after Brain Injury

BRYAN KOLB
JAN CIOE
PRESTON WILLIAMS

The fundamental concept in the emerging field of brain plasticity is that although there is much constancy in brain function and organization across our lifetime, there is remarkable variability as well. This variability reflects the brain's capacity to alter its structure and function in reaction to environmental diversity as well as to perturbations, including injury. Although the term *brain plasticity* is now widely used, it is not easily defined and is used to refer to changes at many levels in the nervous system, ranging from molecular events (such as changes in gene expression) to behavior (e.g., Shaw & McEachern, 2001). The relationship between molecular or cellular changes and behavior is by no means clear and is plagued by the problems inherent in inferring causation from correlation. Nonetheless, a considerable literature is developing, and an understanding of this literature is essential if we are to develop rehabilitation strategies for brain injury. Before we address the plasticity in the injured brain, we must briefly review several key principles of plasticity in the normal brain.

GENERAL PRINCIPLES OF PLASTICITY IN THE NORMAL BRAIN

Changes in the Brain Can Be Shown at Many Levels of Analysis

A change in behavior must certainly result from some change in the brain. The nature of this brain change can be studied at many levels, however. Changes may be inferred from global measures of brain activity, such as the various forms of *in vivo* imaging, but such changes are far removed from the molecular processes that drive them. Global changes presumably reflect synaptic changes, but synaptic changes result from more molecular changes (such as modifications in channels, gene expression, etc.). The problem in studying brain plasticity is to choose a surrogate marker that best suits the question being asked. Changes in calcium channels may be perfect for studying synaptic changes at specific synapses that may be related to simple learning, such as in models like long-term potentiation (e.g., Teyler, 2001), but are impractical for understanding sex differences in language processing. The latter may best be studied by *in vivo* imaging or postmortem analysis of cell morphology (e.g., Jacobs & Scheibel, 1993). But neither level of analysis is "correct." The appropriate level will depend on the research question at hand. In studies of brain injury, the most useful levels have proven to be anatomical (cell morphology and connectivity), physiological (cortical stimulation), and *in vivo* imaging. Each of these levels can be linked to behavioral outcomes in both human and nonhuman studies, whereas more molecular levels have proven to be much more difficult to relate to behavior, especially mental behavior.

The Brain Is Altered by a Wide Range of Experiences

Virtually every experience has the potential to alter the brain, at least briefly. Even a fleeting memory of an event must result from some transient change in brain activity. Although transient changes are interesting in their own right, the enduring changes are most relevant to understanding recovery from injury. It has now been shown that a wide variety of experiences, ranging from general sensory–motor experience to specific exercise to hormones and psychoactive drugs (see Table 2.1), can also produce enduring changes. Most of these studies have used Golgi stain techniques and have demonstrated that experience-dependent changes can be seen in every species of animals tested, ranging from fruit flies to humans (for a review, see Kolb & Whishaw, 1998). Let us consider a couple of examples.

When mammals develop, the brain is influenced by a myriad of chemicals, such as gonadal hormones. Although these hormones have long been known to control the development of the genitals, we now know that they have an important organizing effect on the cerebral hemispheres. For exam-

TABLE 2.1. Factors Affecting the Synaptic Organization of the Normal Brain

Factor	Basic reference
Sensory and motor experience	Greenough and Chang (1989)
Task learning	Greenough and Chang (1989)
Gonadal hormones and stress hormones	Stewart and Kolb (1988)
Psychoactive drugs (e.g., stimulants, tetrahydrocannabinol)	Robinson and Kolb (2004)
Neurotrophic factors (e.g., NGF, bFGF/FGF-2)	Kolb, Gorny, Cote, et al. (1997)
Natural rewards (e.g., social interaction, sex)	Fiorino and Kolb (2003)
Aging	Coleman and Buell (1985)
Stress	McEwen (2005)
Anti-inflammatories (e.g., cyclooxygenase-2 [COX-2] inhibitors)	Silasi and Kolb (2007)
Diet (e.g., choline)	Meck and Williams (2003)
Electrical stimulation	
Kindling	Teskey, Monfils, Silasi, and Young (2006)
Long-term potentiation	Ivanco et al. (2000)
Direct cortical stimulation	Teskey, Flynn, Goertzen, Monfils, and Young (2003)

ple, when we correct for overall brain size in humans, we find that females have a larger dorsolateral prefrontal area than males do, whereas males have a larger orbitofrontal cortex area (OFC) than females do (Goldstein et al., 2001). Curiously, when the morphology of cells in these two regions in rats is compared, we find just the reverse: The cells are more complex in males in the dorsolateral-equivalent region, whereas they are more complex in the OFC of females (Kolb & Stewart, 1991). A similar dissociation between region size and cell morphology can be seen in the posterior speech zone of humans (Jacobs & Scheibel, 1993). The simplest conclusion from areal and morphology comparisons is that gonadal hormones change not only dendritic organization, but probably also neuron number. These morphological changes are generally assumed to reflect sex-related behavioral differences (for a review, see Kolb & Whishaw, 2009).

A second example can be seen in the effects of specific training. When rats are trained to use one paw to reach through a slot for food, there is an increase in dendritic length specific to the contralateral forepaw representation (Kolb, Cioe, & Comeau, 2008; Withers & Greenough, 1989), whereas when they are trained on a visual–spatial maze, there is a specific increase in visual cortex (Greenough & Chang, 1989). Similar changes are not seen when animals simply exercise; however, the neurons need to be actively engaged in cerebral processing for these plastic changes to occur.

A final example can be seen in the effects of psychomotor stimulants. Robinson and Kolb (1997) first showed that treating rats with amphetamine produced increased dendritic length and spine density in the medial prefrontal cortex (mPFC), but had no effect on adjacent sensory–motor regions. Later studies showed that other stimulants, including nicotine, cocaine, and caffeine, produced similar changes in the mPFC (e.g., Brown & Kolb, 2001; Robinson & Kolb, 2004), but nicotine also increased dendritic length and spine density in the motor cortex. The nicotine-induced changes in the motor cortex are intriguing because they suggest that stimulants may be useful in stimulating plasticity after cerebral injury, especially to the motor cortex. We return to this idea later.

Plastic Changes Are Area-Dependent

Although we are tempted to expect plastic changes in neuronal networks to be fairly widespread, it is becoming clear that many experience-dependent changes are highly specific. We have just noted, for example, that rats trained on motor tasks show specific changes in motor cortex, whereas rats trained on visual tasks show specific visual cortical changes. Such task-dependent specific changes are reasonable, in view of the relative localization of functions in the cortex. But not all area-dependent changes are so easily predicted. Let's consider two examples.

We have also noted above that psychomotor stimulants produce increased synaptogenesis in the mPFC. We therefore were surprised to find that the OFC, another prefrontal region that receives very similar inputs to those of the mPFC, showed drug-induced changes that are opposite to those in mPFC (Robinson & Kolb, 2004). Thus, whereas psychomotor stimulants *increased* dendritic length and spine density in the mPFC, they *decreased* the same measures in the OFC. Similarly, whereas morphine *decreased* dendritic length and density in mPFC, morphine *increased* those measures in the OFC (e.g., Robinson & Kolb, 2004). The contrasting effects of these drugs on the two prefrontal regions was certainly unexpected, given the regions' similarity in thalamic and other connections (e.g., Uylings, Groenewegen, & Kolb, 2001). We should recall, however, that there also are differential effects of gonadal hormones on these two prefrontal regions: mPFC neurons have more synaptic space in males, whereas OFC neurons have more space in females (Kolb & Stewart, 1991). Although we do not yet know what such differences mean behaviorally, the differential response of two such similar cortical regions to drugs and hormones must be important in understanding their functions and area-dependent differences in recovery from injury.

Experience-Dependent Changes Interact

Most studies of experience-dependent change in laboratory animals manipulate a single experiential variable at a time and attempt to demonstrate some relationship between the experience and brain plasticity. This is a necessary starting point for research, but as animals travel through life they have an almost infinite number of experiences that could alter brain organization, and these are likely to interact with one another. We attempted to address this issue in a series of studies in which animals received psychoactive drugs before or after placement in complex environments (Hamilton & Kolb, 2005; Kolb, Gorny, Li, Samaha, & Robinson, 2003; Li, Kolb, & Robinson, 2005). We hypothesized that the first experiences might interact in some way with the later experiences, and predicted that prior exposure to the drugs would reduce the effect of later experience in the prefrontal and striatal regions that were affected by the drugs. We also predicted that experience-dependent changes in other cerebral regions, which showed no direct effect of the drugs, would be unaffected by the drugs. To our surprise, prior exposure to amphetamine, cocaine, or nicotine completely blocked the effect of complex housing experience on neurons throughout the cerebrum—including cells in parietal and visual cortex, regions in which the drugs had a negligible direct effect on the structure of these neurons. Prior housing experience also influenced the effect of the drugs, although in this case the drugs were still capable of producing a small synaptic change. We are not certain whether psychoactive drugs are more potent in changing cortical neurons or whether the environment–drug difference simply reflects a difference in the "dose" of each experience. This is a difficult question to address without extensive investigations.

Another example of interactions in experience-dependent changes can be seen in the sexually dimorphic response of cortical and hippocampal neurons to complex housing. Juraska (1990) has shown that whereas occipital cortex neurons show increased dendritic arbor in response to complex housing in males, there are no such changes in females. In contrast, females show increased dendritic arbor in the hippocampus, whereas males do not.

The interactions of different experiences is clearly important in understanding brain plasticity and recovery following cerebral injury. Adults have a lifetime of experiences, including drug experiences, prior to cerebral injury; these experiences must influence not only spontaneous recovery, but also the effectiveness of postinjury treatments. Little is known about these interactions, in either laboratory animals or humans, but it will become an important topic in the coming years. Consider, for example, that McDonald, Craig, and Hong (2010) have shown that although stress and cholinergic depletion individually have little effect on recovery from stroke, the combination of these factors has a huge deleterious effect. One could imagine that preinjury experiences could also prove beneficial for some types of brain injury, although this has proven more difficult to study (e.g., Schulkin, 1989).

THE CASCADE OF NEURODEGENERATIVE CHANGES FOLLOWING BRAIN INJURY

Although we may be able to point to a specific proximal cause of a brain injury, such as a stroke, the final product of brain injury is the result of a cascade of events following the injury. Consider what happens after a stroke in which there is an interruption of the blood supply to one of the cerebral arteries.

The first stage of this type of stroke is a lack of blood (ischemia), which results in subsequent events that progress even if the blood flow is restored. As illustrated in Figure 2.1, there are changes in the ionic balance of the affected regions over the first seconds to minutes, including changes in pH and other properties of the cell membrane. These ionic changes result in a variety of pathological events, including the release of massive amounts of glutamate and the prolonged opening of calcium channels. The open calcium channels allow high levels of calcium to enter the cell. If the cal-

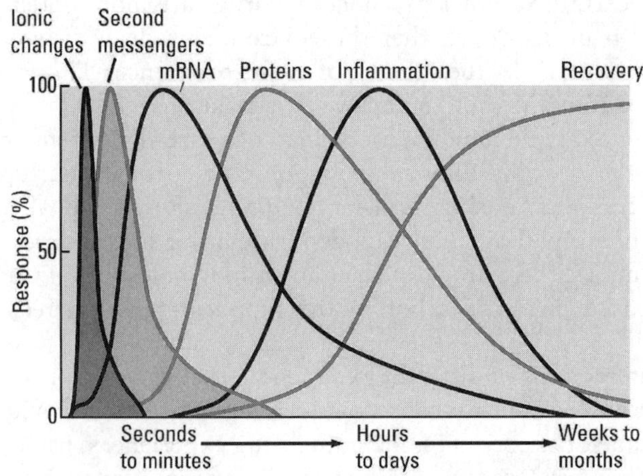

FIGURE 2.1. The cascade of changes taking place after a stroke. In the first seconds to minutes, ionic changes are followed by changes in second messengers and RNA production. These changes are followed by changes in protein production and inflammation, which slowly resolves in hours to days. Recovery follows and takes from weeks to months or years. Adapted from Kolb and Whishaw (2009). Copyright 2009 by Worth. Adapted by permission.

cium levels become too high, there may be toxic effects that result from the instigation of various biochemical pathways. Over the ensuing minutes to hours there is a stimulation of messenger RNA (mRNA), which in turn alters the production of proteins in the neurons; this again may prove toxic to the cells.

One major complication of the stroke is the development of considerable edema (swelling) over the first 24 hours. The edema probably results from both extracellular fluid accumulation, especially in the white matter, and astrocytic swelling (Nieto-Sampedro & Cotman, 1985). Edema is particularly problematic in the brain, because swelling means that there is an increase in volume of the brain, but the skull is not accommodating. Thus the swelling acts to put pressure on the entire brain, which can cause neuronal injury, dysfunction, and death. Luckily, many of the effects of edema are transient, and functions return as the swelling reduces. A good example is seen in the postsurgical recovery of IQ in patients with temporal or frontal lobectomies for the treatment of epilepsy. Milner (1975) reported that IQ had dropped about 15 points when measured 2 weeks after surgery, but that by 1 year IQ had returned to preoperative levels. Although the IQ drop may result from factors in addition to edema, treatment with edema-reducing drugs such as cortisone decreases the IQ drop and speeds up recovery.

The poststroke changes in neuronal functioning also lead to changes in the metabolism and/or glucose utilization of an injured hemisphere that may persist for days. These metabolic changes can have severe effects on brain functioning in otherwise normal tissue, and thus a patient may present with symptoms that are far greater than would be expected from brain scans. It has been shown, for example, that after a cortical stroke there is a drop of about 60% in glucose metabolism throughout the rest of the damaged hemisphere—and, surprisingly, a drop of about 25% in the undamaged hemisphere. These changes in metabolism are likely to form part of what von Monakow called *diaschisis*, which is essentially a form of shock (Pearce, 1994). von Monakow noted that after the brain is injured, not only is localized neural tissue and its function lost, but areas related to the damaged area suffer a sudden withdrawal of excitation or inhibition. Such sudden changes in input can lead to a temporary loss of function both in areas adjacent to an injury and in regions that may be quite distal.

Although neuronal death resulting directly from an injury will occur within 48 hours, there is further neuron death as a result of the changes in blood flow, metabolism, pH, edema, and so on. The secondary cell death can be quite extensive and may even be larger than the cell death resulting directly from the injury itself.

Reparative processes may begin almost immediately after the cell death. Microglia invade the damaged region via the vascular system to act as phagocytes, clearing away degenerative debris—a process that may take months to complete. Astrocytes already lying adjacent to the lesion area enlarge and extend fibrous processes that serve to isolate the surfaces of the injury from the surrounding tissue. Stem cells also may be stimulated to increase division in the subventricular zone and to migrate to the injury, although we do not yet know what function these cells may have. Treatments for cerebral injury can be directed at different targets in the postinjury cascade. For example, drugs can be used to block calcium channels or prevent ionic imbalance. Such drugs are called *neuroprotectants*, because it is hoped that they will protect neurons from the cascade of toxic events that follow an ischemic episode. Much research on neuroprotectants in the latter part of the 20th century showed benefits in laboratory animals, but not in later clinical trials in humans. There are many explanations for the failure of the neuroprotectants, such as inadequate behavioral assessment and confounding factors such as lowered body temperature in the lab animals, but one effect of the failed trials is that drug companies are reluctant to spend money on such drugs. Nonetheless, there are new classes of drugs targeting novel channels. Among these are the transient receptor potential channels, which mediate the response of a cell by increasing or decreasing the selective permeability to particular ions in response to extracellular environmental changes. The key point is that over the next decade a whole new generation of neuroprotectants targeting novel channels is likely to emerge; ideally, these will prove more effective than the first generation of drugs.

Other drugs can be used to stimulate plastic changes in the remaining brain—changes that could potentially underlie functional compensation. These compounds include factors that can stimulate the production of endogenous stem cells (e.g., Kolb et al., 2007) or stimulate the reorganization of existing neuronal networks (e.g., Gonzalez, Gharbawie, & Kolb, 2006).

One important consideration in the immediate postinjury period is what types of activities may actually make cell death worse or interfere with beneficial plastic changes. Nudo and his colleagues have shown, for example, that if monkeys with motor cortex strokes are not forced to use their impaired limbs at least a few hours a day, they show progressive loss of function, essentially because they learn not to use the limbs (*learned nonuse*; see Nudo & Bury, Chapter 4, this volume). But there may be a limit to how much use there can be in the early postinjury period. In the course of studies designed to promote functional recovery after injury, Schallert and his colleagues (e.g., Kozlowski, James, & Schallert, 1996) accidentally found that initiating intense therapy after a stroke made the stroke damage worse. In these studies, rats were fitted with a restraint harness that prevented the animals from using the forelimb ipsilateral to a sensory–motor cortex injury. The idea was to force animals to use the impaired limb and thus, it was hoped, to stimulate recovery. The problem was that the animals wore the harness 24 hours a day, and the continual forced use of the affected limb significantly enlarged the lesion cavity and resulted in a worse functional outcome. Although few human stroke treatments would be so intense, the Schallert et al. studies focus attention on the questions of when therapy should commence and how intense it should be. Answers to both questions remain to be determined.

PLASTICITY IN THE INJURED BRAIN

Changes in neuronal organization after injury can be investigated at many levels, ranging from behavior to molecular changes. We consider various levels in turn.

Behavior

Ultimately, it is behavior that we use to infer that there is some plastic change in the brain. Although it is often thought that behavioral change is obvious, we must emphasize that the science of behavioral analysis after brain injury is at least as difficult as understanding molecular changes. Clinicians have long known that people with brain injuries show improvement in function, but the nature and mechanisms of the mediating processes are poorly understood. One major problem is the absence of a generally accepted definition of *recovery*. It seems rather unlikely that there could ever be a complete return of normal function if there is significant brain injury, but certainly some degree of improvement is quite possible. Another issue is the problem of compensation versus improvement. Consider what we can call "the problem of the three-legged cat." When cats are struck by automobiles, they commonly suffer injury to one of the rear legs. The common veterinary treatment is to remove the injured leg. Such a cat has severe limitations in movement after the surgery, but over a period of months it "recovers" and becomes nearly as agile as before the amputation. The restoration of mobility can be truly impressive, to the point that an observer may not even notice that there are only three legs. But the cat has not "recovered" the lost leg. Rather, the cat has compensated for the loss of the leg.

Many would argue that what is observed after brain injury is virtually always compensation and not recovery. The critical issue is the nature of the behavioral analysis. The majority of behavioral studies, both in humans and in laboratory animals, use what we can call "endpoint" measures rather than detailed analyses of behavior. Consider an example. Piecharka, Kleim, and Whishaw (2005) studied the details of skilled reaching as well as the topographic representation of the motor map in rats with partial or complete lesions of different regions of the pyramidal tract. The rationale of the study is that there is a considerable literature on both humans and laboratory animals suggesting that the pyramidal tract has considerable plasticity, and that the survival of a surprisingly small amount of the tract can mediate restoration of behavior. Piecharka et al. trained rats on a skilled reaching task preoperatively and then studied both the postinjury reaching success and reaching movements before using cortical microstimulation to identify the topographic motor map in the cortex. The animals with partial lesions did not display behavioral deficits, as measured by success scores on the skilled reaching test. Nevertheless, the same animals had qualitative impairments on the details of wrist and digit movements related to grasping and manipulating the food pellets. They were successful in reaching because they had learned to be "three-legged cats." The qualitative deficits were accompanied by a 35% reduction in the size of the cortical representation of the motor maps as mapped electrophysiologically. Thus, although the rats could compensate for the loss of pyramidal fibers, the compensation did not reflect a recovery of the behavior or its underlying neural network. One curious finding is that the reduction of the map was reflected in a shrinkage of the entire map, rather than by a loss of specific fragments of the map. The shrunken but intact motor representation must mean that the motor cortex has undergone considerable reoroganization.

A parallel study of rats with neonatal prefrontal cortex injuries by Williams, Gharbawie, Kolb, and Kleim (2006) found chronic impairments in both endpoint measures and detailed analyses of the animals' movements (known as *kinematic analyses*), which were correlated with shrunken maps in the intact motor cortex (Figure 2.2). The key additional finding in the Williams et al. study was that both rehabilitation training and complex housing were able to improve the reaching success and movement details, as well as to increase the size of the motor map. Once again, the motor representation must have undergone reorganization, but in this case the reorganization was driven by behavioral therapy.

There are several lessons from the Piecharka et al. (2005) and Williams et al. (2006) studies. First, behavior is a sensitive surrogate for plastic changes in the brain. Second, we must be careful in our behavioral analysis, as most functional restitution is likely to be compensation and not recovery per se. Third, behavioral therapies can alter both behavioral outcome and brain plasticity. We can predict that if behavioral therapies prove to be ineffective in stimulating functional improvement, it is probably because the therapy has been ineffective in changing neural circuits in the brain.

Functional Imaging after Cerebral Injury

We have just seen that direct cortical stimulation of the rodent brain can be used to demonstrate functional reorganization after cerebral injury. Although such procedures are possible in human surgical cases, they are

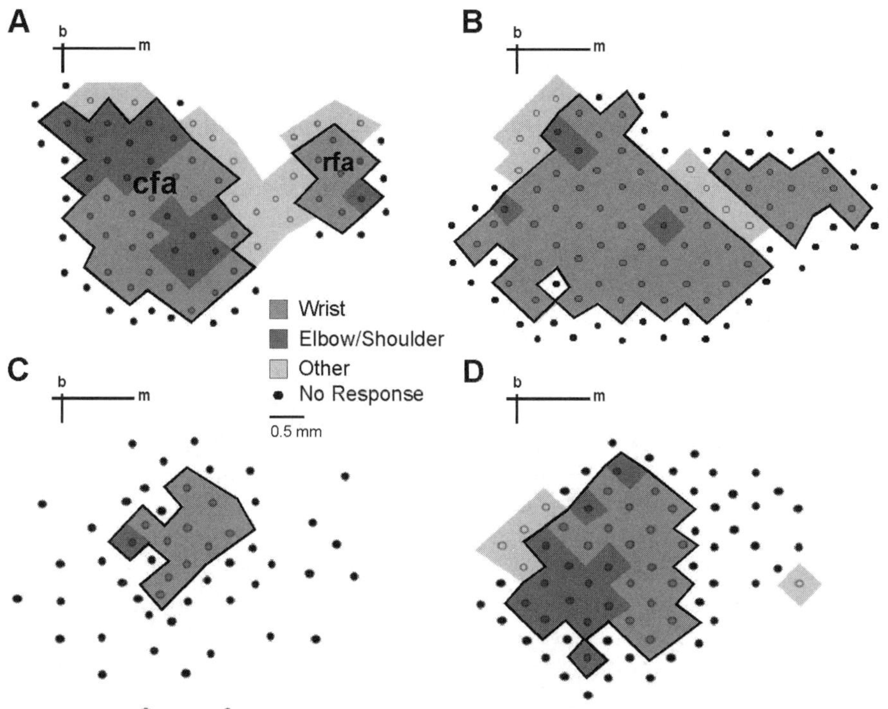

FIGURE 2.2. Forelimb maps in adult rats using intracortical microstimulation (ICMS) in motor cortex. (A) Control map with caudal forelimb area (cfa) and a separate and smaller rostral forelimb area (rfa). (B) Control + complex housing for 1 month in adulthood expanded the representations in cfa. (C) Postnatal day 10 unilateral medial prefrontal cortex (mPFC) lesion decreased the size of cfa, and the rfa was not responsive to microstimulation in the lesion hemisphere. (D) Postnatal day 10 unilateral mPFC lesion + complex Housing for 1 month in adulthood expanded the cfa in the lesion hemisphere. Dots indicate ICMS penetrations, with the corresponding movement produced shown by overlayed shading. Shaded regions outlined in black are distal (wrist; medium shading) and proximal (elbow/shoulder; dark shading) forelimb movements. Regions lightly shaded and not outlined in black are nonforelimb movements (e.g., hindlimb, jaw, neck, vibrissae) (other; light shading) that border or separate the cfa and rfa. Top left of each panel shows reference to the bregmoidal junction (b) and midline (m). Adapted from Williams, Gharbawie, Kolb, and Kleim (2006). Copyright 2006 by Elsevier. Adapted by permission.

generally impractical because of the invasive nature of the procedure. Furthermore, the injuries induced in animal models are different from those typically seen in humans. Nonetheless, it is obviously necessary to study humans using functional imaging techniques, especially positron emission tomograpy, functional magnetic resonance imaging, and transcranial magnetic stimulation. These procedures can be used repeatedly during the weeks and months after stroke to document changes in cerebral activation that might correlate with functional improvement. There have been several reviews of the results of functional imaging studies after stroke, which lead us to several conclusions (see especially reviews by Cramer & Bastings, 2000; Rijntjes & Weiller, 2002).

1. *Behavioral improvement after stroke is associated with an increased recruitment of regions in the damaged hemisphere.* In addition, a larger area of the motor cortex is often activated for a given movement. For example, hand or limb movements often activate regions of the face area, possibly because of intact pyramidal tract fibers leaving the face area. This result is somewhat different from those obtained in the rodent studies discussed above, but is consistent with results of studies in monkeys with focal lesions (e.g., Frost, Barbay, Friel, Plantz, & Nudo, 2003). Later monkey studies have shown the emergence of novel intrinsic motor connections that are likely to underlie the recruitment of additional regions (Dancause et al., 2005).

2. *Reorganization of maps is not restricted to one hemisphere after a unilateral injury, but similar changes occur bilaterally.* Thus, although the performance of a unilateral motor task largely activates only the contralateral cortex, after stroke there is a marked increase in bilateral activation in some patients. It is not known why some patients recruit ipsilateral regions, whereas others recruit contralateral regions, but it is likely that lesion size and location are important factors. For example, patients with disturbances of language may show activation in the complementary tissue in the opposite hemisphere.

3. *There is considerable variability in map changes across stroke victims.* We have noted earlier that the size of lesion in the pyramidal tract of rats is related to the amount of shrinkage in the map, so it seems likely that lesion size is going to be related to variability in map changes. Furthermore, the variability may be related to preinjury differences in map organization, which presumably reflects both genetic differences and preinjury experience. Rijntjes and Weiller (2002) note that the extent of activation of the right hemisphere during language tasks is highly variable, and that the pattern of activation in those people who have shown recovery from Wernicke's aphasia is remarkably similar to the maximal areas of right-hemisphere activation seen in normal brains.

Synaptic Organization after Injury

When neurons lose connections following an injury, retraction and remodeling of dendritic processes ensue. As the brain reorganizes after the injury, there can be an expansion of dendritic fields, although the networks are likely to be rather different (e.g., Steward, 1991). Both behavioral and pharmacological therapies can influence recovery and plasticity by facilitating this dendritic remodeling. For example, when Gonzalez et al. (2006) gave rats strokes to the motor cortex, there was a severe motor deficit associated with drop in dendritic arborization in related cortical areas, such as the ipsilateral anterior cingulate cortex and the contralateral forelimb area (Figure 2.3). When animals were treated with a low dose of a psychomotor stimulant (nicotine), there was an improved functional outcome, and this was associated with enhanced dendritic arborization. The synaptic changes with nicotine were correlated not only with enhanced endpoint measures (i.e., reaching accuracy), but also with changes in kinematic analysis, as illustrated in Figure 2.4. We return to further examples of factors that influence synaptic change after injury below.

Molecular Changes

When there are synaptic changes, there must be changes in gene expression to induce the production of specific proteins. The production of proteins is ultimately controlled by mRNA, so anything that influences the genetic code has the potential to influence reparative processes in the brain. As the Human Genome Project comes to completion, there is a growing interest in applying genomic approaches to the development of new treatments to facilitate recovery from brain injury (Jordan, 2007).

One complexity in understanding genetic changes after brain injury is that the injury itself will induce the postinjury cascade of events discussed earlier, and many of these changes will require the de novo synthesis of genes and proteins (e.g., Ellison, Barone, & Feuerstein, 1999). The alterations in gene expression may or may not be conducive to the creation of new synapses. In the latter case, it may be necessary to develop therapies directed at manipulating gene expression. One difficulty is that there appears to be considerable variability in gene expression after injury. For example, Michael, Byers, and Irwin (2005) analyzed gene expression in pericontusional tissue taken during surgery from four patients with traumatic brain injury and compared it to normal brain tissue resected during the surgical treatment of meningioma. The authors described a wide range of genes differentially expressed after traumatic brain injury, including genes related to both acute and homeostatic response mechanisms. Importantly, however, 55% of the differentially expressed genes were observed in *only one patient.* Given that these differences were not correlated with

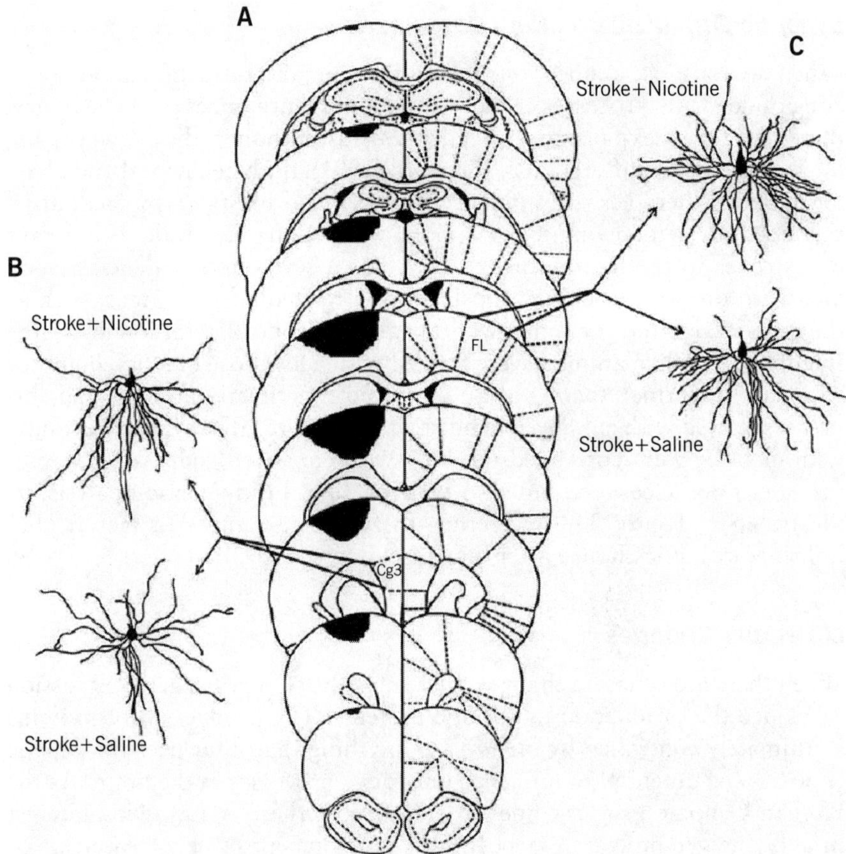

FIGURE 2.3. (A) A diagram of the eight different planes used for infarct measurements, as well as the extension of the lesion in a representative brain. (B and C) Camera lucida drawing of representative layer V pyramidal neurons in cingulate cortex ipsilateral to the lesion (B), or forelimb area in the contralesional hemisphere (C), from a stroke animal treated with nicotine or with saline. In both areas, animals treated with nicotine showed cells with more dendritic branching. Control cells are not shown, because no differences were found between untreated controls and untreated stroke animals.

obvious patient differences such as sex, race, or age, there must be unique factors that contribute to the genetic changes after the injury. Conversely, nearly 50% of the genes were expressed in at least two patients, leading to a list of prime candidates for further study. To date, there have been no studies demonstrating how different therapies can influence the expression of genes, but this is clearly the grist for studies in the future (e.g., Siu, 2010).

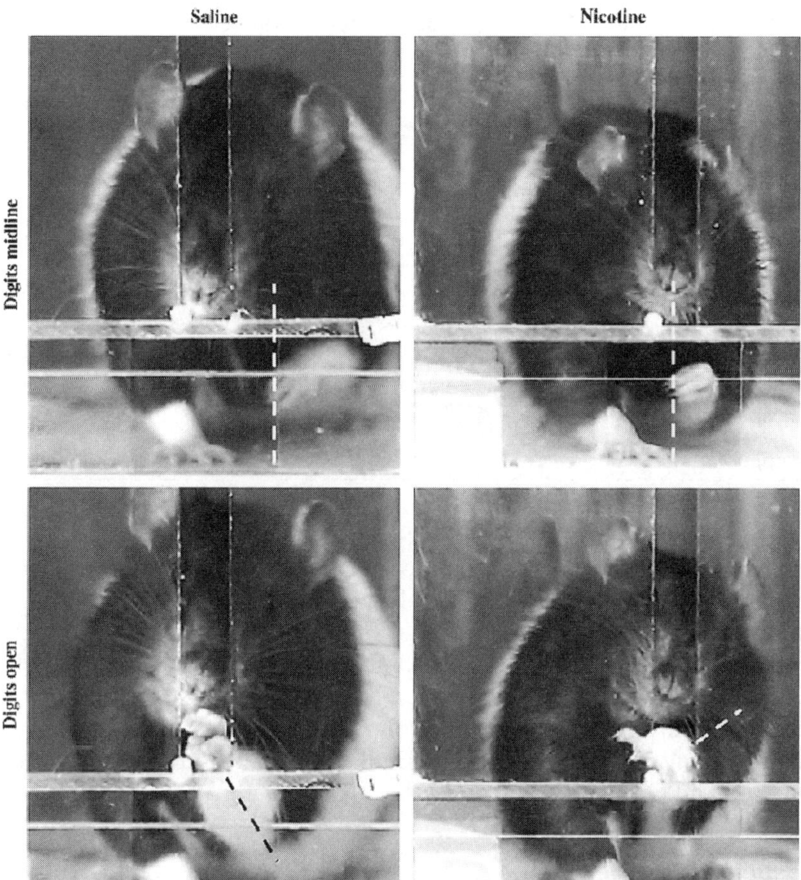

FIGURE 2.4. Illustration of some of the early components of the reach (digits to the midline and digits open) by a stroke (saline) and a stroke + nicotine (nicotine) animal. Note also that the lesion animals that received saline were unable to open the digits properly before grasping the pellet.

FACTORS AFFECTING RECOVERY AND SYNAPTIC PLASTICITY

A key feature of research in behavioral neuroscience is the search for consistency and stability in brain organization and function. As we have seen, however, one characteristic of functional change after cerebral injury is its variability. We have noted earlier, for example, that changes in maps shown by functional imaging studies of brain-injured subjects are variable with respect to ipsilateral and contralateral changes. Similarly, we have seen that

TABLE 2.2. Factors Affecting Recovery of the Injured Brain

Factor	Basic reference
Complex housing	Biernaskie and Corbett (2001)
Olfactory stimulation	Gonzalez et al. (2006)
Psychoactive drugs (e.g., stimulants)	Gonzalez et al. (2006)
Neurotrophic factors (e.g., NGF)	Kolb et al. (1997b)
Mobilization of endogenous stem cells	Kolb et al. (2007)
Anti-inflammatories (e.g., COX-2 inhibitors)	Silasi and Kolb (2007)
Electrical stimulation	Teskey et al. (2004)
Inosine	Chen et al. (2002)
Antibodies to no-go	Papadopoulos et al. (2006)

there are large differences in gene expression after injury. Although some of the postinjury differences are probably due to preinjury experience, various other factors can influence functional outcome. We summarize these factors in Table 2.2. Although space prohibits an extensive review of all these factors, we provide a general overview to give a sense of how some of these factors can influence functional outcome and brain plasticity after cerebral injury in adulthood. For a review of similar research after injury in infancy, see Kolb and Gibb (2007).

Postinjury Experience

Studies of laboratory animals have consistently shown that the single most successful treatment strategy for optimizing functional recovery from various forms of experimental brain damage (including cortical ablation, cortical ischemia, and head trauma) is placing animals in complex, stimulating environments (e.g., Biernaskie & Corbett, 2001; Johansson, 1996; Kolb & Elliott, 1987; Will & Kelche, 1992). Although the mechanism of the beneficial effects of complex housing is not known, it has been hypothesized that the treatment may increase the synthesis of neurotrophic factors, which in turn facilitate synaptic plasticity (e.g., Johansson, 2000). Motor training has been shown to up-regulate trophic factors such as brain-derived neurotrophic factor (BDNF) and basic fibroblast growth factor (bFGF or FGF-2) (see review by Kleim, Jones, & Schallert, 2003), so we might anticipate that rehabilitation training would also be beneficial after cerebral injury. There is some evidence of benefits from repetitive motor training (e.g., Dawson, Howarth, Tarnopolsky, Wong, & Gibala, 2003; Nudo, Wise, SiFuentes,

& Milliken, 1996), and this type of training is often used by physiotherapists. Such treatments have not always been found to be beneficial, however, and the differences may be related to the details of the training (e.g., Witt-Lajeunesse, Cioe, & Kolb, 2011) (see also a metareview of the human literature by Teasell, Bayona, Salter, Hellings, & Bitensky, 2006).

One shortcoming of laboratory studies examining the benefits of behavioral therapies is that we still do not know the best intensity of training or the optimal timing of training. It seems likely, however, that few hours a week will be insufficient. Our hunch is that best practice should include at least 2 hours per day of actual therapy. In fact, there is growing evidence that patients who are placed in a dedicated stroke unit, rather than treated on an outpatient basis, are likely to show a better outcome. A stroke unit will have a variety of professional rehabilitation therapists working together and providing stimulation for much of the waking day. There is also evidence that constraint-induced therapy (see Morris & Bickle, Chapter 7, this volume) is most effective if it lasts several hours per day.

Pharmacological Therapies

The purpose of pharmacological therapies is to facilitate plastic changes in the injured brain that will support functional improvement. For example, psychomotor stimulants such as amphetamine or nicotine are known to stimulate changes in cortical and subcortical circuits in the normal brain (e.g., Lena & Changeux, 1999; Robinson & Kolb, 2004). Given the power of these agents in stimulating plastic changes in the brain, it is hypothesized that administering these compounds after injury will stimulate plastic changes that support functional improvement, and there is growing evidence supporting this idea. We have noted above that nicotine facilitates recovery from motor stroke and does so by leading to synaptic changes in remaining motor regions, and that these changes are correlated with both qualitative and quantitative changes in behavior. Amphetamine has also been shown to be beneficial (e.g., Feeney & Sutton, 1987; Goldstein, 2003) but has had mixed success clinically. We have compared the effects of amphetamine on recovery from focal versus more extensive strokes. The main finding is that whereas amphetamine is effective in producing both synaptic change and behavioral improvement after focal cortical injuries, there is little benefit after large middle cerebral occlusions (Moroz & Kolb, 2005). In contrast, nicotine still has some benefit after larger strokes. One important difference between the drugs is that nicotine produces more widespread effects on cortical circuitry than amphetamine does (Robinson & Kolb, 2004); this difference may account for the added benefits of nicotine after cerebral injury. We note, parenthetically, that the effect of nicotine is studied by giving animals nicotine alone and not in conjunction with smoke and other contaminants related to taking nicotine by smoking tobacco. It seems likely that postinjury smoking will not be the ideal treatment, especially after stroke.

Neurotrophic Factors

Basic neurobiological research over the past decade has shown that several proteins have the property of stimulating neurogenesis as well as synaptogenesis, both during development and in adulthood. These compounds have generated considerable interest because of their potential for treatment of dementing diseases as well as recovery from injuries (e.g., Hefti, 1997).

The first neurotrophic factor to be described was nerve growth factor (NGF) so it was logical to begin looking at the potential benefits of growth factors by using NGF to treat laboratory animals with brain injuries. A study by Kolb, Cote, Gorny, Ribeiro-da-Silva, and Cuello (1997b) showed that NGF produced about 20% increases in the dendritic arborization and spine density in cortical pyramidal neurons in otherwise normal animals. A subsequent study showed that rats with large cortical strokes showed about a 20% decrease in dendritic arborization in the remaining motor regions, and that this was completely reversed by NGF (Kolb, Cote, Ribeiro-daSilva, & Cuello, 1997a). Although the results of this study were compelling, the difficulty with NGF as a potential treatment is that it is expensive and does not pass the blood–brain barrier. One advantage of FGF-2 is that it does pass the blood–brain barrier. Furthermore, FGF-2 is particularly interesting because psychomotor stimulants transiently increase FGF-2 (Flores & Stewart, 2000). Preliminary studies (Kawamata, Speliotes, & Finklestein, 1996) suggested that administration of FGF-2 after stroke could stimulate functional improvement, although the effects were small and task-dependent. Later studies (Witt-Lajeunesse et al., 2011) are intriguing because although FGF-2 alone had a minimal effect on recovery from motor cortex injury, FGF-2 was remarkably effective in stimulating functional improvement when given in combination with rehabilitation training or complex housing. Furthermore, the functional improvement was correlated with increased synaptogenesis in the remaining motor regions.

A further aspect of the actions of neurotrophic factors is that their endogenous production is potentiated by experience (e.g., Kolb, Forgie, Gibb, Gorny, & Rowntree, 1998). Thus it is possible that one mechanism whereby experience facilitates functional recovery is by increasing the endogenous production of neurotrophic factors, which in turn stimulate synaptic changes. For example, allowing animals to run spontaneously in running wheels (or explore complex environments) can increase levels of growth factors, stimulate neurogenesis, increase resistance to brain injury, and improve learning and mental performance (Cotman & Berchtold, 2002). Little is known, however, about the optimal timing or intensity of exercise needed to maximally enhance behavioral outcome or neuronal plasticity.

Brain Tissue Transplants and Stem Cell Induction

Although the idea of transplanting either embryonic neurons or stem cells has been actively studied over the past 20 years, there is little evidence that either strategy will be effective for repairing damage to complex neural circuits like the neocortex. Even in patients with Parkinson's disease who receive embryonic dopaminergic cells, the general finding is that relief from symptoms is minor or only short-lived (e.g., Polgar, Morris, Reilly, Bilney, & Sanberg, 2003). The difficulties with the transplants in humans may be that they do not grow sufficiently in the large human brain, they are not adequately incorporated into brain circuitry, and they are subject to the same disease process that is causing the original loss of dopamine cells.

There is, however, another approach to neuron replacement: using growth factors to stimulate endogenous stem cells. There are now many reports that stem cell activity is up-regulated after cerebral injury, but the major problem is that the cells do not migrate to the perilesional region in sufficient numbers to affect behavioral change. Recently, Kolb et al. (2007) used a combination of a growth factor (epidermal growth factor, or EGF) known to simulate stem cell production *in vivo* with the later application of erythropoietin (EPO), a factor that stimulates stem cells to adopt a neuronal phenotype. The intraventricular infusion of EGF and EPO promoted substantial regeneration of the damaged cerebral cortex and reversed motor impairments in a rat stroke model (Figure 2.5). Although the regenerated tissue was poorly organized and the cells were simple, the tissue played some role in the functional recovery, although perhaps an indirect one. Thus, when the tissue was removed, the behavioral advantage slowly dissipated over a 2-week period. Had the tissue been directly responsible for the recovery, we would have expected an immediate behavioral loss after tissue removal; however, the slow behavioral loss implies that the tissue had some indirect effect on the behavior, perhaps by releasing growth factors that facilitated the function of cells in the perilesional region. The EGF and EPO results are exciting, but there are still many unanswered questions about the precise mechanism of the behavioral benefits.

POSTSCRIPT

When the brain is injured, there are both degenerative and reparative changes over the ensuing hours, days, and even months. The degenerative changes may act to produce nonspecific effects of the brain injury, such as the loss of synapses in widespread regions of the injured hemisphere. The

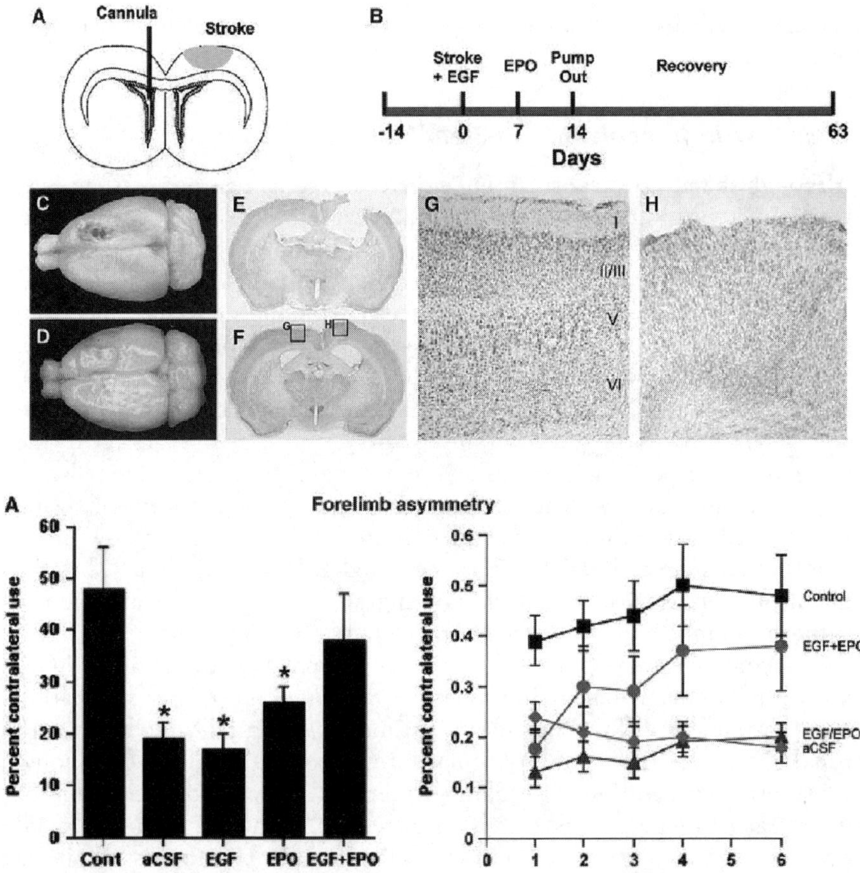

FIGURE 2.5. (Top) EGF + EPO infusions lead to tissue regeneration in the motor cortex after focal stroke. (A, B) Experimental paradigm. Devascularizing lesion on day 0 was following by EGF and/or EPO infusion via an intraventricular cannula in the contralateral hemisphere beginning on poststroke day 7. EGF was infused for 7 days, followed by EPO for 7 days. (C, D) Dorsal photographs of lesion brains (42 days after stroke), infused with either cerebrospinal fluid (CSF) + CSF (C) or EGF + EPO (D). The stroke produced a chronic cavity, whereas treatment with EGF + EPO led to the development of newly generated cortical tissue. (E–H) Coronal cresyl-violet-stained sections showing the lesion cavity in a CSF + CSF lesion brain (E) and an EGF + EPO lesion brain (F). The lesion cavity is filled with tissue in the latter brain. The intact hemisphere of the EGF + EPO brain has clear lamination characteristic of motor cortex (G), but there is no obvious organization in the newly generated cortical tissue and a complete absence of a layer I (H). (Bottom) Stroke-induced motor deficits recover EGF + EPO infusions. (Left panels) Summaries of the behavioral effects after 6 weeks of postinjury recovery. Rats treated with EGF + EPO showed better function on forelimb asymmetry. Adapted from Kolb et al. (2007). Copyright 2007 by Nature Publishing Group. Adapted by permission.

reparative changes that follow may reverse some of the nonspecific degenerative changes, but without either experiential, physiological, or pharmacological assistance, the spontaneous reparative changes do not generally lead to significant behavioral restitution. As we learn more about the principles of brain plasticity in laboratory animals and human subjects, we should be in a better position to develop novel treatments to facilitate behavioral compensation, and perhaps even some recovery, after cortical injury.

REFERENCES

Biernaskie, J., & Corbett, D. (2001). Enriched rehabilitative training promotes improved forelimb motor function and enhanced dendritic growth after focal ischemic injury. *Journal of Neuroscience, 21*, 5272–5280.

Brown, R. W., & Kolb, B. (2001). Nicotine sensitization increases dendritic length and spine density in the nucleus accumbens and cingulate cortex. *Brain Research, 899*(1–2), 94–100.

Chen, P., Goldberg, D., Kolb, B., Lanser, M., & Benowitz, L. (2002) Axonal rewiring and improved function induced by inosine after stroke. *Proceedings of the National Academy of Sciences USA, 99*(13), 9031–9036.

Coleman, P. D., & Buell, S. J. (1985). Regulation of dendritic extent in developing and aging brain. In C. W. Cotman (Ed.), *Synaptic plasticity* (pp. 311–333). New York: Guilford Press.

Cotman, C. W., & Berchtold, N. C. (2002). Exercise: A behavioral intervention to enhance brain health and plasticity. *Trends in Neurosciences, 25*(6), 295–301.

Cramer, S. C., & Bastings, E. P. (2000). Mapping clinically relevant plasticity after stroke. *Neuropharmacology, 39*, 842–851.

Dancause, N., Barbay, S., Frost, S. B., Plautz, E. J., Chen, D., Zoubina, E. V., et al. (2005). Extensive cortical rewiring after brain injury. *Journal of Neuroscience, 25*, 10167–10179.

Dawson, K. D., Howarth, K. R., Tarnopolsky, M. A., Wong, N. D., & Gibala, M. J. (2003). Short-term training attenuates muscle TCA cycle expansion during exercise in women. *Journal of Applied Physiology, 95*, 999–1004.

Ellison, J. A., Barone, F. C., & Feuerstein, G. Z. (1999). Matrix remodeling after stroke: De novo expression of matrix proteins and integrin receptors. *Annals of the New York Academy of Sciences, 890*, 204–222.

Feeney, D. M., & Sutton, R. L. (1987). Pharmacotherapy for recovery of function after brain injury. *Critical Reviews in Neurobiology, 3*, 135–197.

Fiorino, D., & Kolb, B. (2003). Sexual experience leads to long-lasting morphological changes in male rat prefrontal cortex, parietal cortex, and nucleus accumbens neurons. *Society for Neuroscience Abstracts, 29*, 402.3.

Flores, C., & Stewart, J. (2000). Changes in astrocytic basic fibroblast growth factor expression during and after prolonged exposure to escalating doses of amphetamine. *Neuroscience, 98*, 287–293.

Frost, S. B., Barbay, S., Friel, K. M., Plautz, E. J., & Nudo, R. J. (2003). Reorganization of remote cortical regions after ischemic brain injury: A potential substrate for stroke recovery. *Journal of Neurophysiology, 89,* 3205–3214.

Goldstein, J. M., Seidman, L. J., Horton, N. J., Makris, N., Kennedy, D. N., Caviness, V. S., Jr., et al. (2001). Normal sexual dimorphism of the adult human brain assessed by in vivo magnetic resonance imaging. *Cerebral Cortex, 11,* 490–497.

Goldstein, L. B. (2003). Amphetamines and related drugs in motor recovery after stroke. *Physical Medicine and Rehabilitative Clinics of North America, 14,* S125–S134.

Gonzalez, C. L. R., Gharbawie, O. A., & Kolb, B. (2006). Chronic low-dose administration of nicotine facilitates recovery and synaptic change after focal ischemia in rats. *Neuropharmacology, 50*(7), 777–787.

Greenough, W. T., & Chang, F. F. (1989). Plasticity of synapse structure and pattern in the cerebral cortex. In A. Peters & E. G. Jones (Eds.), *Cerebral cortex* (Vol. 7, pp. 391–440). New York: Plenum Press.

Hamilton, D., & Kolb, B. (2005). Nicotine, experience, and brain plasticity. *Behavioral Neuroscience, 119*(2), 355–365.

Hefti, F. (1997). Pharmacology of neurotrophic factors. *Annual Review of Pharmacology and Toxicology, 37,* 239–267.

Ivanco, T., Racine, R. J., & Kolb, B. (2000). The morphology of layer III pyramidal cells is altered following induction of LTP in somatomotor cortex. *Synapse, 37,* 16–22.

Jacobs, B., & Scheibel, A. B. (1993). A quantitative dendritic analysis of Wernicke's area in humans. I. Lifespan changes. *Journal of Comparative Neurology, 327,* 383–396.

Johansson, B. B. (1996). Functional outcome in rats transferred to an enriched environment 15 days after focal brain ischemia. *Stroke, 27,* 324–326.

Johansson, B. B. (2000). Brain plasticity and stroke rehabilitation: The Willis lecture. *Stroke, 31,* 223–230.

Jordan, B. D. (2007). Genetic influences on outcome following traumatic brain injury. *Neurochemical Research, 32,* 905–915.

Juraska, J. (1990). The structure of the rat cerebral cortex: Effects of gender and environment. In B. Kolb & R. C. Tees (Eds.), *Cerebral cortex of the rat* (pp. 483–506). Cambridge, MA: MIT Press.

Kawamata, T., Speliotes, E. K., & Finklestein, S. P. (1997). The role of polypeptide growth factors in recovery from stroke. *Advances in Neurology, 73,* 377–382.

Kleim, J. A., Jones, T. A., & Schallert, T. (2003). Motor enrichment and the induction of plasticity before or after brain injury. *Neurochemistry Research, 28,* 1757–1769.

Kolb, B., Cioe, J., & Comeau, W. (2008). Contrasting effects of motor and visual learning tasks on dendritic arborization and spine density in rats. *Neurobiology of Learning and Memory, 90,* 295–300.

Kolb, B., Cote, S., Ribeiro-da-Silva, A., & Cuello, A. C. (1997a). NGF stimulates recovery of function and dendritic growth after unilateral motor cortex lesions in rats. *Neuroscience, 76,* 1139–1151.

Kolb, B., & Elliott, W. (1987). Recovery from early cortical damage in rats: II.

Effects of experience on anatomy and behavior following frontal lesions at 1 or 5 days of age. *Behavioural Brain Research, 26*, 47–56.

Kolb, B., Forgie, M., Gibb, R., Gorny, G., & Rowntree, S. (1998). Age, experience, and the changing brain. *Neuroscience and Biobehavioral Reviews, 22*, 143–159.

Kolb, B., & Gibb, R. (2007). Brain plasticity and recovery from early cortical injury. *Developmental Psychobiology, 49*, 107–118.

Kolb, B., Gorny, G., Cote, S., Ribeiro-da-Silva, A., & Cuello, A. C. (1997b). Nerve growth factor stimulates growth of cortical pyramidal neurons in young adult rats. *Brain Research, 751*, 289–294.

Kolb, B., Gorny, G., Li, Y., Samaha, A. N., & Robinson, T. E. (2003). Amphetamine or cocaine limits the ability of later experience to promote structural plasticity in the neocortex and nucleus accumbens. *Proceedings of the National Academy of Sciences USA, 100*(18), 10523–10528.

Kolb, B., Morshead, C., Gonzalez, C., Kim, N., Shingo, T., & Weiss, S. (2007). Growth factor-stimulated generation of new cortical tissue and functional recovery after stroke damage to the motor cortex of rats. *Journal of Cerebral Blood Flow and Metabolism, 27*(5), 983–997.

Kolb, B., & Stewart, J. (1991). Sex-related differences in dendritic branching of cells in the prefrontal cortex of rats. *Journal of Neuroendocrinology, 3*, 95–99.

Kolb, B., & Whishaw, I. Q. (1998). Brain plasticity and behavior. *Annual Review of Psychology, 49*, 43–64.

Kolb, B., & Whishaw, I. Q. (2009). *Fundamentals of human neuropsychology* (6th Ed.). New York: Worth.

Kozlowski, D. A., James, D. C., & Schallert, T. (1996). Use-dependent exaggeration of neuronal injury after unilateral sensorimotor cortex lesions. *Journal of Neuroscience, 16*, 4776–4786.

Lena, C., & Changeux, J. P. (1999). The role of beta 2-subunit-containing nicotinic acetylcholine receptors in the brain explored with a mutant mouse. *Annals of the New York Academy of Sciences, 868*, 611–616.

Li, Y., Kolb, B., & Robinson, T. E. (2005). Psychostimulant drugs alter the effect of complex housing on synaptic plasticity in CA1 pyramidal neurons. *Society for Neuroscience Abstracts, 31*, 1032.4.

McDonald, R. J., Craig, L. A., & Hong, N. S. (2010). The etiology of age-related dementia is more complicated than we think. *Behavioural Brain Research, 214*, 3–11.

McEwen, B. S. (2005). Glucocorticoids, depression, and mood disorders: Structural remodeling in the brain. *Metabolism, 54*(5, Suppl. 1), 20–23.

Meck, W. H., & Williams, C. L. (2003). Metabolic imprinting of choline by its availability during gestation: Implications for memory and attentional processing across the lifespan. *Neuroscience and Biobehavioral Reviews, 27*, 385–399.

Michael, D. B., Byers, D. M., & Irwin, L. N. (2005). Gene expression following traumatic brain injury in humans: Analysis by microarray. *Journal of Clinical Neuroscience, 12*, 284–290.

Milner, B. (1975). Psychological aspects of focal epilepsy and its neurosurgical management. *Advances in Neurology, 8*, 299–321.

Moroz, I. A., & Kolb, B. (2005). Amphetamine facilitates recovery of skilled reaching following cortical devascularization in the rat. *Society for Neuroscience Abstracts, 31*, 835–839.

Nieto-Sampedro, M., & Cotman, C. W. (1985). Growth factor induction and temporal order in central nervous system repair. In C. W. Cotman (Ed.), *Synaptic plasticity* (pp. 407–456). New York: Guilford Press.

Nudo, R. J., Wise, B. M., SiFuentes, F., & Milliken, G. W. (1996). Neural substrates for the effects of rehabilitative training on motor recovery after ischemic infarct. *Science, 272*(5269), 1791–1794.

Papadopoulos, C., Tsai, S.-Y., Cheatwood, J. L., Bollnow, M. R., Kolb, B., & Schwab, M. (2006). Dendritic plasticity in the adult rat following middle cerebral artery occlusion and nogo-A neutralization. *Cerebral Cortex, 16*(4), 529–536.

Pearce, J. M. (1994). Von Monakow and diaschisis. *Journal of Neurology, Neurosurgery, and Psychiatry, 57*, 197.

Piecharka, D. M., Kleim, J. A., & Whishaw, I. Q. (2005). Limits on recovery in the corticospinal tract of the rat: Partial lesions impair skilled reaching and the topographic representation of the forelimb in motor cortex. *Brain Research Bulletin, 66*, 203–211.

Polgar, S., Morris, M. E., Reilly, S., Bilney, B., & Sanberg, P. R. (2003). Reconstructive neurosurgery for Parkinson's disease: A systematic review and preliminary meta-analysis. *Brain Research Bulletin, 60*, 1–24.

Rijntjes, M., & Weiller, C. (2002). Recovery of motor and language abilities after stroke: The contribution of functional imaging. *Progress in Neurobiology, 66*, 109–122.

Robinson, T. E., & Kolb, B. (1997). Persistent structural adaptations in nucleus accumbens and prefrontal cortex neurons produced by prior experience with amphetamine. *Journal of Neuroscience, 17*, 8491–8498.

Robinson, T. E., & Kolb, B. (2004). Structural plasticity associated with drugs of abuse. *Neuropharmacology, 47*(Suppl. 1), 33–46.

Schulkin, J. (Ed.). (1989). *Preoperative events: Their effects on behavior following brain damage.* Hillsdale, NJ: Erlbaum.

Shaw, C. A., & McEachern, J. C. (Eds.). (2001). *Toward a theory of neuroplasticity.* Philadelphia: Psychology Press.

Silasi, G., & Kolb, B. (2007). Chronic inhibition of cyclooxygenase-2 induced dendritic hypertrophy and limited functional improvement following motor cortex stroke. *Neuroscience, 144*, 1160–1168.

Siu, D. (2010). A new way of targeting to treat nerve injury. *International Journal of Neuroscience, 120*, 1–10.

Steward, O. (1991). Synapse replacement on coretical neurons following denervatin. In A. Peters & E. G. Jones (Eds.), *Cerebral cortex* (Vol. 9, pp. 81–132). New York: Plenum Press.

Stewart, J., & Kolb, B. (1988). The effects of neonatal gonadectomy and prenatal stress on cortical thickness and asymmetry in rats. *Behavioral and Neural Biology, 49*, 344–360.

Teasell, R., Bayona, N., Salter, K., Hellings, C., & Bitensky, J. (2006). Progress in clinical neurosciences: Stroke recovery and rehabilitation. *Canadian Journal of Neurological Sciences, 33*, 357–364.

Teskey, G. C., Flynn, C., Goertzen, C. D., Monfils, M. H., & Young, N. A. (2003). Cortical stimulation improves skilled forelimb use following a focal ischemic infarct in the rat. *Neurological Research, 25*, 794–800.

Teskey, G. C., Monfils, M. N., Silasi, G., & Kolb, B. (2006). Neocortical kindling is associated with opposing alterations in dendritic morphology in neocortical layer V and striatum from neocortical layer III. *Synapse, 59*, 1–9.

Teyler, T. J. (2001). LTP and the superfamily of synaptic plasticities. In C. A. Shaw & J. C. McEachern (Eds.), *Toward a theory of neuroplasticity* (pp. 101–117). Philadelphia: Psychology Press.

Uylings, H., Groenewegen, H., & Kolb, B. (2003). Does the rat have a prefrontal cortex? *Behavioural Brain Research, 146*, 3–17.

Will, B., & Kelche, C. (1992). Environmental approaches to recovery of function from brain damage: A review of animal studies (1981 to 1991). In F. D. Rose & D. A. Johnson (Eds.), *Recovery from brain damage: Reflections and directions* (pp. 79–104). New York: Plenum Press.

Williams, P. T., Gharbawie, O. A., Kolb, B., & Kleim, J. A. (2006). Experience-dependent amelioration of motor impairments in adulthood following neonatal medial frontal lesions in rats is accompanied by motor map expansion. *Neuroscience, 141*(3), 1315–1326.

Withers, G. S., & Greenough, W. T. (1989). Reach training selectively alters dendritic branching in subpopulations of layer II–III pyramids in rat motor–somatosensory forelimb cortex. *Neuropsychologia, 27*, 61–69.

Witt-Lajeunesse, A., Cioe, J., & Kolb, B. (2011). *Rehabilitative experience interacts with bFGF to facilitate functional improvement after motor cortex injury*. Manuscript submitted for publication.

CHAPTER 3

Experience-Dependent Changes in Nonhumans

THERESA A. JONES

This chapter focuses on evidence from animal models supporting a critical role for experience in shaping reorganization of the damaged brain. Decades of research have shown that the brain's neural and non-neuronal cells are constantly undergoing changes—changes that permit animals, including humans, to learn and adapt to an ever-changing environment (Churchill et al., 2002). This is one reason why one should not underestimate the importance of behavioral experience in recovery from brain damage. Another reason is that brain damage places the brain in an especially dynamic state as it undergoes the process of reorganization. Some have suggested that this state rivals and, in some sense, recapitulates that found during brain development (Carmichael, 2006; Cramer & Chopp, 2000). Like development, this dynamic state is also extraordinarily sensitive to behavioral experience (Table 3.1); this raises the possibility of using manipulations of experience to improve function by shaping the very course of the reorganization. This possibility is supported by research manipulating the environments of rodents and other animals, as well as by studies of more directed "rehabilitative" training approaches. Other research indicates that experience can be both good and bad for functional outcome. It seems safe to say that we are mostly beyond the stage of establishing that experience *does* matter, and are now working on trying to understand precisely *how* it matters by probing the nature of the interaction between experience and functional reorganization. Such an understanding is likely to be key for

TABLE 3.1. Examples of Behavioral Influences on Injury-Induced Brain Changes

Injury-induced event	Direction	Finding
Tissue loss	+	Forced forelimb use increased tissue loss near sensory–motor cortex lesions (Kozlowski et al., 1996). Major stress increased tissue loss after cerebral infarcts (Kirkland et al., 2008).
Tissue loss	–	Constraint-induced movement-like therapy decreased tissue loss after striatal hemorrhage (DeBow et al., 2003).
Cell death	+	Early EC exaggerated postischemic hippocampal neuron death (Farrell et al., 2001).
Cell death	–	Forced forelimb use decreased loss of dopamine neurons in a model of Parkinson's disease (Tillerson et al., 2001).
Growth factors	+	Delayed exercise increased BDNF after traumatic brain injury (Griesbach et al., 2004b).
Growth factors	–	Too-early exercise decreased BDNF and other plasticity-related proteins after traumatic brain injury (Griesbach et al., 2004a).
Reactive astrocytes	+	Forced forelimb use increased astrocytic reactions to callosal denervation (Bury et al., 2000b).
Axonal sprouting	+	Axonal prouting after nigrostriatal damage depended on behavioral asymmetries (Morgan et al., 1983).
Dendritic growth	+	Dendritic growth contralateral to sensory–motor cortex lesions depended on behavioral asymmetries (Jones & Schallert, 1994).
Synaptogenesis	+	Motor skills training increased cortical lesion-induced synaptogenesis (Jones et al., 1999).
Neurogenesis	+	EC increased SVZ neurogenesis after cortical infarct (Komitova et al., 2005a).
Neurogenesis	–	Exercise decreased SGZ neurogenesis after cortical infarct (Komitova et al., 2005b).
Cortical functional activity	+	Skilled reach training increased movement representations near cortical infarcts (Nudo et al., 1996).

Note. This table illustrates two points: (1) Many degenerative and regenerative processes are sensitive to behavioral experience, and (2) the nature of the effect varies with dose and timing of the behavioral manipulation and with severity and type of injury, among other factors. +, increased compared to controls; –, decreased compared to controls; EC, environmental complexity; BDNF, brain-derived neurotrophic factor; SVZ, subventricular zone; SGZ, subgranular zone.

attempts to use behavioral manipulations, alone and in combination with other treatment approaches, to optimize functional outcome. This topic requires an appreciation of the way brains adapt to brain damage, and I briefly review this adaptation next.

INJURY-INDUCED NEURAL PLASTICITY

Brain injury is an event that nervous systems may have long evolved to cope with, because, in the right circumstances, it induces a dramatic and highly orchestrated counteroffensive (reviewed in Carmichael, 2006; Kelley & Steward, 1997). Even when an injury is relatively small, there are widespread inflammatory, neurotoxic, and degenerative pressures. Neurons in diverse regions lose some of their synapses as connected neurons die. If the injury is too severe, and too many neural connections are lost in connected brain regions, the neurons there may also die. This is because the connections of a neuron help it to survive by contributing prosurvival molecules and by maintaining healthy levels of activity. These contributions may become even more important for neurons that have been metabolically challenged or exposed to toxic substances, as happens near an ischemic infarct. However, the degenerative pressures also serve as the stimulus for the counteroffensive.

In response to partial denervation, remaining axons sprout and form new synaptic connections. This phenomenon, known as *reactive synaptogenesis*, was first extensively studied in denervated hippocampus (e.g., Matthews, Cotman, & Lynch, 1976; reviewed in Cotman & Anderson, 1988), but has since been established to occur in a great many other parts of the brain; thus it seems reasonable to assume that it can happen in most brain regions that lose some input (e.g., Dancause et al., 2005; Riban & Chesselet, 2006; Serfaty, Campello-Costa, & Linden, 2005). What happens is that as axonal processes of dying neurons begin to degenerate, glial cells are called upon to clear degenerating debris. They also contribute to the production of numerous growth- and survival-promoting molecules (*neurotrophins*), which cause remaining axons in the vicinity to sprout and begin to form new connections (Kelley & Steward, 1997). After ischemic injury, molecules that normally keep wayward axons at bay (presumably to reduce the formation of inappropriate neural connections) may be transiently inhibited to contribute to this growth-permissive environment (Benowitz & Carmichael, 2010; Carmichael et al., 2005; Hobohm et al., 2005). Although this sequence is sometimes referred to as "synapse replacement," the recipients of the new connections are hardly standing by, passively awaiting the new inputs. The partially denervated neurons begin to express new genes; some of these help them survive the damage, and others help them change their cytoskeletons so that dendrites are restructured in orchestration with the formation of their new synaptic inputs (Deller et al., 2006; Hamori, 1990; Murphy & Corbett, 2009). The fine structure of synaptic connections is also changed. In many denervated regions, there is the appearance of synapses that have the structural characteristics related to greater synaptic efficacy (Jones, 1999; Marrone, LeBoutillier, & Petit, 2004; McNeill, Brown, Hogg, Cheng, & Meshul, 2003). There are also major changes in neural activity and excitability, which can be long-lasting after the injury (Brown, Aminoltejari, Erb, Winship, & Murphy, 2009; Di Filippo et al., 2008; Witte, Bidmon, Schiene, Redecker, & Hagemann, 2000).

Another tactic in the counteroffensive is the generation of new neurons. The adult mammalian brain has two *germinal zones*, which produce new cells throughout life: the *subgranular zone* (SGZ) of the hippocampus, and the *subventricular zone* (SVZ), which lies adjacent to the lateral ventricles. Precursors to neurons are generated in each zone in close association with microvasculature, in what is known as the *neurovascular niche* (Alvarez-Buylla & Lim, 2004). The growth-permissive environment induced by the injury is thought to enhance the cell production in these zones (Greenberg & Jin, 2006; Ohab, Fleming, Blesch, & Carmichael, 2006), and indeed enhanced production has been documented in diverse injury models, including ischemia (Gotts & Chesselet, 2005; Ramaswamy, Goings, Soderstrom, Szele, & Kozlowski, 2005; reviewed in Lichtenwalner & Parent, 2006). This phenomenon has been primarily studied in rodents, but it also occurs in Old World monkeys (macaque; Tonchev, Yamashima, & Chaldakov, 2007), and new neurons have been found near ischemic damage in the cortex of humans (Jin et al., 2006). As in the intact brain, newly generated cells in the SGZ travel a short distance to become neurons in the dentate gyrus after ischemia (e.g., Liu, Solway, Messing, & Sharp, 1998). Neural precursors from the SVZ travel a longer distance to become olfactory neurons in intact animals, and these cells have also been found to migrate into the striatum and neocortex near an injury (Arvidsson, Collin, Kirik, Kokaia, & Lindvall, 2002; Gotts & Chesselet, 2005; Parent, Vexler, Gong, Derugin, & Ferriero, 2002). Molecules released by remodeling tissue appear to call new neurons to injured tissue (Ohab et al., 2006). However, in rats, few of the new neurons in striatum and cortex survive long (e.g., Arvidsson et al., 2002). Gotts and Chesselet (2005) carefully examined the newly generated cells in the region bordering a cortical infarct and found that most developed into a type of glial cell (oligodendroglia). This may seem disappointing, but one should keep in mind that glial cells have many critical roles in neural and synaptic function and are well-established mediators of brain restructuring and synaptic plasticity (reviewed in Jones & Greenough, 2002).

Is the counteroffensive beneficial for behavioral function? Many correlative data indicate that it can be (reviewed in Benowitz & Carmichael,

2010). In hippocampus, the time course of reactive synaptogenesis is correlated with functional outcome (Steward, Loesche, & Horton, 1977). Traumatic brain injury that results in significant diffuse axonal injury is linked with impaired sprouting responses and poorer recovery (Phillips & Reeves, 2001; Reeves, Zhu, Povlishock, & Phillips, 1997). Ischemic damage to neocortex results in more sprouting in the denervated striatum than suction ablation damage, and rats with ischemic lesions have better functional outcome (Carmichael & Chesselet, 2002; Uryu, MacKenzie, & Chesselet, 2001; see also Voorhies & Jones, 2002). Treatments that promote greater axonal sprouting improve functional outcome (e.g., Zhang et al., 2010). In adult animals, a growth-inhibiting substance, Nogo, is normally produced by myelin and limits the sprouting that would be possible in a younger animal. Blocking Nogo-A in rodents and monkeys greatly increases sprouting and improves functional recovery (Emerick & Kartje, 2004; Freund et al., 2006). Providing substances that promote neurogenesis (Greenberg & Jin, 2006) and migration of immature neurons (Ohab et al., 2006) improves functional outcome after cortical infarcts. Manipulations of behavioral experience that enhance neurogenesis have also been found to improve functional outcome, as discussed below. However, it is highly unlikely that every example of neural plasticity after brain damage is functionally beneficial. Some changes may be detrimental or have mixed effects on functional outcome (e.g., Hsu & Jones, 2006; Neumann-Haefelin et al., 1998). Thus it is important to better understand specific relationships between these processes of neuronal adaptation and behavioral function. Given that the neuronal adaptation also varies with injury type (e.g., stroke vs. traumatic brain injury; Phillips & Reeves, 2001), it is also important to investigate these interactions in multiple injury models.

All together, these processes take time. In rodents, the neural responses to injury may take months or more to resolve (reviewed in Carmichael, 2006; Wieloch & Nikolich, 2006; Winship & Murphy, 2009). The time course varies with age (it tends to take longer in older animals; Anderson, Scheff, & DeKosky, 1986; Li & Carmichael, 2006) and also probably varies with injury severity, locus, and type (Phillips & Reeves, 2001). There is nevertheless a clear sequence to the events, and the ability to influence them with external manipulations is likely to be greatest at earlier postinjury time points (Murphy & Corbett, 2009). The time-dependent nature of the reactive changes also means that it is unwise to assume that a therapy that improves function at one time will be optimal at another, as discussed below.

The existence of such amazing injury-triggered plasticity also, of course, raises the possibility of using manipulations of behavioral experience to drive this plasticity in a beneficial direction and to increase it when it is deficient.

INJURY–EXPERIENCE INTERACTIONS IN REACTIVE PLASTICITY

Investigation of a type of reactive plasticity in neocortex in rats has revealed a major way in which behavior can influence neural restructuring. In rats, the forelimb representation region of the motor cortex of either hemisphere is connected via transcallosal projections. When the cortex of one hemisphere is damaged by a small lesion or ischemic infarct (Figure 3.1), the contralateral cortex undergoes degeneration of axonal projections, reactive changes in glia, increases in growth factor expression, growth of dendritic processes, and formation of new and different types of synapses (Adkins, Voorhies, & Jones, 2004; Allred & Jones, 2008a, 2009; Jones, 1999; Jones et al., 2003; Jones, Hawrylak, Klintsova, & Greenough, 1998). This process resembles many aspects of reactive synaptogenesis reported in other models, but the dendrites and synapses actually increase in quantity, compared to levels found in the same brain region in intact animals. Synapses also increase in quantity, although this takes longer (~1 month; Jones,

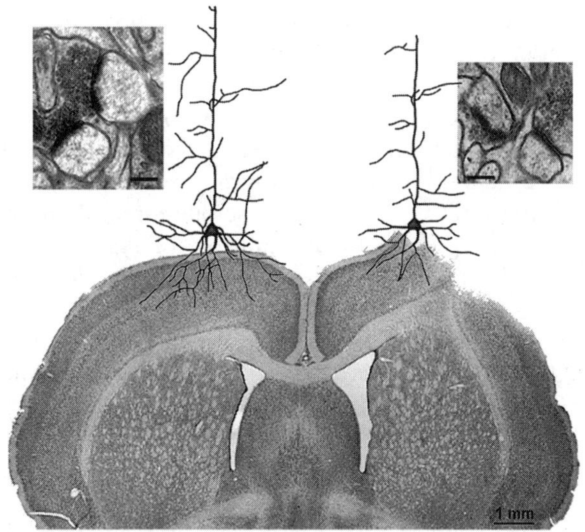

FIGURE 3.1. Unilateral infarct in the right sensory–motor cortex, viewed in a coronal section of the rat forebrain. Dendritic growth and synaptogenesis in the contralateral motor cortex are related to compensation with the less affected forelimb. Neural plasticity in the damaged hemisphere can be driven with motor training to mediate better function in the impaired limb. Inserts are electron micrographs of motor cortical synapses. The author thanks Dr. J. E. Hsu for help in creating this figure. Scale bars = 250 nm.

Kleim, & Greenough, 1996). In a manner reminiscent of brain development, both dendrites and synapses seem to be overproduced and then partially eliminated.

One could view this cortical restructuring as merely another example of reactive plasticity if it were not for the co-occurrence of dramatic behavioral changes. Rats use their forepaws for postural support and in dexterous ways for handling food and other objects, somewhat like squirrels. After unilateral sensory–motor cortex lesions, these behaviors are impaired in the contralateral forelimb; with no prompting from the experimenter, rats spontaneously begin to use the less affected (ipsilateral to the lesion) forelimb more and in different ways to compensate for the deficits (Jones & Schallert, 1992; Schallert, Kozlowski, Humm, & Cocke, 1997; Whishaw, 2000).

It is well documented that experience with one forelimb can drive changes in the motor cortex of adult rats (Monfils, Plautz, & Kleim, 2005), and my colleagues and I wondered how increased reliance on the less affected forelimb contributed to the restructuring in the cortex contralateral to the lesion. Huston and colleagues had previously found that sprouting in the nigrostriatal system after unilateral lesions was dependent upon behavioral asymmetries in rats (Huston, Morgan, & Steiner, 1987; Morgan, Huston, & Pritzel, 1983). We hypothesized that the neuronal growth contralateral to the lesion was dependent upon a lesion–behavior interaction (Jones & Schallert, 1992). Several findings are consistent with this hypothesis. First, if animals are prevented from using their less affected forelimb after unilateral lesions, the growth is reduced (Jones & Schallert, 1994). Second, if animals are forced to use one forelimb more (by placing them in limb-restricting vests), there is only a subtle growth of spines in the cortex opposite this limb. In contrast, major spine and dendrite addition is found when animals forced to use one limb that also have partial split-brain procedures that create degeneration of transcallosal fibers (Adkins, Bury, & Jones, 2002; Bury et al., 2000a). Finally, if degeneration and behavioral asymmetries are uncoupled in time, there is little dendritic growth (Jones & Allred, 2004). Thus it appears that lesion-induced degeneration enhances the propensity of neurons in the contralateral cortex to grow new synapses and dendrites in response to relevant behavioral pressures.

Does this have any functional relevance? Rats with small electrolytic or ischemic sensory–motor cortex lesions are better able to learn a new task of manual dexterity (skilled reaching) with the less affected limb than intact animals are (Allred, Maldonado, Hsu, & Jones, 2005; Bury & Jones, 2002; Hsu & Jones, 2005; see also Bury & Jones, 2004; Glazewski, Benedetti, & Barth, 2007)—an effect that is found despite the presence of some impairments in this forelimb (Hsu & Jones, 2006). This paradoxical functional enhancement most likely facilitates the development of new ways of using the less affected limb to compensate for impairments. However, this is an example of neural plasticity that probably has mixed effects on functional outcome, because greater reliance on, and learning with, the less affected limb may exacerbate disuse of the impaired limb. As discussed more fully below, it may also limit adaptive plasticity in the affected hemisphere (Allred & Jones, 2008a).

These findings support the sensitivity of reactive plasticity to behavioral experience. They also point to a category of experiences that influence brain restructuring—that is, "self-taught" behavioral changes occurring in the absence of any overt interventions. This provides yet another reason to understand experience–injury interactions. In the absence of behavioral interventions, an animal's experiences may drive brain plasticity in a direction that is suboptimal and possibly even maladaptive for functional outcome. Thus it seems quite urgent for us to obtain a better understanding of these interactions, so that appropriate behavioral interventions can be used. Research on the effects of environmental manipulation serves as a foundation for this line of inquiry.

EFFECTS OF ENVIRONMENTAL COMPLEXITY AFTER BRAIN DAMAGE

Housing laboratory animals in a complex ("enriched") environment can have powerful effects on brain function and structure. In the typical study of environmental complexity (EC), rats live in social groups of six or more in an environment containing different objects that can be explored and manipulated, and that are changed regularly (Figure 3.2). In most standard laboratory environments, rats live in a simple cage alone or with a few cage mates. As originally noted by Hebb (1949) over 60 years ago, EC rats seem better able to "profit by new experience" (p. 298; see also Black, Jones, Nelson, & Greenough, 1997; Rosenzweig & Bennett, 1996). EC-housed rats are superior at solving mazes and outperform rats from standard housing on many measures of learning and perceptual function (e.g., Greenough, Wood, & Madden, 1972; Tees, Buhrmann, & Hanley, 1990; Woodcock & Richardson, 2000).

The brains of animals housed for a period of time in EC have more dendrites, synapses, vasculature, and glial processes than do those of animals housed in standard-cage conditions (reviewed in Black et al., 1997; Grossman, Churchill, Bates, Kleim, & Greenough, 2002). Brain weight and cortical thickness are also increased (Bennett, Diamond, Krech, & Rosenzweig, 1964). Structural changes are preceded by changes in gene expression (Wallace et al., 1995). The magnitudes of EC brain effects tend to be large. For example, rats housed in EC for 30 days beginning at weaning have 25% more synapses in the visual cortex than rats housed alone in standard laboratory cages do (Turner & Greenough, 1985). The neuronal

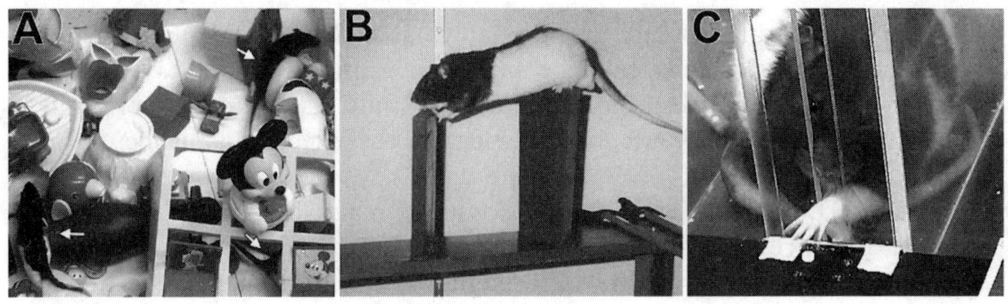

FIGURE 3.2. Examples of rodent behavioral manipulations. (A) Rats (arrows) in a complex environment; (B) rats traversing an obstacle of the acrobatic task; and (C) rats performing the skilled reaching task.

plasticity is quite notable in the neocortex, but neuroplastic effects have been reported in numerous other brain regions, including striatum (Comery, Shah, & Greenough, 1995) and cerebellum (Floeter & Greenough, 1979). Changes are also evident in the structure of cortical synapses, which increase in size, in complexity, and in their coverage by the fine processes of astrocytes (Jones & Greenough, 2002; Jones, Klintsova, Kilman, Sirevaag, & Greenough, 1997; Sirevaag & Greenough, 1985). EC housing also enhances neurogenesis in the dentate gyrus of the hippocampus (Kempermann, Kuhn, & Gage, 1997; Nilsson, Perfilieva, Johansson, Orwar, & Eriksson, 1999). The effects of EC tend to be greatest when it is initiated at young ages, and there are some age-dependent differences in the patterns of neuronal growth (Kolb, Forgie, Gibb, Gorny, & Rowntree, 1998; Kolb, Gibb, & Gorny, 2003); nevertheless, the brain effects are robust in mature and aging animals (Green, Greenough, & Schlumpf, 1983; Kobayashi, Ohashi, & Ando, 2002), and EC can offset aging-related cognitive deficits (Kramer, Bherer, Colcombe, Dong, & Greenough, 2004).

Because EC housing has such a major beneficial effect on brain structure and function in intact animals, it is perhaps not surprising that it also leads animals to fare better after brain injury. In studies spanning half a century, it has been found that animals housed in EC have superior functional outcome after many different types and loci of brain injury, compared to rats in standard housing (e.g., Schwartz, 1964; reviewed in Greenough, Fass, & DeVoogd, 1976; Johansson, 2000; Schallert, Leasure, & Kolb, 2000). Will, Galani, Kelche, and Rosenzweig (2004) provide an excellent review of the literature on this topic. For example, housing rats in EC after unilateral middle cerebral artery occlusions greatly improves recovery from deficits in spatial learning (Dahlqvist, Ronnback, Bergstrom, Soderstrom, & Olsson, 2004; Sonninen, Virtanen, Sivenius, & Jolkkonen, 2006) and sensory and motor function (Ohlsson & Johansson, 1995).

What is improved by EC? In a series of studies, Rose and colleagues found that EC housing is particularly useful for improving behavioral compensation and response substitution, rather than "true" recovery of function (Rose, Davey, & Attree, 1993; Rose, Davey, Love, & Dell, 1987; Rose, Dell, Love, & Davey, 1988; see also Knieling, Metz, Antonow-Schlorke, & Witte, 2009). This is consistent with the idea that EC promotes the capacity for future learning (Greenough et al., 1976; Hebb, 1949) and, in the case of animals recovering from brain damage, the capacity for "relearning" and for adopting alternative task strategies. EC housing also affords more opportunity for complex motor activities, which can be thought of as a type of motor rehabilitative therapy. It is also promotes physical activity, which itself has functional benefits. In intact rats, running is associated with angiogenesis, increases in neurotrophins, and other plastic changes in the hippocampus, cerebellum, and neocortex (reviewed in Kleim, Jones, & Schallert, 2003b; Vaynman & Gomez-Pinilla, 2005). Exercise *prior* to brain injury can have a major neuroprotective effect (Ding et al., 2006). Voluntary running can also improve cognitive function when initiated after traumatic brain injury in rats, although, as discussed below, it can have detrimental effects when initiated too early after injury (Griesbach, Gomez-Pinilla, & Hovda, 2004a; Griesbach, Hovda, Molteni, Wu, & Gomez-Pinilla, 2004b).

Understanding the mechanisms underlying EC-induced functional improvements after brain damage is an inherently complex issue, because they can be expected to vary with the type and size of brain injury and the timing of its onset (see Will et al., 2004, for a discussion of this issue). How animals behave in the environment also varies with the severity and type of the injury (see Jones et al., 1998, for a discussion of this issue). Nevertheless, many studies have found that EC promotes greater neural plasticity after brain damage. For example, EC housing increases dendrites and spines in the motor cortex contralateral to cerebral infarcts (Biernaskie & Corbett, 2001; Johansson & Belichenko, 2002). Xerri, Zennou-Azougui, and Coq (2003) found that small lesions of the somatosensory cortex lead to loss and fragmentation of uninjured receptive fields surrounding the lesion, but that EC partially spares animals from this effect. Several studies have found that EC enhances postinjury neurogenesis (reviewed in Komitova, Johansson, & Eriksson, 2006), although the effect varies across studies with different injury locations (Komitova, Mattsson, Johansson, & Eriksson, 2005a; Nygren, Wieloch, Pesic, Brundin, & Deierborg, 2006)—as might be predicted if, for example, the magnitude of degeneration near germinal zones interacts with EC to influence cell proliferation.

What relevance does this animal research on complex housing have for human rehabilitation efforts? After all, the "standard-cage" condition in rats is arguably unnatural (Würbel, 2001), and perhaps humans should be viewed as typically living in complex environments. To the extent that humans can be considered to live in EC, this work strongly suggests that it is critical to avoid impoverishment of experience after brain injury. Interventions may be needed to counter the tendency of functional deficits resulting from brain injury to reduce the social, cognitive, and physical complexity of an individual's experience. One obvious way that experience can become impoverished is through the disuse of impaired modalities.

MALADAPTIVE BEHAVIORAL INFLUENCES

Experiences can be both good and bad for functional recovery. An example of a maladaptive change is the tendency for animals, including humans, to disuse impaired extremities—a phenomenon termed *learned nonuse* by Taub and colleagues (Taub, Uswatte, Mark, & Morris, 2006; see also Morris & Bickel, Chapter 7, this volume). Like humans, rats with unilateral cerebral injury reduce use of impaired extremities and rely more on less affected extremities for a variety of species-typical daily activities, including food-handling behavior and postural support. Because maintenance of normal neuronal function is use-dependent, disuse of the impaired body side may contribute to its dysfunction and limit opportunities for adaptive neural reorganization in the damaged hemisphere (reviewed in Kleim & Jones, 2008). Recent research in rats suggests another contributor to this dysfunction. Allred et al. (2005) found that a brief (10-day) period of motor training focused on the less affected forelimb after unilateral ischemic lesions of the sensory–motor cortex worsened function in the impaired forelimb and limited the ability to improve its function later through rehabilitative training. Furthermore, it reduced the ability to activate neurons in the peri-infarct cortex with later training of the impaired limb (Allred & Jones, 2006, 2008b). Disruption of the cortical connections between the injured and uninjured hemispheres attenuated the effects of training the less affected limb (Allred, Cappellini, & Jones, 2010). These findings are consistent with the idea that unilateral brain injury unbalances competitive interactions between the hemispheres (e.g., Rushmore, Valero-Cabre, Lomber, Hilgetag, & Payne, 2006; Ward & Cohen, 2004), and they indicate that behavioral experiences can contribute to this in a manner that limits functionally beneficial restructuring in the damaged hemisphere. Behavioral interventions, such as focused training of impaired extremities, are likely to be needed to counter these effects.

Too much activity early after a brain injury can also be maladaptive for functional outcome. Rats placed in vests that force the use of the impaired forelimb for the first 7 days after unilateral sensory–motor cortex lesions have worsened function in this limb and increased injury extent (Kozlowski, James, & Schallert, 1996; Schallert et al., 1997; see also

Risedal, Zeng, & Johansson, 1999). Tissue loss can be further exaggerated in rats that are moved from group housing to social isolation at the time of the injury (Woodlee & Schallert, 2006) and excessive social instability early after injury also impairs recovery (Silasi, Hamilton, & Kolb, 2008). Furthermore, early forced *disuse* of the impaired limb extends the time window of vulnerability to later overuse (Leasure & Schallert, 2004). Early voluntary exercise can also have maladaptive effects after brain damage. Griesbach and colleagues found that rats permitted to exercise voluntarily in running wheels during the first 6 days after traumatic brain injury had reduced expression of plasticity-related molecules in hippocampus. In contrast, delayed voluntary exercise improved function and enhanced expression of some of the same molecules (Griesbach et al., 2004a, 2004b; see also Ploughman et al., 2007). It is important to note that these studies involved a major amount of activity initiated very early after the injury. The forced-forelimb-use procedure involves continuous restriction of one forelimb and no other rehabilitative training, which is markedly different from constraint-induced movement therapy (CIMT) in humans (reviewed by Morris & Bickel, Chapter 7, this volume). When provided with access to running wheels, rats tend to exercise a great deal. In the study by Griesbach (2004b), rats averaged more than 800 wheel rotations (~800 meters) per night in the 6 days after a traumatic brain injury. Furthermore, the influence of early activity varies with injury type. As reviewed in Woodlee and Schallert (2006), forced activity in models of Parkinson's disease can protect neurons in the substantia nigra from dying, but only if the activity is initiated before or shortly after the onset of the degeneration.

ANIMAL MODELS OF REHABILITATIVE TRAINING

Part of the reason why housing rats in EC may be so effective in improving function is that the manipulation is intensive and complex. Indeed, more specific training approaches tend not to have as dramatic an effect on behavioral function as EC (Will et al., 2004). However, EC is not a very precise manipulation of behavioral experience, because it is difficult to control what the animals do in the environment. Furthermore, some injuries limit the propensity of animals to engage with the environment (Jones et al., 1998), and more targeted manipulations are likely to be necessary to improve severely impaired behavioral modalities.

In rats and monkeys, motor skill training after brain injury has been found to improve motor function and to drive major neuroplastic changes in remaining tissue (Nudo, 2007; see also Nudo & Bury, Chapter 4, this volume). In one manipulation, acrobatic training, rats are trained to traverse a series of challenging obstacles (Figure 3.2B), whereas exercised controls simply run back and forth in a straight alley. In intact animals, acquisition of this task results in major cellular, structural, and functional changes in the motor cortex and cerebellum (e.g., Black, Isaacs, Anderson, Alcantara, & Greenough, 1990; Kleim, Lussnig, Schwarz, Comery, & Greenough, 1996). Training rats on this task daily for a month after focal lesions of the sensory–motor cortex improved the coordinated use of the forelimbs and enhanced synaptogenesis in the motor cortex contralateral to the lesion (Jones, Chu, Grande, & Gregory, 1999). However, functional improvements were primarily found in the less affected forelimb (ipsilateral to the injury), and there was a failure to find significant dendritic and synaptic changes in regions of the remaining cortex of the damaged hemisphere after the training (Chu & Jones, 2000), so it seemed that acrobatic training was primarily effective in improving compensation with the less affected body side.

Skilled reaching (aka *reaching to grasp*) (Figure 3.2C) has been used to investigate the neural changes resulting from motor rehabilitation focused on the impaired upper extremity after unilateral brain damage (Nudo, 2007). In skilled reaching, rats or monkeys are trained to reach through an opening to grasp palatable food pellets. Errors in aiming or grasping result in missing or dropping the pellets. In rats, the movements used to perform this task have major homologies to those used by humans (Foroud & Whishaw, 2006; Whishaw et al., 2002), and intact animals learning the task undergo well-characterized neuroplastic changes in the primary motor cortex (reviewed in Adkins, Boychuk, Remple, & Kleim, 2006). After unilateral cortical lesions, extensive training in skilled reaching improves reaching function and promotes reorganization of peri-infarct cortex. This was demonstrated in a landmark study by Nudo and colleagues in squirrel monkeys (Nudo, Wise, SiFuentes, & Milliken, 1996; see also Nudo & Bury, Chapter 4). Small infarcts of the hand representation of the motor cortex result in a loss of movement representations in remaining cortex surrounding the infarcts. Training the monkeys in skilled reaching for 25 days prevented this loss and, in some monkeys, caused an expansion of the hand representation into territory previously eliciting elbow and shoulder movements. Similarly, training rats in skilled reaching improves function and promotes reorganization of remaining motor cortex after unilateral lesions of the forelimb representation region of the motor cortex (Castro-Alamancos & Borrel, 1995; Conner, Chiba, & Tuszynski, 2005; Ramanathan, Conner, & Tuszynski, 2006).

The time when training begins is an important variable in its efficacy. In monkeys, if reach training is delayed until 1 month after cortical infarcts, it is less effective than earlier training in sparing the loss of movement representations (Barbay et al., 2005). Training initiated 1 month after cerebral infarcts in rats is less effective in improving function and enhancing dendritic growth than is training initiated at 5 days (Biernaskie, Chernenko, & Corbett, 2004). It may be that when training onset is delayed, combining it with other treatment approaches (discussed below) will be especially important. Of course, animals maintain their ability to learn throughout the lifespan; although delayed behavioral manipulations may miss the opportunity to shape early phases of reactive plasticity, the ability to use behavior to drive functionally beneficial plasticity should remain indefinitely. Consistent with this, Williams, Gharbawie, Kolb, and Kleim (2006) found that in rats with neonatal frontal cortex injuries, EC or reach training initiated in adulthood improved motor performance and increased the size of motor maps in remaining cortex.

Most animal models of targeted rehabilitative training have focused on motor skills, and there has been relatively little parallel research in animals using targeted manipulations of cognitive or other experiences as therapies after brain damage (if one considers EC and exercise to be nontargeted). This is despite the fact that such function is a major focus of rodent research in intact animals. It seems likely that this will receive greater attention as this field continues to advance, given that there are many tools available for measuring and manipulating such functions as episodic and working memory, spatial learning, visual and auditory discrimination, and perceptual skill learning in rodents (see MacLellan et al., 2009). Even some aspects of speech and oral–motor impairment can be studied in rats. Rats can be trained in tongue and mouth movements (Gaggermos et al., 2009). Furthermore, they communicate through ultrasonic vocalizations. Newly developed methods for quantifying how these vocalizations change after CNS injury raise the possibility of modeling some aspects of rehabilitative speech and language training in rats (Ciucci et al., 2007, 2009).

COMBINING REHABILITATIVE TRAINING WITH OTHER THERAPIES

Although rehabilitative training clearly improves function, it has often been found to be insufficient to normalize it. Performance improvements resulting from postinjury reach training in monkeys and rats are related to the adoption of compensatory movement patterns for completing the task (e.g., Alaverdashvili & Whishaw, 2010; Friel & Nudo, 1998; Nudo & Bury, Chapter 4; Whishaw, 2000). Furthermore, significant improvements may require weeks or months of effortful training. This leads to the question of how one might improve rehabilitative training efficacy by combining it with other treatments.

The combination of pharmacological manipulations and behavioral training has been under investigation for decades (Barbay & Nudo, 2009; Goldstein, 2003; Nudo, 2006). Among the most extensively studied approach is the combination of repeated D-amphetamine administration with motor training after brain damage, including training rats to walk on a narrow beam (Feeney & Sutton, 1988) and to perform skilled reaching tasks (Adkins & Jones, 2005). Although D-amphetamine has had mixed success in human studies (e.g., Gladstone et al., 2006), it nevertheless provides an important proof of concept for combining behavioral manipulations with other treatment approaches. As noted by others, these mixed results also indicate the need to better understand how to translate animal research dose, timing, and other parameters to clinical trial designs (Barbay & Nudo, 2009; Goldstein, 2009). Other promising approaches are combining training with administration of substances that promote neuronal survival and growth (Puurunen, Jolkkonen, Sirvio, Haapalinna, & Sivenius, 2001) and with substances that block the activity of growth-inhibitory substances (Emerick & Kartje, 2004).

Another approach is to combine rehabilitative training with electrical stimulation of residual tissue in the hope of facilitating experience-dependent neural plasticity, which is impaired near ischemic damage (Jablonka, Witte, & Kossut, 2007). In rats and monkeys with motor cortical infarcts, electrical stimulation of remaining regions of the cortex during daily rehabilitative training in skilled reaching markedly improves functional outcome over that obtained with training alone. The functional improvements are linked to an increased density of dendrites (Adkins, Hsu, & Jones, 2008; Adkins-Muir & Jones, 2003), increased movement representations (Kleim et al., 2003a; Plautz et al., 2003), and enhanced evoked potentials (Teskey, Flynn, Goertzen, Monfils, & Young, 2003) in the stimulated cortex, compared to training alone (see also Carmel et al., 2010). These animal studies used electrodes implanted below the skull and more work is needed to determine how the effectiveness of this stimulation approach varies with stroke size and location (see Plow, Carey, Nudo, & Pascual-Leone, 2008). There is also mounting support for the potential of noninvasive transcranial magnetic and direct current stimulation for enhancing the effects of rehabilitative training (Bolognini, Pascual-Leone, & Fregni, 2009; Hummel & Cohen, 2006).

Behavioral manipulations themselves may serve to facilitate rehabilitative training. CIMT is a major example of this (again, see Morris & Bickel, Chapter 7). In this approach, subjects typically wear a mitt on the less affected hand for many waking hours, and also undergo intensive training focused on the impaired limb. In addition to improving motor function, CIMT can enhance functional activation in the stroke-affected hemisphere (Taub et al., 2006). A rat model of CIMT has been found to improve functional outcome and to reduce injury extent after striatal hemorrhagic injury (DeBow, Davies, Clarke, & Colbourne, 2003; Maclellan, Grams, Adams, & Colbourne, 2005). Behavioral manipulations are also coming to be viewed as core strategies for optimizing other treatment approaches (Johansson, 2000), including the use of exogenous stem cells and brain tissue grafts (Dobrossy & Dunnett, 2005).

CONCLUSIONS

At this point, there should be no doubt that experience *does* matter. We have obtained a wealth of information about how brains reorganize after brain damage and how this is influenced by experience. We are beginning to understand the neural mechanisms of rehabilitation's efficacy and how to combine rehabilitation with other treatment approaches. But it also appears that we are just now in the earliest stages of asking the questions needed to determine how best to manipulate experience to improve outcome. This requires a better understanding of how behavioral intervention effects vary with different types of experiences, injuries, time periods, ages, and preexisting conditions. This may seem hopelessly complex, but looking back at the dramatic advances made in the field of brain plasticity in just the last two decades provides a basis for optimism that we will learn how to maximize the potential of behavioral manipulations to heal the damaged brain.

REFERENCES

Adkins, D. L., Boychuk, J., Remple, M. S., & Kleim, J. A. (2006). Motor training induces experience-specific patterns of plasticity across motor cortex and spinal cord. *Journal of Applied Physiology, 101*(6), 1776–1782.

Adkins, D. L., Bury, S. D., & Jones, T. A. (2002). Laminar-dependent dendritic spine alterations in the motor cortex of adult rats following callosal transection and forced forelimb use. *Neurobiology of Learning and Memory, 78*(1), 35–52.

Adkins, D. L., & Jones, T. A. (2005). D-amphetamine enhances skilled reaching after ischemic cortical lesions in rats. *Neuroscience Letters, 380*(3), 214–218.

Adkins, D. L., Voorhies, A. C., & Jones, T. A. (2004). Behavioral and neuroplastic effects of focal endothelin-1 induced sensorimotor cortex lesions. *Neuroscience, 128*(3), 473–486.

Adkins-Muir, D. L., & Jones, T. A. (2003). Cortical electrical stimulation combined with rehabilitative training: Enhanced functional recovery and dendritic plasticity following focal cortical ischemia in rats. *Neurological Research, 25*(8), 780–788.

Alaverdashvili, M., & Whishaw, I. Q. (2010). Compensation aids skilled reaching in aging and in recovery from forelimb motor cortex stroke in the rat. *Neuroscience, 167*(1), 21–30.

Allred, R. P., Cappellini, C. H., & Jones, T. A. (2010). The "good" limb makes the "bad" limb worse: Experience-dependent interhemispheric disruption of functional outcome after cortical infarcts in rats. *Behavioral Neuroscience, 124*(1), 124–132.

Allred, R. P., & Jones, T. A. (2006). Training the "good" forelimb after unilateral sensorimotor cortex lesions worsens function of the impaired forelimb and alters perilesion neuroplasticity. *Society for Neuroscience Abstracts, 32*, 582–584.

Allred, R. P., & Jones, T. A. (2008a). Experience—A double edged sword for restorative neural plasticity after brain damage. *Future Neurology, 3*, 189–198.

Allred, R. P., & Jones, T. A. (2008b). Maladaptive effects of learning with the less-affected forelimb after focal cortical infarcts in rats. *Experimental Neurology, 210*(1), 172–181.

Allred, R. P., Maldonado, M. A., Hsu, J. E., & Jones, T. A. (2005). Training the "less-affected" forelimb after unilateral cortical infarcts interferes with functional recovery of the impaired forelimb in rats. *Restorative Neurology and Neuroscience, 23*(5–6), 297–302.

Alvarez-Buylla, A., & Lim, D. A. (2004). For the long run: Maintaining germinal niches in the adult brain. *Neuron, 41*(5), 683–686.

Anderson, K. J., Scheff, S. W., & DeKosky, S. T. (1986). Reactive synaptogenesis in hippocampal area CA1 of aged and young adult rats. *Journal of Comparative Neurology, 252*(3), 374–384.

Arvidsson, A., Collin, T., Kirik, D., Kokaia, Z., & Lindvall, O. (2002). Neuronal replacement from endogenous precursors in the adult brain after stroke. *Nature Medicine, 8*(9), 963–970.

Barbay, S., & Nudo, R. J. (2009). The effects of amphetamine on recovery of function in animal models of cerebral injury: A critical appraisal. *NeuroRehabilitation, 25*(1), 5–17.

Barbay, S., Plautz, E. J., Friel, K. M., Frost, S. B., Dancause, N., Stowe, A. M., et al. (2005). Behavioral and neurophysiological effects of delayed training following a small ischemic infarct in primary motor cortex of squirrel monkeys. *Experimental Brain Research*, 1–11.

Bennett, E. L., Diamond, M. C., Krech, D., & Rosenzweig, M. R. (1964). Chemical and anatomical plasticity of brain. *Science, 146*, 610–619.

Benowitz, L. I., & Carmichael, S. T. Promoting axonal rewiring to improve outcome after stroke. *Neurobiology of Disease, 37*(2), 259–266.

Biernaskie, J., Chernenko, G., & Corbett, D. (2004). Efficacy of rehabilitative experience declines with time after focal ischemic brain injury. *Journal of Neuroscience, 24*(5), 1245–1254.

Biernaskie, J., & Corbett, D. (2001). Enriched rehabilitative training promotes improved forelimb motor function and enhanced dendritic growth after focal ischemic injury. *Journal of Neuroscience, 21*(14), 5272–5280.

Black, J. E., Isaacs, K. R., Anderson, B. J., Alcantara, A. A., & Greenough, W. T. (1990). Learning causes synaptogenesis, whereas motor activity causes angiogenesis, in cerebellar cortex of adult rats. *Proceedings of the National Academy of Sciences USA, 87*(14), 5568–5572.

Black, J. E., Jones, T. A., Nelson, C. A., & Greenough, W. T. (1997). Neuronal plasticity and the developing brain. In J. D. Noshpitz, N. Alessi, J. T. Coyle, S. I. Harrison, & S. Eth (Eds.), *Handbook of child and adolescent psychiatry: Vol. 6. Basic psychiatric treatment and science* (pp. 31–53). New York: Wiley.

Bolognini, N., Pascual-Leone, A., & Fregni, F. (2009). Using non-invasive brain stimulation to augment motor training-induced plasticity. *Journal of Neuroengineering and Rehabilitation, 6*, 8.

Brown, C. E., Aminoltejari, K., Erb, H., Winship, I. R., & Murphy, T. H. (2009). In vivo voltage-sensitive dye imaging in adult mice reveals that somatosensory maps lost to stroke are replace over weeks by new structural and functional circuits with prolonged modes of activation within both the peri-infarct zone and distant sites. *Journal of Neuroscience, 29*(6), 1719–1734.

Bury, S. D., Adkins, D. L., Ishida, J. T., Kotzer, C. M., Eichhorn, A. C., & Jones, T. A. (2000). Denervation facilitates neuronal growth in the motor cortex of rats in the presence of behavioral demand. *Neuroscience Letters, 287*(2), 85–88.

Bury, S. D., Eichhorn, A. C., Kotzer, C. M., & Jones, T. A. (2000b). Reactive astrocytic responses to denervation in the motor cortex of adult rats are sensitive to manipulations of behavioral experience. *Neuropharmacology, 39*(5), 743–755.

Bury, S. D., & Jones, T. A. (2002). Unilateral sensorimotor cortex lesions in adult rats facilitate motor skill learning with the "unaffected" forelimb and training-induced dendritic structural plasticity in the motor cortex. *Journal of Neuroscience, 22*(19), 8597–8606.

Bury, S. D., & Jones, T. A. (2004). Facilitation of motor skill learning by callosal denervation or forced forelimb use in adult rats. *Behavioural Brain Research, 150*(1–2), 43–53.

Carmel, J. B., Berrol, L. J., Brus-Ramer, M., & Martin, J. H. Chronic electrical stimulation of the intact corticospinal system after unilateral injury restores skilled locomotor control and promotes spinal axon outgrowth. *Journal of Neuroscience, 30*(32), 10918–10926.

Carmichael, S. T. (2006). Cellular and molecular mechanisms of neural repair after stroke: Making waves. *Annals of Neurology, 59*(5), 735–742.

Carmichael, S. T., Archibeque, I., Luke, L., Nolan, T., Momiy, J., & Li, S. (2005). Growth-associated gene expression after stroke: Evidence for a growth-promoting region in peri-infarct cortex. *Experimental Neurology, 193*(2), 291–311.

Carmichael, S. T., & Chesselet, M. F. (2002). Synchronous neuronal activity is a signal for axonal sprouting after cortical lesions in the adult. *Journal of Neuroscience, 22*(14), 6062–6070.

Castro-Alamancos, M. A., & Borrel, J. (1995). Functional recovery of forelimb response capacity after forelimb primary motor cortex damage in the rat is due to the reorganization of adjacent areas of cortex. *Neuroscience, 68*(3), 793–805.

Chu, C. J., & Jones, T. A. (2000). Experience-dependent structural plasticity in cortex heterotopic to focal sensorimotor cortical damage. *Experimental Neurology, 166*(2), 403–414.

Churchill, J. D., Galvez, R., Colcombe, S., Swain, R. A., Kramer, A. F., & Greenough, W. T. (2002). Exercise, experience and the aging brain. *Neurobiology of Aging, 23*(5), 941–955.

Ciucci, M., Ma, T. S., Fox, C., Kane, J. R., Ramig, L., & Schallert, T. (2007). Qualitative changes in ultrasonic vocalization in rats after unilateral dopamine depletion or haloperidol. *Behavioural Brain Research, 182*(2), 284–289.

Comery, T. A., Shah, R., & Greenough, W. T. (1995). Differential rearing alters spine density on medium-sized spiny neurons in the rat corpus striatum: Evidence for association of morphological plasticity with early response gene expression. *Neurobiology of Learning and Memory, 63*(3), 217–219.

Conner, J. M., Chiba, A. A., & Tuszynski, M. H. (2005). The basal forebrain cholinergic system is essential for cortical plasticity and functional recovery following brain injury. *Neuron, 46*(2), 173–179.

Cotman, C. W., & Anderson, K. J. (1988). Synaptic plasticity and functional stabilization in the hippocampal formation: Possible role in Alzheimer's disease. *Advances in Neurology, 47*, 313–335.

Cramer, S. C., & Chopp, M. (2000). Recovery recapitulates ontogeny. *Trends in Neurosciences, 23*(6), 265–271.

Dahlqvist, P., Ronnback, A., Bergstrom, S. A., Soderstrom, I., & Olsson, T. (2004). Environmental enrichment reverses learning impairment in the Morris water maze after focal cerebral ischemia in rats. *European Journal of Neuroscience, 19*(8), 2288–2298.

Dancause, N., Barbay, S., Frost, S. B., Plautz, E. J., Chen, D., Zoubina, E. V., et al. (2005). Extensive cortical rewiring after brain injury. *Journal of Neuroscience, 25*(44), 10167–10179.

DeBow, S. B., Davies, M. L., Clarke, H. L., & Colbourne, F. (2003). Constraint-induced movement therapy and rehabilitation exercises lessen motor deficits and volume of brain injury after striatal hemorrhagic stroke in rats. *Stroke, 34*(4), 1021–1026.

Deller, T., Bas Orth, C., Vlachos, A., Merten, T., Del Turco, D., Dehn, D., et al. (2006). Plasticity of synaptopodin and the spine apparatus organelle in the rat fascia dentata following entorhinal cortex lesion. *Journal of Comparative Neurology, 499*(3), 471–484.

Di Filippo, M., Tozzi, A., Costa, C., Belcastro, V., Tantucci, M., Picconi, B., et al. (2008). Plasticity and repair in the post-ischemic brain. *Neuropharmacology, 55*(3), 353–362.

Ding, Y. H., Mrizek, M., Lai, Q., Wu, Y., Reyes, R., Jr., Li, J., et al. (2006). Exercise preconditioning reduces brain damage and inhibits TNF-alpha receptor expression after hypoxia/reoxygenation: An in vivo and in vitro study. *Current Neurovascular Research, 3*, 263–271.

Dobrossy, M. D., & Dunnett, S. B. (2005). Optimising plasticity: Environmental and training associated factors in transplant-mediated brain repair. *Reviews in the Neurosciences, 16*(1), 1–21.

Emerick, A. J., & Kartje, G. L. (2004). Behavioral recovery and anatomical plasticity in adult rats after cortical lesion and treatment with monoclonal antibody IN-1. *Behavioural Brain Research, 152*(2), 315–325.

Farrell, R., Evans, S., & Corbett, D. (2001). Environmental enrichment enhances recovery of function but exacerbates ischemic cell death. *Neuroscience, 107*(4), 585–592.

Feeney, D. M., & Sutton, R. L. (1988). Catecholamines and recovery of function after brain damage. In B. A. Sabel & D. Stein (Eds.), *Pharmacological approaches to the treatment of brain and spinal cord injury* (pp. 121–142). New York: Plenum Press.

Floeter, M. K., & Greenough, W. T. (1979). Cerebellar plasticity: Modification of Purkinje cell structure by differential rearing in monkeys. *Science, 206*(4415), 227–229.

Foroud, A., & Whishaw, I. Q. (2006). Changes in the kinematic structure and non-kinematic features of movements during skilled reaching after stroke: A Laban movement analysis in two case studies. *Journal of Neuroscience Methods, 158*(1), 137–149.

Freund, P., Schmidlin, E., Wannier, T., Bloch, J., Mir, A., Schwab, M. E., et al. (2006). Nogo-A-specific antibody treatment enhances sprouting and functional recovery after cervical lesion in adult primates. *Nature Medicine, 12*(7), 790–792.

Friel, K. M., & Nudo, R. J. (1998). Recovery of motor function after focal cortical injury in primates: Compensatory movement patterns used during rehabilitative training. *Somatosensory and Motor Research, 15*(3), 173–189.

Gladstone, D. J., Danells, C. J., Armesto, A., McIlroy, W. E., Staines, W. R., Graham, S. J., et al. (2006). Physiotherapy coupled with dextroamphetamine for rehabilitation after hemiparetic stroke: A randomized, double-blind, placebo-controlled trial. *Stroke, 37*(1), 179–185.

Glazewski, S., Benedetti, B. L., & Barth, A. L. (2007). Ipsilateral whiskers suppress experience-dependent plasticity in the barrel cortex. *Journal of Neuroscience, 27*(14), 3910–3920.

Goldstein, L. B. (2003). Amphetamines and related drugs in motor recovery after stroke. *Physical Medicine and Rehabilitation Clinics of North America, 14*(1, Suppl.), S125–134, x.

Goldstein, L. B. (2009). Amphetamine trials and tribulations. *Stroke, 40*(3, Suppl.), S133–S135.

Gotts, J. E., & Chesselet, M. F. (2005). Migration and fate of newly born cells after focal cortical ischemia in adult rats. *Journal of Neuroscience Research, 80*(2), 160–171.

Green, E. J., Greenough, W. T., & Schlumpf, B. E. (1983). Effects of complex or isolated environments on cortical dendrites of middle-aged rats. *Brain Research, 264*(2), 233–240.

Greenberg, D. A., & Jin, K. (2006). Growth factors and stroke. *NeuroRx, 3*(4), 458–465.

Greenough, W. T., Fass, B., & DeVoogd, T. J. (1976). The influence of experience on recovery following brain damage in rodents: Hypotheses based on development research. In R. N. Walsh & W. T. Greenough (Eds.), *Environments as therapy for brain dysfunction* (pp. 10–50). New York: Plenum Press.

Greenough, W. T., Wood, W. E., & Madden, T. C. (1972). Possible memory storage differences among mice reared in environments varying in complexity. *Behavioral Biology, 7*(5), 717–722.

Griesbach, G. S., Gomez-Pinilla, F., & Hovda, D. A. (2004a). The upregulation of plasticity-related proteins following TBI is disrupted with acute voluntary exercise. *Brain Research, 1016*(2), 154–162.

Griesbach, G. S., Hovda, D. A., Molteni, R., Wu, A., & Gomez-Pinilla, F. (2004b). Voluntary exercise following traumatic brain injury: Brain-derived neurotrophic factor upregulation and recovery of function. *Neuroscience, 125*(1), 129–139.

Grossman, A. W., Churchill, J. D., Bates, K. E., Kleim, J. A., & Greenough, W. T. (2002). A brain adaptation view of plasticity: Is synaptic plasticity an overly limited concept? *Progress in Brain Research, 138*, 91–108.

Guggenmos, D. J., Barbay, S., Bethel-Brown, C., Nudo, R. J., & Stanford, J. A. (2009). Effects of tongue force training on orolingual motor cortical representation. *Behavioural Brain Research, 201*(1), 229–232.

Hamori, J. (1990). Morphological plasticity of postsynaptic neurones in reactive synaptogenesis. *Journal of Experimental Biology, 153*, 251–260.

Hebb, D. O. (1949). *The organization of behavior: A neuropsychological theory.* New York: Wiley.

Hobohm, C., Gunther, A., Grosche, J., Rossner, S., Schneider, D., & Bruckner, G. (2005). Decomposition and long-lasting downregulation of extracellular matrix in perineuronal nets induced by focal cerebral ischemia in rats. *Journal of Neuroscience Research, 80*(4), 539–548.

Hsu, J. E., & Jones, T. A. (2005). Time-sensitive enhancement of motor learning with the less-affected forelimb after unilateral sensorimotor cortex lesions in rats. *European Journal of Neuroscience, 22*(8), 2069–2080.

Hsu, J. E., & Jones, T. A. (2006). Contralesional neural plasticity and functional changes in the less-affected forelimb after large and small cortical infarcts in rats. *Experimental Neurology, 201*(2), 479–494.

Hummel, F. C., & Cohen, L. G. (2006). Non-invasive brain stimulation: A new strategy to improve neurorehabilitation after stroke? *Lancet Neurology, 5*(8), 708–712.

Huston, J. P., Morgan, S., & Steiner, H. (1987). Plasticity in crossed efferents from the substantia nigra as related to behavioral reorganization. In J. S. Schneider & T. L. Lidksy (Eds.), *Basal ganglia and behavior: Sensory aspects of motor functioning* (pp. 89–102). Bern: Hans Huber.

Jablonka, J. A., Witte, O. W., & Kossut, M. (2007). Photothrombotic infarct impairs experience-dependent plasticity in neighboring cortex. *NeuroReport, 18*(2), 165–169.

Jin, K., Wang, X., Xie, L., Mao, X. O., Zhu, W., Wang, Y., et al. (2006). Evidence for stroke-induced neurogenesis in the human brain. *Proceedings of the National Academy of Sciences USA, 103*(35), 13198–13202.

Johansson, B. B. (2000). Brain plasticity and stroke rehabilitation. The Willis lecture. *Stroke, 31*(1), 223–230.

Johansson, B. B., & Belichenko, P. V. (2002). Neuronal plasticity and dendritic spines: effect of environmental enrichment on intact and postischemic rat brain. *Journal of Cerebral Blood Flow and Metabolism, 22*(1), 89–96.

Jones, T. A. (1999). Multiple synapse formation in the motor cortex opposite unilateral sensorimotor cortex lesions in adult rats. *Journal of Comparative Neurology, 414*(1), 57–66.

Jones, T. A., & Allred, R. P. (2004). Dendritic growth in the cortex opposite unilateral sensorimotor cortex lesions in rats is inhibited by prior transection of the corpus callosum. *Society for Neuroscience Abstracts, 30*, 681.617.

Jones, T. A., Bury, S. D., Adkins-Muir, D. L., Luke, L. M., Allred, R. P., & Sakata, J. T. (2003). Importance of behavioral manipulations and measures in rat models of brain damage and brain repair. *ILAR Journal, 44*(2), 144–152.

Jones, T. A., Chu, C. J., Grande, L. A., & Gregory, A. D. (1999). Motor skills training enhances lesion-induced structural plasticity in the motor cortex of adult rats. *Journal of Neuroscience, 19*(22), 10153–10163.

Jones, T. A., & Greenough, W. T. (2002). Behavioral experience-dependent plasticity of glial–neuronal interactions. In A. Volterra, P. Magistretti, & P. G. Haydon (Eds.), *Glia in synaptic transmission* (pp. 248–265). New York: Oxford University Press.

Jones, T. A., Hawrylak, N., Klintsova, A. Y., & Greenough, W. T. (1998). Brain damage, behavior, rehabilitation, recovery, and brain plasticity. *Mental Retardation and Developmental Disabilities Research Reviews, 4*, 231–237.

Jones, T. A., Kleim, J. A., & Greenough, W. T. (1996). Synaptogenesis and dendritic growth in the cortex opposite unilateral sensorimotor cortex damage in adult rats: A quantitative electron microscopic examination. *Brain Research, 733*(1), 142–148.

Jones, T. A., Klintsova, A. Y., Kilman, V. L., Sirevaag, A. M., & Greenough, W. T. (1997). Induction of multiple synapses by experience in the visual cortex of adult rats. *Neurobiology of Learning and Memory, 68*(1), 13–20.

Jones, T. A., & Schallert, T. (1992). Overgrowth and pruning of dendrites in adult rats recovering from neocortical damage. *Brain Research, 581*(1), 156–160.

Jones, T. A., & Schallert, T. (1994). Use-dependent growth of pyramidal neurons after neocortical damage. *Journal of Neuroscience, 14*(4), 2140–2152.

Kelley, M. S., & Steward, O. (1997). Injury-induced physiological events that may modulate gene expression in neurons and glia. *Reviews in the Neurosciences, 8*(3–4), 147–177.

Kempermann, G., Kuhn, H. G., & Gage, F. H. (1997). More hippocampal neurons in adult mice living in an enriched environment. *Nature, 386*(6624), 493–495.

Kirkland, S. W., Coma, A. K., Colwell, K. L., & Metz, G. A. (2008). Delayed recovery and exaggerated infarct size by post-lesion stress in a rat model of focal cerebral stroke. *Brain Research, 1201*, 151–160.

Kleim, J. A., Bruneau, R., VandenBerg, P., MacDonald, E., Mulrooney, R., & Pocock, D. (2003a). Motor cortex stimulation enhances motor recovery and reduces peri-infarct dysfunction following ischemic insult. *Neurological Research, 25*(8), 789–793.

Kleim, J. A., & Jones, T. A. (2008). Principles of experience-dependent neural plasticity: Implications for rehabilitation after brain damage. *Journal of Speech, Language, and Hearing Research, 51*(1), S225–S239.

Kleim, J. A., Jones, T. A., & Schallert, T. (2003b). Motor enrichment and the induction of plasticity before or after brain injury. *Neurochemical Research, 28*(11), 1757–1769.

Kleim, J. A., Lussnig, E., Schwarz, E. R., Comery, T. A., & Greenough, W. T. (1996). Synaptogenesis and Fos expression in the motor cortex of the adult rat after motor skill learning. *Journal of Neuroscience, 16*(14), 4529–4535.

Knieling, M., Metz, G. A., Antonow-Schlorke, I., & Witte, O. W. (2009). Enriched environment promotes efficiency of compensatory movements after cerebral ischemia in rats. *Neuroscience, 163*(3), 759–769.

Kobayashi, S., Ohashi, Y., & Ando, S. (2002). Effects of enriched environments with different durations and starting times on learning capacity during aging in rats assessed by a refined procedure of the Hebb–Williams maze task. *Journal of Neuroscience Research, 70*(3), 340–346.

Kolb, B., Forgie, M., Gibb, R., Gorny, G., & Rowntree, S. (1998). Age, experience and the changing brain. *Neuroscience and Biobehavioral Reviews, 22*(2), 143–159.

Kolb, B., Gibb, R., & Gorny, G. (2003). Experience-dependent changes in dendritic arbor and spine density in neocortex vary qualitatively with age and sex. *Neurobiology of Learning and Memory, 79*(1), 1–10.

Komitova, M., Johansson, B. B., & Eriksson, P. S. (2006). On neural plasticity, new neurons and the postischemic milieu: An integrated view on experimental rehabilitation. *Experimental Neurology, 199*(1), 42–55.

Komitova, M., Mattsson, B., Johansson, B. B., & Eriksson, P. S. (2005a). Enriched environment increases neural stem/progenitor cell proliferation and neurogenesis in the subventricular zone of stroke-lesioned adult rats. *Stroke, 36*(6), 1278–1282.

Komitova, M., Zhao, L. R., Gido, G., Johansson, B. B., & Eriksson, P. (2005b). Postischemic exercise attenuates whereas enriched environment has certain enhancing effects on lesion-induced subventricular zone activation in the adult rat. *European Journal of Neuroscience, 21*(9), 2397–2405.

Kozlowski, D. A., James, D. C., & Schallert, T. (1996). Use-dependent exaggeration of neuronal injury after unilateral sensorimotor cortex lesions. *Journal of Neuroscience, 16*(15), 4776–4786.

Kramer, A. F., Bherer, L., Colcombe, S. J., Dong, W., & Greenough, W. T. (2004). Environmental influences on cognitive and brain plasticity during aging. *Journals of Gerontology Series A: Biological Sciences and Medical Sciences, 59*(9), M940–M957.

Leasure, J. L., & Schallert, T. (2004). Consequences of forced disuse of the impaired forelimb after unilateral cortical injury. *Behavioural Brain Research, 150*(1–2), 83–91.

Li, S., & Carmichael, S. T. (2006). Growth-associated gene and protein expression in the region of axonal sprouting in the aged brain after stroke. *Neurobiology of Disease, 23*(2), 362–373.

Lichtenwalner, R. J., & Parent, J. M. (2006). Adult neurogenesis and the ischemic forebrain. *Journal of Cerebral Blood Flow and Metabolism, 26*(1), 1–20.

Liu, J., Solway, K., Messing, R. O., & Sharp, F. R. (1998). Increased neurogenesis in the dentate gyrus after transient global ischemia in gerbils. *Journal of Neuroscience, 18*(19), 7768–7778.

Maclellan, C. L., Grams, J., Adams, K., & Colbourne, F. (2005). Combined use of a cytoprotectant and rehabilitation therapy after severe intracerebral hemorrhage in rats. *Brain Research, 1063*(1), 40–47.

MacLellan, C. L., Langdon, K. D., Churchill, K. P., Granter-Button, S., & Corbett, D. (2009). Assessing cognitive function after intracerebral hemorrhage in rats. *Behavioural Brain Research, 198*(2), 321–328.

Marrone, D. F., LeBoutillier, J. C., & Petit, T. L. (2004). Changes in synaptic ultrastructure during reactive synaptogenesis in the rat dentate gyrus. *Brain Research, 1005*(1–2), 124–136.

Matthews, D. A., Cotman, C., & Lynch, G. (1976). An electron microscopic study of lesion-induced synaptogenesis in the dentate gyrus of the adult rat: II. Reappearance of morphologically normal synaptic contacts. *Brain Research, 115*(1), 23–41.

McNeill, T. H., Brown, S. A., Hogg, E., Cheng, H. W., & Meshul, C. K. (2003). Synapse replacement in the striatum of the adult rat following unilateral cortex ablation. *Journal of Comparative Neurology, 467*(1), 32–43.

Morgan, S., Huston, J. P., & Pritzel, M. (1983). Effects of reducing sensory–motor feedback on the appearance of crossed nigro-thalamic projections and recovery from turning induced by unilateral substantia nigra lesions. *Brain Research Bulletin, 11*(6), 721–727.

Murphy, T. H., & Corbett, D. (2009). Plasticity during stroke recovery: From synapse to behaviour. *Nature Reviews Neuroscience, 10*(12), 861–872.

Neumann-Haefelin, T., Staiger, J. F., Redecker, C., Zilles, K., Fritschy, J. M., Mohler, H., et al. (1998). Immunohistochemical evidence for dysregulation of the GABAergic system ipsilateral to photochemically induced cortical infarcts in rats. *Neuroscience, 87*(4), 871–879.

Nilsson, M., Perfilieva, E., Johansson, U., Orwar, O., & Eriksson, P. S. (1999). Enriched environment increases neurogenesis in the adult rat dentate gyrus and improves spatial memory. *Journal of Neurobiology, 39*(4), 569–578.

Nudo, R. J. (2006). Plasticity. *NeuroRx, 3*(4), 420–427.

Nudo, R. J. (2007). Postinfarct cortical plasticity and behavioral recovery. *Stroke, 38*(2, Suppl.), 840–845.

Nudo, R. J., Wise, B. M., SiFuentes, F., & Milliken, G. W. (1996). Neural substrates for the effects of rehabilitative training on motor recovery after ischemic infarct. *Science, 272*(5269), 1791–1794.

Nygren, J., Wieloch, T., Pesic, J., Brundin, P., & Deierborg, T. (2006). Enriched environment attenuates cell genesis in subventricular zone after focal ischemia in mice and decreases migration of newborn cells to the striatum. *Stroke, 37*(11), 2824–2829.

Ohab, J. J., Fleming, S., Blesch, A., & Carmichael, S. T. (2006). A neurovascular niche for neurogenesis after stroke. *Journal of Neuroscience, 26*(50), 13007–13016.

Ohlsson, A. L., & Johansson, B. B. (1995). Environment influences functional outcome of cerebral infarction in rats. *Stroke, 26*(4), 644–649.

Parent, J. M., Vexler, Z. S., Gong, C., Derugin, N., & Ferriero, D. M. (2002). Rat forebrain neurogenesis and striatal neuron replacement after focal stroke. *Annals of Neurology, 52*(6), 802–813.

Phillips, L. L., & Reeves, T. M. (2001). Interactive pathology following traumatic brain injury modifies hippocampal plasticity. *Restorative Neurology and Neuroscience, 19*(3–4), 213–235.

Plautz, E. J., Barbay, S., Frost, S. B., Friel, K. M., Dancause, N., Zoubina, E. V., et al. (2003). Post-infarct cortical plasticity and behavioral recovery using concurrent cortical stimulation and rehabilitative training: A feasibility study in primates. *Neurological Research, 25*(8), 801–810.

Ploughman, M., Granter-Button, S., Chernenko, G., Attwood, Z., Tucker, B. A., Mearow, K. M., et al. (2007). Exercise intensity influences the temporal profile of growth factors involved in neuronal plasticity following focal ischemia. *Brain Research, 1150*, 207–216.

Plow, E. B., Carey, J. R., Nudo, R. J., & Pascual-Leone, A. (2009). Invasive cortical stimulation to promote recovery of function after stroke: A critical appraisal. *Stroke, 40*(5), 1926–1931.

Puurunen, K., Jolkkonen, J., Sirvio, J., Haapalinna, A., & Sivenius, J. (2001). Selegiline combined with enriched-environment housing attenuates spatial learning deficits following focal cerebral ischemia in rats. *Experimental Neurology, 167*(2), 348–355.

Ramanathan, D., Conner, J. M., & Tuszynski, M. H. (2006). A form of motor cortical plasticity that correlates with recovery of function after brain injury. *Proceedings of the National Academy of Sciences USA, 103*(30), 11370–11375.

Ramaswamy, S., Goings, G. E., Soderstrom, K. E., Szele, F. G., & Kozlowski, D. A. (2005). Cellular proliferation and migration following a controlled cortical impact in the mouse. *Brain Research, 1053*(1–2), 38–53.

Reeves, T. M., Zhu, J., Povlishock, J. T., & Phillips, L. L. (1997). The effect of combined fluid percussion and entorhinal cortical lesions on long-term potentiation. *Neuroscience, 77*(2), 431–444.

Riban, V., & Chesselet, M. F. (2006). Region-specific sprouting of crossed corticofugal fibers after unilateral cortical lesions in adult mice. *Experimental Neurology, 197*(2), 451–457.

Risedal, A., Zeng, J., & Johansson, B. B. (1999). Early training may exacerbate brain damage after focal brain ischemia in the rat. *Journal of Cerebral Blood Flow and Metabolism, 19*(9), 997–1003.

Rose, F. D., Davey, M. J., & Attree, E. A. (1993). How does environmental enrichment aid performance following cortical injury in the rat? *NeuroReport, 4*(2), 163–166.

Rose, F. D., Davey, M. J., Love, S., & Dell, P. A. (1987). Environmental enrichment and recovery from contralateral sensory neglect in rats with large unilateral neocortical lesions. *Behavioural Brain Research, 24*(3), 195–202.

Rose, F. D., Dell, P. A., Love, S., & Davey, M. J. (1988). Environmental enrichment and recovery from a complex go/no-go reversal deficit in rats following large unilateral neocortical lesions. *Behavioural Brain Research, 31*(1), 37–45.

Rosenzweig, M. R., & Bennett, E. L. (1996). Psychobiology of plasticity: Effects of training and experience on brain and behavior. *Behavioural Brain Research, 78*(1), 57–65.

Rushmore, R. J., Valero-Cabre, A., Lomber, S. G., Hilgetag, C. C., & Payne, B. R. (2006). Functional circuitry underlying visual neglect. *Brain, 129*(Pt. 7), 1803–1821.

Schallert, T., Kozlowski, D. A., Humm, J. L., & Cocke, R. R. (1997). Use-dependent structural events in recovery of function. *Advances in Neurology, 73*, 229–238.

Schallert, T., Leasure, J. L., & Kolb, B. (2000). Experience-associated structural events, subependymal cellular proliferative activity, and functional recovery after injury to the central nervous system. *Journal of Cerebral Blood Flow and Metabolism, 20*(11), 1513–1528.

Schwartz, S. (1964). Effect of neocortical lesions and early environmental factors on adult rat behavior. *Journal of Comparative and Physiological Psychology, 57*, 72–77.

Serfaty, C. A., Campello-Costa, P., & Linden, R. (2005). Rapid and long-term plasticity in the neonatal and adult retinotectal pathways following a retinal lesion. *Brain Research Bulletin, 66*(2), 128–134.

Silasi, G., Hamilton, D. A., & Kolb, B. (2008). Social instability blocks functional restitution following motor cortex stroke in rats. *Behavioural Brain Research, 188*(1), 219–226.

Sirevaag, A. M., & Greenough, W. T. (1985). Differential rearing effects on rat visual cortex synapses: II. Synaptic morphometry. *Brain Research, 351*(2), 215–226.

Sonninen, R., Virtanen, T., Sivenius, J., & Jolkkonen, J. (2006). Gene expression profiling in the hippocampus of rats subjected to focal cerebral ischemia and enriched environment housing. *Restorative Neurology and Neuroscience, 24*(1), 17–23.

Steward, O., Loesche, J., & Horton, W. C. (1977). Behavioral correlates of denervation and reinnervation of the hippocampal formation of the rat: Open field activity and cue utilization following bilateral entorhinal cortex lesions. *Brain Research Bulletin, 2*(1), 41–48.

Taub, E., Uswatte, G., Mark, V. W., & Morris, D. M. (2006). The learned nonuse phenomenon: implications for rehabilitation. *Europa Medicophysica, 42*(3), 241–256.

Tees, R. C., Buhrmann, K., & Hanley, J. (1990). The effect of early experience on water maze spatial learning and memory in rats. *Developmental Psychobiology, 23*(5), 427–439.

Teskey, G. C., Flynn, C., Goertzen, C. D., Monfils, M. H., & Young, N. A. (2003). Cortical stimulation improves skilled forelimb use following a focal ischemic infarct in the rat. *Neurological Research, 25*(8), 794–800.

Tillerson, J. L., Cohen, A. D., Philhower, J., Miller, G. W., Zigmond, M. J., & Schallert, T. (2001). Forced limb-use effects on the behavioral and neurochemical effects of 6-hydroxydopamine. *Journal of Neuroscience, 21*(12), 4427–4435.

Tonchev, A. B., Yamashima, T., & Chaldakov, G. N. (2007). Distribution and phenotype of proliferating cells in the forebrain of adult macaque monkeys after transient global cerebral ischemia. *Advances in Anatomy, Embryology and Cell Biology, 191*, 1–106.

Turner, A. M., & Greenough, W. T. (1985). Differential rearing effects on rat visual cortex synapses: I. Synaptic and neuronal density and synapses per neuron. *Brain Research, 329*(1–2), 195–203.

Uryu, K., MacKenzie, L., & Chesselet, M. F. (2001). Ultrastructural evidence for differential axonal sprouting in the striatum after thermocoagulatory and aspiration lesions of the cerebral cortex in adult rats. *Neuroscience, 105*(2), 307–316.

Vaynman, S., & Gomez-Pinilla, F. (2005). License to run: Exercise impacts functional plasticity in the intact and injured central nervous system by using neurotrophins. *Neurorehabilitation and Neural Repair, 19*(4), 283–295.

Voorhies, A. C., & Jones, T. A. (2002). The behavioral and dendritic growth effects of focal sensorimotor cortical damage depend on the method of lesion induction. *Behavioural Brain Research, 133*(2), 237–246.

Wallace, C. S., Withers, G. S., Weiler, I. J., George, J. M., Clayton, D. F., & Greenough, W. T. (1995). Correspondence between sites of NGFI-A induction and sites of morphological plasticity following exposure to environmental complexity. *Brain Research. Molecular Brain Research, 32*(2), 211–220.

Ward, N. S., & Cohen, L. G. (2004). Mechanisms underlying recovery of motor function after stroke. *Archives of Neurology, 61*(12), 1844–1848.

Whishaw, I. Q. (2000). Loss of the innate cortical engram for action patterns used in skilled reaching and the development of behavioral compensation following motor cortex lesions in the rat. *Neuropharmacology, 39*(5), 788–805.

Whishaw, I. Q., Suchowersky, O., Davis, L., Sarna, J., Metz, G. A., & Pellis, S. M. (2002). Impairment of pronation, supination, and body co-ordination in reach-to-grasp tasks in human Parkinson's disease (PD) reveals homology to deficits in animal models. *Behavioural Brain Research, 133*(2), 165–176.

Wieloch, T., & Nikolich, K. (2006). Mechanisms of neural plasticity following brain injury. *Current Opinion in Neurobiology, 16*(3), 258–264.

Will, B., Galani, R., Kelche, C., & Rosenzweig, M. R. (2004). Recovery from brain injury in animals: Relative efficacy of environmental enrichment, physical exercise or formal training (1990–2002). *Progress in Neurobiology, 72*(3), 167–182.

Williams, P. T., Gharbawie, O. A., Kolb, B., & Kleim, J. A. (2006). Experience-dependent amelioration of motor impairments in adulthood following neonatal medial frontal cortex injury in rats is accompanied by motor map expansion. *Neuroscience, 141*(3), 1315–1326.

Winship, I. R., & Murphy, T. H. (2009). Remapping the somatosensory cortex after stroke: Insight from imaging the synapse to network. *Neuroscientist, 15*(5), 507–524.

Witte, O. W., Bidmon, H. J., Schiene, K., Redecker, C., & Hagemann, G. (2000). Functional differentiation of multiple perilesional zones after focal cerebral ischemia. *Journal of Cerebral Blood Flow and Metabolism, 20*(8), 1149–1165.

Woodcock, E. A., & Richardson, R. (2000). Effects of environmental enrichment on rate of contextual processing and discriminative ability in adult rats. *Neurobiology of Learning and Memory, 73*(1), 1–10.

Woodlee, M. T., & Schallert, T. (2006). The impact of motor activity and inactivity on the brain. *Current Directions in Psychological Science, 15*(4), 203–206.

Würbel, H. (2001). Ideal homes?: Housing effects on rodent brain and behaviour. *Trends in Neurosciences, 24*(4), 207–211.

Xerri, C., Zennou-Azougui, Y., & Coq, J. O. (2003). Neuroprotective effects on somatotopic maps resulting from piracetam treatment and environmental enrichment after focal cortical injury. *ILAR Journal, 44*(2), 110–124.

Zhang, Y., Xiong, Y., Mahmood, A., Meng, Y., Liu, Z., Qu, C., et al. Sprouting of corticospinal tract axons from the contralateral hemisphere into the denervated side of the spinal cord is associated with functional recovery in adult rat after traumatic brain injury and erythropoietin treatment. *Brain Research, 1353*, 249–257.

CHAPTER 4

Motor and Sensory Reorganization in Primates

RANDOLPH J. NUDO
SCOTT BURY

In the 1980s a fundamental change in our thinking about cortical plasticity occurred, spurred by innovative neurophysiological studies by Michael Merzenich at the University of California at San Francisco, Jon Kaas at Vanderbilt University, and others (Buonomano & Merzenich, 1998). Although it had been known for many years that functional plasticity occurs in the cerebral cortex of developing animals, these ground-breaking studies demonstrated that the topographic organization of the representation of skin surfaces in the somatosensory cortex of adult monkeys is modifiable as a result of peripheral nerve injury, disuse, or behavioral training. Subsequently, parallel studies were conducted in other sensory areas of the cerebral cortex, as well as in the motor cortex of experimental animals and in humans. All of these studies have provided strong support for the notion that plasticity of cortical maps is a general trait of cerebral cortex even in mature animals, and that rules of temporal coincidence and behavioral context drive emergent properties of cortical modules, regardless of their specific cortical location.

If we assume that map plasticity and behavioral abilities are interrelated, as they appear to be, these studies have enormous importance for our understanding of the process of recovery after central and peripheral nervous system injury. Topographic maps can be tracked over time in individual animals, and thus can be used as biological markers of recovery. Furthermore, by examining cellular and molecular correlates of map change, we may achieve a fuller understanding of the neural mechanisms underlying neuroplasticity, and ultimately may be able to control these mechanisms for rehabilitative purposes.

The notion that input and output properties in cortical sensory and motor areas are plastic throughout life is now widely accepted, and is generalizable across all cortical regions. With respect to relevance for rehabilitation, most studies have focused on the primary motor cortex (M1), primarily because (1) it is often affected by clinical stroke, due to its blood supply by the middle cerebral artery; (2) the clinical effects of stroke in M1 are often devastating (hemiparesis); and (3) the close link between neurons in M1 and motoneurons in the spinal cord via the corticospinal tract allows the relationship between cortical physiology and motor behavior to be examined at various levels of analysis.

But the function of the motor cortex cannot be understood in isolation. Skilled motor behavior requires continuous integration of somatosensory (proprioceptive and cutaneous) inputs with motor output programs. The intimacy of the motor and somatosensory systems is clearly illustrated by the rich connectivity between parietal cortical regions and frontal motor regions. Therefore, to illustrate many of the principles of neuroplasticity, especially as they apply to the field of neurorehabilitation, this chapter focuses on both somatosensory and motor cortices. Though rodent models of plasticity have been invaluable to our understanding of mechanisms at the cellular and synaptic levels, especially with regard to the rodent barrel cortex system, this chapter concentrates primarily on nonhuman primate studies. The differentiation of primate somatosensory and motor areas and their rich intracortical connectivity is unique in these species. Thus the study of plasticity in nonhuman primates may offer numerous advantages for understanding the brain's recovery processes in humans.

PLASTICITY IN SOMATOSENSORY CORTEX

The receptor sheet for each sensory modality is represented in the cerebral cortex in a topographic manner. For example, the representation of visual space is transferred from locations on the retina to primary visual cortex (V1) in a highly organized, site-specific manner. The arrangement of frequency-specific locations along the basilar membrane within the cochlea is maintained in a tonotopic fashion within the primary auditory cortex. The distribution of cutaneous sensory receptors across skin surfaces is represented as skin surface (or body) maps in the primary somatosensory cortex (S1), which includes separate body maps in areas 3b, 1, and 2. Distortions in magnification of specific receptor locations are largely related to the density of receptors in the periphery. Thus the hand and the face, especially the digit tips and the lips, are represented in the cerebral cortex in relatively larger expanses of cortical space.

Although the sensory examples in this chapter are limited to the topographic organization of cutaneous inputs within S1 area 3b, other properties of sensory information are also represented in discrete functional modules throughout primary, secondary, and tertiary sensory regions. For example, area 3b displays segregation of slowly adapting and rapidly adapting inputs. As one examines the functional organization of secondary stages of sensory processing, such as topographic organization within somatosensory area 1, receptive fields of individual neurons become more complex; hence topographic organization with respect to body surface topography is not as precise as that in area 3b. But in area 1, functional domains are segregated based on selectivity for pressure, vibration, and flutter (Friedman, Chen, & Roe, 2004)—in other words, higher-level processing of specific submodalities of somatosensory stimuli. Plasticity in these higher-order aspects of somatosensory organization has rarely, if ever, been explored systematically.

The details of receptotopic organization in the cerebral cortex are highly dynamic throughout life. One early demonstration of this principle was the remodeling of somatosensory representations in area 3b after peripheral nerve injury. Transecting the median nerve in a monkey deprives the cortex of cutaneous input from the glabrous skin surfaces of digits (D1–D3, or thumb, index, and middle fingers; Figure 4.1). However, this cortical territory does not simply become silent. Neurons in the D1–D3 territory become responsive to inputs from adjacent skin surfaces, such as the dorsal skin surfaces of D3 and the palmar surfaces (Merzenich et al., 1983). Since similar experiments in rats have demonstrated that much of the deprived cortex becomes responsive to other somatosensory inputs almost immediately (Barbay, Peden, Falchook, & Nudo, 1999), it is likely that such rapid, injury-induced plasticity is largely due to what is called *unmasking*. That is, preexisting inputs exist in an overlapping zone in the cortex, but normally these inputs are not expressed. Through a process that is just beginning to be understood, the latent synaptic connections become unmasked. It is likely that unmasking occurs at multiple levels of the somatosensory system (spinal cord, dorsal column nuclei, thalamus, and cortex), and that unmasking at lower levels is maintained and perhaps amplified at cortical levels due to progressive divergence of inputs. Then during the ensuing weeks, representational maps become more defined in precise topographic order (see also Jain, Qi, Collins, & Kaas, 2008).

Thus it is likely that at least two processes are involved in the alteration of receptive fields of deprived somatosensory cortex. The immediate unmasking phenomena cannot be explained on the basis of neuroanatomical sprouting. Instead, there must be a change in the efficacy of existing synapses, allowing subthreshold inputs to be expressed. The expression of

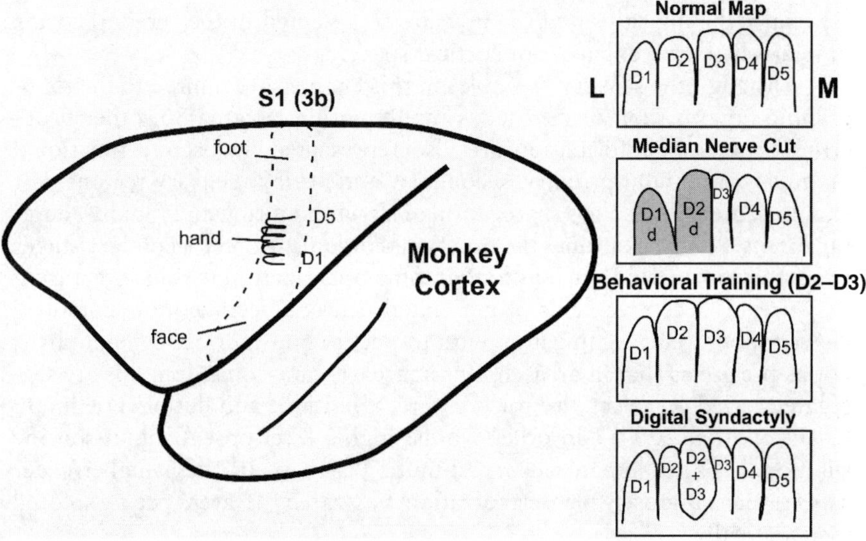

FIGURE 4.1. Representation of the body in primary somatosensory cortex (S1) of a nonhuman primate. Skin surfaces of the hand are normally represented in an orderly progression from thumb (digit 1, or D1) laterally to little finger (D5) medially. After peripheral deafferentation (median nerve cut), behavioral training, or digital syndactyly, S1 hand representations become distorted, reflecting the new patterns of inputs generated by the manipulation. Shaded area indicates dorsal (hairy) skin surfaces that assume novel locations after median nerve cut.

inputs from ascending fibers arriving in the cerebral cortex is largely controlled by inhibitory interneurons that utilize gamma-aminobutyric acid, subtype a (GABAa) as a neurotransmitter. GABAa receptor binding in layer IV of adult monkey area 3b is reduced in the deprived cortex within hours of peripheral nerve injury, and this reduction persists for at least several weeks, if not permanently (Garraghty, Arnold, Wellman, & Mowery, 2006; Wellman, Arnold, Garman, & Garraghty, 2002). This result is consistent with the long-held belief that peripheral nerve transaction results in disinhibition of tonically suppressed inputs.

In the second phase, lasting at least several weeks, the remainder of the deprived cortex gradually becomes responsive to other inputs from adjacent skin surfaces. It is likely that dendritic sprouting plays a role in this longer-term alteration in reorganizational maps (Hickmott & Steen, 2005). Systematic change occurs in dendritic arborization of layer II–III pyramidal and layer IV spiny stellate cells. There appears to be a progressive expansion of distal, but not proximal, regions of the dendritic trees of both basal and apical dendrites (Churchill, Tharp, Wellman, Sengelaub, &

Garraghty, 2004). It is also now known that blockade of the *N*-methyl-D-aspartate (NMDA) receptor at the time of peripheral nerve injury has no effect on the immediate stage of unmasking, but prevents the second phase of reorganization from occurring. Interestingly, NMDA receptor blockade has no apparent effect on the organization of normal area 3b cortex, or on the topography of injury-induced reorganized 3b (Myers, Churchill, Muja, & Garraghty, 2000). However, by 1 month after injury, GABAb receptor binding is reduced, and alpha-amino-3-hydroxy-5-methyl-4-isoxazole propionic acid (AMPA) receptor binding is increased. Comparisons have been made between topographic changes in somatosensory cortex and changes in the hippocampus during long-term potentiation, or LTP (Garraghty et al., 2006).

These early changes after peripheral nerve injury appear to be limited to several hundred microns. However, after years of deafferentation, cortical reorganization can occur over distances of 1 cm or more. Thus, after cervical and thoracic dorsal roots are severed in adult monkeys, depriving the cortex of its normal input from arm and hand, the neurons in the deprived territory in S1 become responsive to stimulation of the face when examined more than 10 years later (Pons et al., 1991).

Remodeling of S1 hand representations also occurs as an experience-dependent process during the development of skilled use of the hand. For example, when adult monkeys are trained to regulate contact on a rotating plate with only two digit tips, the representations of the contacted digits in S1 become enlarged, and receptive field size decreases (Jenkins, Merzenich, & Recanzone, 1990) (Figure 4.1). Parallel findings have been reported in humans. For example, in Braille readers, the index finger is represented over a larger cortical territory (Pascual-Leone & Torres, 1993).

The shaping of precise topography in somatosensory cortex is maintained dynamically, based on temporal correlation of inputs. Since receptors in the skin that are located in neighboring territories (e.g., the same digit tip) are typically stimulated together in time, their inputs arrive at cortical neurons in S1 at precisely the same time. According to Hebbian plasticity models, coincident inputs should allow cortical neurons with different inputs (i.e., from different receptors) to fire together. Of course, fibers innervating receptors on the same digit tip tend to align in their trajectory along peripheral nerves, and this topography is maintained throughout the ascending lemniscal pathway. But what if inputs from two different fingers are artificially linked in time? This situation exists in an experimental procedure called *digital syndactyly*, in which the skin of two adjacent fingers is sutured together. This greatly increases the probability that receptors on the two digits will be activated simultaneously. Following several weeks of syndactyly, the somatosensory representations are greatly altered (Figure 4.1). Neurons in S1 become responsive to both digits (Allard, Clark, Jenkins, & Merzenich, 1991; Clark, Allard, Jenkins, & Merzenich, 1988).

This is highly unusual in normal S1 (at least in area 3b. where the topography is most precise). where neurons are responsive to only one digit. Local horizontal corticocortical connections are probably involved in emergence of multidigit receptive fields (Zarzecki et al., 1993). This digital syndactyly paradigm provides support for the temporal correlation hypothesis.

Temporal correlation of inputs may drive specific forms of experience-dependent plasticity in S1. When monkeys are trained to respond to stimulus sequences on different digits, many neurons in S1 display multiple-digit receptive fields, some on all the stimulated digits (Wang, Merzenich, Sameshima, & Jenkins, 1995). Interestingly, this phenomenon appears to be restricted to the cortex, as thalamic neurons display only single-digit receptive fields. From studies tracking receptive fields in monkeys with implanted electrode arrays during the training of a cross-digit discrimination task, it is now known that one-digit receptive fields are converted to two-digit receptive fields across 3–4 weeks of behavioral training (Blake, Strata, Kempter, & Merzenich, 2005). Behavioral training may change the excitability of cortical neurons, presumably changing subthreshold inputs into suprathreshold inputs.

It is important to point out that context-dependent reinforcement is critical for such plasticity to occur in cortical neurons of adult animals. That is, simple exposure to sensory stimuli causes little or no long-lasting change in receptive field properties. This principle was illustrated in a set of studies in which both somatosensory and auditory stimuli were presented to animals. The animals were rewarded for discriminating physical properties of only one of the modalities. Receptive field plasticity was seen in cortex corresponding to the relevant sensory modality, but not in that corresponding to the irrelevant modality (Recanzone, Merzenich, & Schreiner, 1992).

Because somatosensory map enlargement has consistently been associated with improved behavioral performance, this dynamic process is considered adaptive. Under certain conditions, experience-dependent plasticity in somatosensory cortex can be maladaptive. For example, monkeys trained on highly repetitive somatosensory discrimination tasks display a breakdown in the normal topographic map in S1. Double-digit receptive fields are common, reminiscent of the results after digital syndactyly. After several weeks of repetitive use, monkeys appear to have problems placing their hands on the experimental manipulandum.

Could the mechanism underlying the deficits displayed by monkeys in this highly repetitive task be similar to those in the human conditions known as *focal dystonias* (Altenmüller & Jabusch, 2010; Byl, Merzenich, & Jenkins, 1996)? Dystonias are disorders characterized by sustained involuntary muscle contractions resulting in abnormal movements or postures. Dystonic movements are associated with abnormal patterns of electromyographic activity, involving co-contraction of antagonist muscles and overflow into extraneous muscles. Focal dystonias, such as blepharospasm (eyelids), torticollis (neck), and writer's cramp (hand), affect a limited subset of muscles. Other types of focal dystonias include typist's cramp, pianist's cramp, and musician's cramp. Such occupational dystonias tend to be quite task-specific, and are only evident during certain postures and/or joint movement combinations. In the case of the primate model developed by Byl and colleagues, monkeys engaged in a repetitive motor task (digital grasp) while weak vibratory stimuli were delivered to the hand that engaged widespread digital surfaces. After several weeks of repetitive practice, the monkeys' motor performance deteriorated: They began to have difficulty in making complete contact with or removing the hand from the handpiece. Examination of the somatosensory cortex of these monkeys revealed that the representations of the fingers were substantially altered. The boundaries between individual finger representations were degraded, representing a seemingly maladaptive form of cortical plasticity.

Similar findings have been obtained in neuroimaging studies of somatosensory cortex in human subjects with focal hand dystonia. For example, in dystonic musicians, magnetic source imaging reveals a similar degrading of the boundaries between the finger representations (Elbert et al., 1998). Thus a putative hypothesis to explain the neural basis for at least certain types of focal hand dystonia has emerged: Heavy hand use, especially in highly attended, skilled activities, is accompanied by synchronous inputs from multiple skin surfaces at unusually high rates, resulting in degradation of the normal somatosensory cortex topography. The abnormal somatosensory processing, in turn, leads to development of sensory–motor abnormalities. Consistent with this hypothesis, recent studies have revealed that spatial and temporal tactile discrimination is also impaired in focal hand dystonia. Human study participants who experienced musician's dystonia were found to have similarly disorganized S1 maps. Treating these individuals with a splinting technique designed to reestablish independent digit sensation and movement resulted in a return of S1 maps to the normal orderly segregation of digits (Candia, Wienbruch, Elbert, Rockstroh, & Ray, 2003). It is possible that in certain highly skilled, highly repetitive tasks, temporally correlated inputs drive cortical network connectivity in aberrant ways, resulting in sensory–motor dysfunction.

When we consider the large number of paradigms demonstrating that the adult somatosensory cortex is plastic, it is not surprising that somatosensory organization is altered by cortical injury, as might occur in stroke. After small, ischemic lesions that destroy single-digit representations in S1 of adult monkeys, the destroyed representation reemerges in the adjacent cortical territory (Xerri, Merzenich, Peterson, & Jenkins, 1998). Neuroimaging studies in human stroke survivors suggest that structural plasticity accompanies somatosensory cortical reorganization. Cortical areas that undergo changes in activation response to tactile stimuli show increased cortical thickness (Schaechter, Moore, Connell, Rosen, & Dijkhuizen, 2006).

SKILL-DEPENDENT PLASTICITY IN THE PRIMATE MOTOR CORTEX

Although the majority of our understanding of the relationship between behavior and motor cortex organization comes from rodent studies, the use of nonhuman primates has provided some of the most valuable knowledge. Primates possess several unique advantages over rodents, including differentiated motor and sensory cortices, which can be subdivided into smaller regions similar to human sensory–motor cortical organization (Nudo & Frost, 2007). This allows for the study of the differential contribution of various subregions to motor learning, and allows for a more direct comparison to human studies. Furthermore, it allows for an understanding of how these subregions are functionally integrated through their extensive network of intracortical connections. In addition, primates possess the ability to perform complex behavioral tasks, especially those that require the use of fine digit manipulation. This digital dexterity is, with few exceptions, unrivaled in the animal kingdom (Heffner & Masterton, 1983); it is ideal for studying the acquisition of motor skills, as well as allowing for a large degree of control and detail in the design of behavioral training and testing paradigms.

The term *motor learning* is not rigidly defined in most experimental models, but instead is thought of as a form of procedural learning that encompasses such elements as skill acquisition and motor adaptation. More specific is *motor skill learning* itself: It is often described as the modification of the temporal and spatial organization of muscle synergies, which result in smooth, accurate, and consistent movement sequences (Hammond, 2002). Functional magnetic resonance imaging studies in humans have led to the hypothesis that motor skill learning is a two-stage process (Ungerleider, Doyon, & Karni, 2002). The first stage is rapid, and results in within-session decreases in neural activity. The second, slower stage results in increases and expansion of activity in M1.

While it is evident that numerous brain areas are involved in the production of complex motor movements, M1 has long been implicated in the acquisition and performance of skilled motor behaviors. Although M1 was originally believed to be involved in the activation of complex motor reflexes (Sherrington, 1912), subsequent advances in electrophysiological techniques revealed that movements could be elicited through electrical stimulation of the precentral gyrus (Fritsch & Hitzig, 1870). On the basis of these early findings, John Hughlings Jackson (1884) hypothesized that movement control was somatotopically organized. This hypothesis was later confirmed when more systematic cortical stimulation studies were used to develop a somatotopic map of the precentral gyrus (Penfield & Rasmussen, 1950; Woolsey et al., 1952).

The development of the more sophisticated *intracortical microstimulation* (ICMS) technique in the late 1960s by Asanuma and colleagues allowed for derivation at a much higher spatial resolution of maps within M1, which in turn revealed a more complex and dynamic cortical map organization, including the presence of columnar organization (Asanuma, 1975). The ICMS technique typically consists of applying a volley of short-duration cathodal pulses at a high frequency while using very weak currents ($\leq$60 μA), thus allowing for relatively little spread of cortical excitation. This higher spatial resolution revealed that while M1 is grossly somatotopically organized, discrete cortical areas consist of a montage of representations of individual muscles and movements, which are repeated and highly overlapping. As shown by ICMS mapping experiments that define movements evoked by the lowest possible current levels, motor map organization resembles a fractured mosaic of movement representations, overlaid over a gross somatotopic representation.

It is well known that a subset of corticospinal neurons make monosynaptic contact with motoneurons in the spinal cord (and thus are called *corticomotoneuronal* cells). Spike-triggered averaging techniques in awake primates reveal that individual corticomotoneuronal cells can facilitate up to four or five motoneuron pools (Fetz, Cheney, & German, 1976). This provides further evidence of the divergence in the anatomical projections from cortex to spinal cord, and challenges the notion that functional organization in motor cortex is based on muscle-specific domains. Direct neuroanatomical evidence refuting muscle-specific domains in motor cortex has been provided in more recent research. Rabies viruses can be used as transneuronal retrograde markers. Injecting a virus into a single muscle results in retrograde transport of the virus to the cell bodies in the spinal cord motoneuron pool. There, the virus replicates and is picked up by terminal arbors that innervate the motoneurons. In turn, the virus is retrogradely transported back to second-order neurons in the cerebral cortex, red nucleus, and other locations. At the appropriate survival time, postmortem analysis reveals the location of corticospinal neurons that contain the virus. Thus these neurons represent corticomotoneuronal cells that project to the specific motoneuron pool of interest. Combining results of injections into various forelimb muscles of different animals reveals that the cortical neurons influencing the various forelimb muscles are completely interspersed and overlapping (Rathelot & Strick, 2006). Thus the motor cortex can be viewed as containing a shared neural substrate for motor control of the hand. The highly overlapping and divergent architecture provides an ideal substrate for flexibility in outputs to the spinal cord.

Since the advent of ICMS, numerous studies have expanded our understanding of the relationship between motor maps and motor skill learning. Several general principles of motor map organization have been demonstrated that are thought to underlie the motor cortex's ability to encode motor skills (Monfils, Plautz, & Kleim, 2005). First, as mentioned above, motor maps are fractionated, in that they contain multiple, overlapping representations of movements. Second, adjacent areas within cortical motor maps are highly interconnected via a dense network of intracortical fibers. Third, these maps are extremely dynamic and can be modulated by a number of intrinsic and extrinsic stimuli. Together, these characteristics provide a framework that facilitates the acquisition of novel muscle synergies, at least in part, through changes in the intracortical connectivity of individual movement representations.

However, the dynamic nature of motor maps belies the issue of stable neural connections that must be maintained to respond to environmental demands and retain acquired motor skills. Within the cortex, this balance is thought to be achieved through interactions of the excitatory and inhibitory connections of pyramidal cells and local inhibitory networks (Aroniadou & Keller, 1993; Huntley & Jones, 1991; Lowel & Singer, 1992). This in turn requires an internal mechanism that is capable of shifting this balance toward strengthening relevant synaptic connections. Horizontal fiber connections have been shown to arise from excitatory pyramidal neurons and allow for the coactivation of adjacent and nonadjacent cortical columns. In addition to activating excitatory pyramidal cells, they also generate inhibitory responses via the activation of GABAergic interneurons (Jones, 1993). Furthermore, the activity of these horizontal fibers has been shown to be mediated by both LTP and long-term depression between distant motor cortical areas (Hess & Donoghue, 1994, 1996). Together, these horizontal fiber characteristics provide a mechanism capable of facilitating the activation of multiple novel muscle synergies that are required for motor skill acquisition, while likewise providing a mechanism, via inhibitory processes, of motor map stability that is required to maintain stable neural representations in response to irrelevant (i.e., untrained) environmental events.

The plasticity of M1 and premotor cortical areas in relation to the acquisition of motor skills, specifically in nonhuman primates, has been a primary focus of recent neurophysiological studies. In addition to having larger brains than rodents do, primates possess well-differentiated motor regions. For example, whereas rodents possess two motor representations of the distal forelimb (caudal and rostral forelimb areas, respectively), all nonhuman primate species studied to date possess at least five separate motor representations of the distal musculature: M1; dorsal and ventral premotor cortex (PMd and PMv, respectively); the supplementary motor area (SMA); and the cingulate motor areas (Dancause, Duric, Barbay,

Frost, Stylianou, & Nudo, 2008; Nudo & Frost, 2007). In particular, certain primate species, such as the squirrel monkey (*Saimiri sciureus*), possess a relatively flat, unfissured frontoparietal cortex (in comparison to other primate species), which allows for more precise electrode placement during ICMS procedures.

As employed in recent plasticity studies in motor cortex of nonhuman primates, the ICMS protocol utilizes glass microeletrodes (10- to 20-μm tips) filled with 3.5 M NaCl. Current is delivered through a platinum wire inserted in the stimulating electrode. The stimulus consists of 13 cathodal, monophasic 200-microsecond pulses delivered at 350 Hz, with a maximum current of 30 μA. The electrode is lowered perpendicular to the surface of the cortex to a depth of 1,750 μm, which targets layer V of the cortex, the location of the corticospinal cell bodies. Current levels required for evoking overt movements in anesthetized animals are lowest at this depth. Electrode penetrations are made at 250-μm increments and recorded on a digital picture of the cortical surface (see Figure 4.2). This procedure allows for the derivation of high-resolution maps of motor cortical movement representations with negligible damage to the tissue, thus allowing for repeated mapping procedures within the same subject. Typically, baseline maps are derived prior to behavioral training. These maps consist of digit and wrist/distal forelimb movement representations, bordered medially,

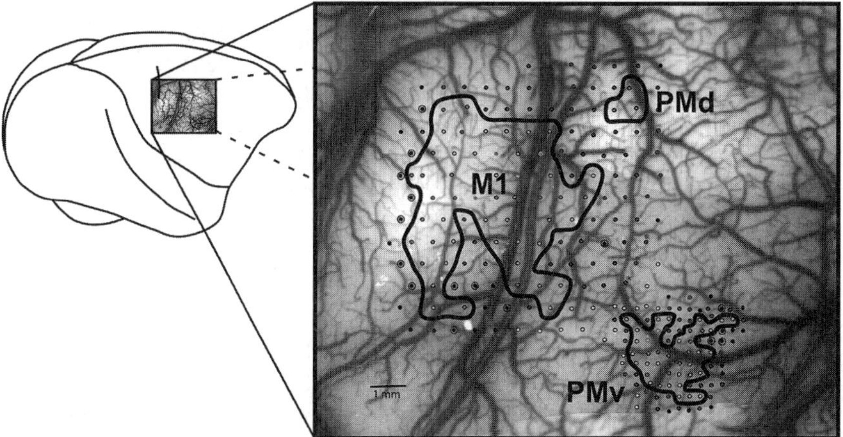

FIGURE 4.2. Results of a typical intracortical microstimulation (ICMS) mapping experiment in squirrel monkey motor cortex (M1). Dots indicate microelectrode penetration sites that are placed 250–500 μm apart. Curved boundary encompasses electrode sites where ICMS within layer V evokes movements of the distal forelimb (fingers, thumb, wrist, forearm). Inset shows outline of squirrel monkey brain and location of mapping experiment. Scale bar = 1 mm. M1, primary motor cortex; PMd, dorsal premotor cortex; PMv, ventral premotor cortex.

rostrally, and laterally by proximal shoulder representations. The caudal border is composed of somatosensory cortex (area 3a), and thus movements are rarely evoked at the current intensities employed in these studies (maximum of 30 μA).

To examine the relationship between motor skill learning and changes in motor map representations, a manual dexterity task is often utilized. The apparatus consists of a Plexiglas board that is attached to front of the monkeys' home cage. The board contains five food wells of different sizes; the largest is large enough got a monkey to insert its entire hand, while only one or two digits can be inserted into the smallest well. Small, flavored food pellets are placed in the wells one at a time. Although initial performance on the task is typically very poor, the monkeys are quite adept and can become very skilled on the task, retrieving 500–600 pellets per day within 1–2 weeks.

Utilizing manual dexterity training in combination with ICMS maps has been crucial in demonstrating the dynamic relationship between motor skill learning and cortical map plasticity. The first study that directly examined this relationship used varying behaviorally demanding tasks to selectively activate specific components of motor maps (Nudo, Milliken, Jenkins, & Merzenich, 1996). This study used three monkeys trained on the manual dexterity task to retrieve food pellets by using primarily digit and wrist movements. A fourth subject was trained to use its wrist and forearm to receive pellets by turning a rotatable eye bolt. Training continued for approximately 10–11 days, sufficient for an asymptotic level of performance to be reached. Posttraining ICMS mapping revealed training-induced changes in motor map topography that directly reflected the demands of the particular behavioral task (Figure 4.3). Thus monkeys trained on the manual dexterity task showed an increase in digit representations and corresponding reduction in wrist and shoulder representations compared to pretraining maps, while the monkey trained to turn the eye bolt exhibited the opposite effects—an increase in wrist and forearm representations at the expense of digit representations.

In addition, an increase in ICMS-evoked multijoint movements was observed. These movements consisted of simultaneous executions of digit and wrist or proximal movements at low ICMS thresholds, and were only observed after training on the digit use intensive manual dexterity task. Both before and after training, thresholds for evoking multijoint responses were significantly lower than those for single-joint responses. These results imply that behaviorally relevant simultaneous or sequential movements may become associated in the motor cortex through repeated activation. We have presented a temporal correlation hypothesis in the section on somatosensory plasticity to describe the results of digital syndactyly; it is possible that this hypothesis is generalizable to motor cortex as well. Thus muscle and joint synergies used in complex, skilled motor actions may be

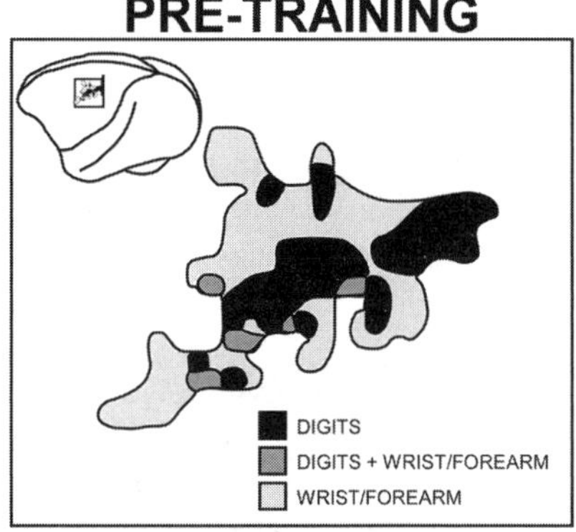

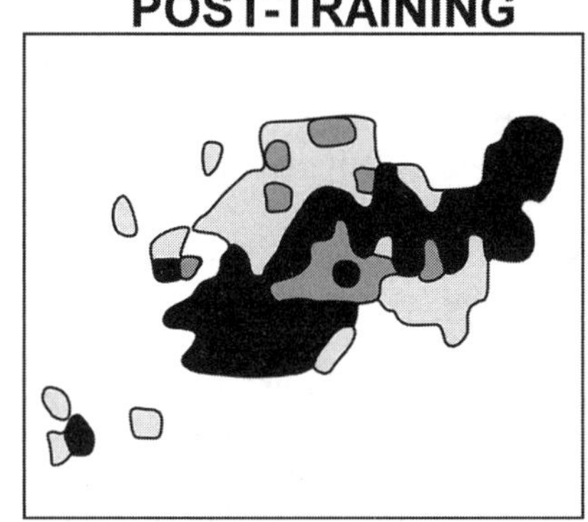

FIGURE 4.3. Effects of digital dexterity training on motor representations in M1. After 10–12 days of training on a task requiring skilled use of the hand (pellet retrieval), ICMS-derived representations of digits (black areas) expanded significantly. In addition, specific joint combinations used in the task (e.g., digit flexion + wrist extension) expanded their representations (dark grey). Such multijoint modules after skill training may reflect the emergence of specific muscle and joint synergies.

supported by alterations in local networks within the motor cortex. As skilled tasks become more stereotyped in timing of sequential joint movements, functional modules emerge in the cortex to link the outputs of different motoneuron pools.

These findings lead to the question of what aspects of motor skill learning drive the observed changes in map representations. Given that in the previously described experiments, subjects were trained repeatedly on the same motor skills task, it is possible that increased muscle activity alone produced the observed changes in map representations. In research designed to address this issue, a group of monkeys was trained exclusively on either the largest or the smallest well in the digital dexterity task. The rationale in this design is that the largest well allows for simple multidigit movements for pellet retrieval; a subject is not required to develop novel skilled digit movements, since simply grasping for food is a normal part of its daily home cage behavior, and this is already part of its behavioral repertoire. Retrieving a food pellet from a small well, in contrast, requires a monkey to manipulate one to two digits to retrieve the pellet; this is considerably harder, given that squirrel monkeys lack monosynaptic corticospinal projections to motoneurons, which probably limits individuation of digit movements (Lemon & Griffiths, 2005). Compared to pretraining maps, monkeys trained in large-well pellet retrieval did not show an expansion of the digit representation, while those trained in small-well retrieval did exhibit an expansion of the digit representation (Plautz, Milliken, & Nudo,

2000). These findings strongly suggest that an increase in motor activity in the absence of motor skill acquisition is insufficient to drive neurophysiological changes in the motor cortex. Similar findings have been obtained in research examining pellet retrieval versus bar pressing in rodents. Rats that learned to retrieve pellets from a rotating platform displayed more distal movements in their motor maps. This expansion was associated with significant synaptogenesis (Kleim, Barbay, & Nudo, 1998; Kleim et al., 2002).

The hypothesis that Hebbian-like changes in intracortical synaptic connections link different cortical neurons to form functional modules has gained further support from a study in the motor cortex of adult macaque monkeys. This study demonstrated that the output properties of motor cortex neurons can be altered by artificially coupling neuronal discharge patterns (Jackson, Mavoori, & Fetz, 2006). Electrodes were implanted in the motor cortex of monkeys, and two sites were selected on the basis of their response to ICMS. ICMS produced different movements at the two sites, which were located 1–2 mm apart. Then spike discharges were recorded from one site (site 1) and used to stimulate the second site (site 2) with a predetermined delay. When ICMS was used to determine the output properties of the two sites a few weeks later, it was found that site 2 acquired the properties of site 1: The ICMS-evoked movements were identical. This study provides further support for the notion that temporal correlation of inputs and outputs drives the emergence of coupling among motor cortex modules.

INJURY-INDUCED PLASTICITY IN MOTOR CORTEX

Deficits in motor function are common in numerous neurological conditions. However, the adult central nervous system (CNS) retains an impressive capacity to recover and adapt following injury. Such so-called "spontaneous" (or "natural") recovery occurs after spinal cord injury, traumatic brain injury, and stroke. Therefore, a basic understanding of the mechanisms that underlie spontaneous recovery of function is the initial step in the development of modulatory therapies that may improve recovery rates and endpoints.

The progression of recovery itself can be thought of as processes of reinstatement and relearning of lost functions, as well as of adaptation and compensation with spared, residual functions. Thus it follows that the neurophysiological mechanisms that support learning in the intact cortex should mediate motor relearning and adaptation in the injured brain. Numerous studies over the last century and a half have provided substantial evidence to support the role of neural plasticity in functional recovery, both spontaneous and directed.

Cortical lesion studies provided some of the earliest evidence of representational map plasticity. Early attempts to observe the effects of motor cortical lesions were unsuccessful, most likely due to the coarse nature of surface-mapping techniques used in the early 20th century. Then Glees and Cole (1950) performed studies in nonhuman primates that examined the effects of motor map reorganization following removal of the thumb representation. These studies showed the reemergence of the thumb representation in the adjacent, undamaged M1. The advent of ICMS and its relatively high spatial resolution has since provided extensive evidence on the extent and nature of motor cortex reorganization in response to injury.

Nudo and Milliken (1996) utilized ICMS techniques to examine the effects of cortical injury of motor map organization. Whereas many cortical injury and functional recovery studies at that time employed large ablations of the entire M1, Nudo and Milliken performed small focal ischemic lesions of the distal forelimb representation, which allowed for the examination of motor representations in intact, adjacent cortical areas. It might be argued that such small cortical lesions are not very clinically relevant, as most strokes are much more widespread, often involve both cortical and subcortical structures, and result in more severe and longer-lasting deficits. However, this model was developed not to mimic clinical stroke per se, but to create a highly reproducible, focal lesion in neurophysiologically characterized tissue in order to determine the adaptive responses in adjacent, intact tissue.

Following a baseline mapping procedure using ICMS, an ischemic infarct was created via bipolar electrocoagulation of the vascular bed within the area of interest. In most cases, this involved all or part of the M1 hand area. In initial studies, after an infarct affecting approximately one-third of the M1 hand area, adult squirrel monkeys were allowed to recover spontaneously for several weeks, at which time the cortex was remapped. Results showed that while the monkeys demonstrated significant functional recovery with the impaired limb by 2 months, the representational maps of the distal forelimb retracted. They were replaced by an expansion of proximal shoulder and elbow representations, indicating a further loss of digit representation than that initially caused by the lesion itself. It is important to note that this was not a further loss of tissue, but a change in function within the spared, adjacent tissue from distal to proximal movement representations.

These findings presented some interesting new questions, especially in relation to the initial findings by Glee and Cole (1950). Whereas the Glee and Cole studies predicted a reemergence of the lost digit representation, the Nudo and Milliken (1996) study actually showed a seemingly maladaptive plastic response in the further loss of cortex devoted to digit representations. However, given the extensive functional recovery observed in these animals, the map changes seem to support the development of potential compensatory strategies utilizing unaffected cortical tissue (in this case, shoulder and elbow areas). Numerous studies in both primates and rats have suggested that behavioral compensation may underlie functional plasticity (Goldberger, 1972; Whishaw, Pellis, Gorny, & Pellis, 1991). Also, it is well known in human stroke that compensatory movements of the trunk are employed during reaching (Cirstea & Levin, 2000). In the case of the study above, the combination of the increased disuse of the impaired digits with the increased use of proximal digits could explain the shift in map topography.

The various regions of the sensory–motor cortex of mammalian brains are densely interconnected via reciprocal neural pathways. Thus an injury that impairs M1 should likewise lead to a disruption of the entire sensory–motor network. Since the development of compensatory behaviors and involvement of uninjured M1 were thought to contribute to spontaneous recovery in the previously described experiments, it follows that intact motor areas outside of M1 may also contribute to recovery. In addition to M1, the frontal cortex contains several areas that contribute to skilled motor behaviors in primates; as noted earlier, these areas include the PMv, PMd, and SMA. All of these possess reciprocal connections with M1, contain numerous corticospinal neurons, and contain complete hand representations. Thus it is plausible that following an injury to M1, the remaining, intact motor areas provide some role in functional recovery, via intracortical connectivity with other cortical regions and/or their direct corticospinal projection pathways.

To begin to explore the possibility that spontaneous recovery could be mediated by premotor cortical areas, our lab has been examining both physiological and anatomical changes in these regions following ischemic insults to M1. Experiments by Liu and Rouiller (1999) showed in nonhuman primates that inactivation of premotor cortex with the GABAergic agonist muscimol following an M1 ischemic lesion reinstated behavioral deficits. This reinstatement was not observed with inactivation of the perilesional, or contralateral, cortex. Thus it follows that if premotor cortex is capable of compensating for the loss of motor function following an M1 injury, physiological changes should accompany this recovery. In adult squirrel monkeys, ICMS mapping techniques were used to characterize representational maps of both M1 and PMv, before and after experimental ischemic infarcts that destroyed at least 50% of the M1 hand representation (Frost, Barbay, Friel, Plautz, & Nudo, 2003). All subjects showed an increased hand representation in PMv, specifically in digit, wrist, and forearm sites. Furthermore, the amount of PMv expansion was correlated with the amount of the M1 hand representation that was destroyed. In other words, the more complete the M1 hand area lesion, the greater the compensatory reorganization in PMv (Figure 4.4).

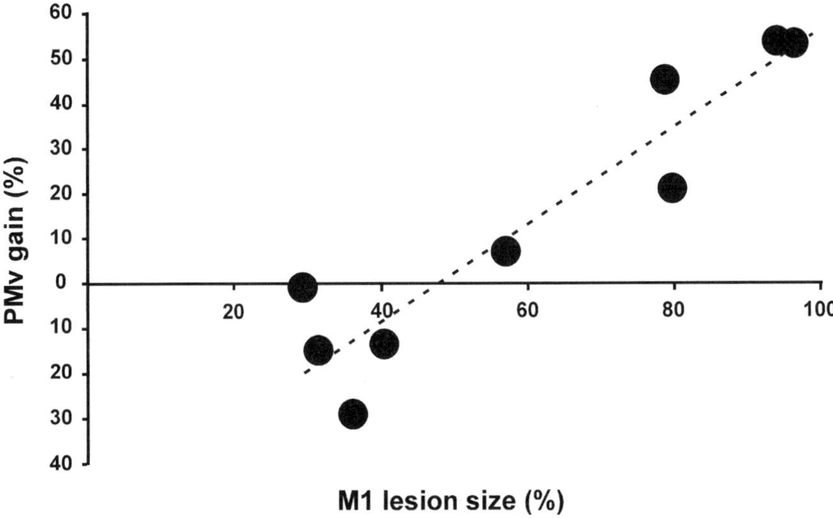

FIGURE 4.4. Relationship between size of lesion in M1 and increase in motor representation in premotor cortex (PMv). The percentages refer to the proportion of the M1 hand representation that was destroyed by an experimental cortical infarct in squirrel monkeys. Note that as lesion sizes exceed 50% of the M1 hand representation, hand representations in PMv expand in a linear fashion.

Interestingly, when lesions were smaller than 50% of the M1 hand area, the PMv hand representation decreased in size (Figure 4.4). Thus, across the entire spectrum of M1 infarcts of varying sizes, the linear relationship is maintained. This result occurred despite the fact that some of these subtotal M1 hand area lesions nonetheless destroyed nearly the entire terminal field of PMv–M1 connections. What possible compensatory changes in the neuronal network could account for proportional gains in premotor hand areas, but losses with very small lesions? This phenomenon is reminiscent of Lashley's (1929, 1930) classic description of the relationship between cerebral mass and behavioral change. According to this hypothesis, lesion size is generally assumed to be associated with the severity of deficits, whereas lesion location is related to the specificity of deficits. Lashley also proposed the concept of *equipotentiality*, suggesting that each portion of a given cortical area is able to encode or produce behavior normally controlled by the entire area. If so, after smaller lesions, the surviving M1 tissue could potentially subserve the recovery of function. In that case, reorganization in distant, interconnected cortical areas would be a more "passive" process resulting from the loss of intracortical connections. This reorganization could be compared to a "sustained diaschisis" of PMv.

After larger lesions, reorganization of the adjacent tissue may not suffice for normal motor execution. Thus learning-associated reorganization may need to take place elsewhere, resulting in greater PMv expansion. Accordingly, in rats, the contralesional cortex is thought to be involved in behavioral recovery only after large lesions (Biernaskie, Szymanska, Windle, & Corbett, 2005). Our current set of data similarly suggests that lesion size is a major factor involved in initiating some of the vicarious processes that purportedly play a role in recovery from CNS lesions.

To further explore what mechanism may underlie these changes in PMv, we have examined the anatomical reorganization of axonal projections within the motor cortex to see whether it parallels the reorganization in PMv. There is ample evidence that synaptogenesis occurs in the peri-infarct zone after a cortical injury in rats (Stroemer, Kent, & Hulsebosch, 1995). In addition, recent studies in the rodent barrel-field cortex have shown axonal sprouting over relatively short distances (Carmichael, 2003). However, long-distance sprouting of corticocortical pathways has not been observed. We found that 5 months after an ischemic injury to the M1 hand representation, most intracortical connection patterns of the PMv remained intact (Dancause et al., 2005). This was despite the fact that the major intracortical target of PMv was destroyed by this procedure. However, when compared to uninjured control monkeys, the M1-lesioned monkeys showed a remarkable proliferation of novel PMv terminal projections in S1, specifically in the hand representations of areas 1 and 2. Likewise, this somatosensory area had a significant increase in the number of retrogradely labeled cell bodies, indicating an increase in reciprocal projections from S1 to PMv. In addition, intracortical axonal projections from PMv significantly altered their trajectory near the site of the lesion.

This finding is particularly interesting, given the direct intracortical connections between M1 and S1, as well as the presence of direct corticospinal projections originating from PMv. One hypothesis is that the postinjury sprouting represents a repair strategy of the sensory–motor cortex to reengage the motor areas with somatosensory areas. In intact brains, M1 receives input from various regions of the parietal lobe, which supply cutaneous and proprioceptive information that is largely segregated in the M1 hand area—cutaneous information arriving in the posterior portion of M1, and proprioceptive information arriving in the more anterior portion. The functional importance of this somatosensory input can be appreciated from studies employing discrete lesions in these subregions in M1. Lesions in the posterior M1 hand area lesions result in behavioral deficits akin to those seen after S1 lesions. These deficits appear to be similar to sensory agnosia, in which an animal reaches for food items, but does not appear to know whether the item is actually in the hand. In contrast, anterior M1 hand area lesions result in deficits in metrics of the reach, perhaps indicating the disruption of proprioceptive information in the motor cortex (Friel et al., 2005). One lesson from these studies is that the motor cortex cannot be considered solely as a motor structure. Deficits result from sensory–motor disconnection in addition to disruption of motor output. Thus, after M1 injury, there is a substantial reduction of somatosensory input to motor areas. Perhaps the novel connection between PMv and S1 is an attempt by the cortical motor systems to reconnect with somatosensory input. However, it is not yet known whether this connection is functional, or, if it is, whether it is adaptive or maladaptive. An alternative hypothesis is that the new pathway represents an aberrant connection that interferes with behavioral recovery. Additional studies are needed to determine the functional consequences of blocking or enhancing this pathway.

It is likely that this phenomenon of intracortical sprouting of remote pathways interconnected with the injured zone is not a unique event. It is more likely that many structures, both cortical and subcortical, that are normally connected with the injured tissue undergo substantial physiological and anatomical aterations. For instance, all of the other cortical motor areas (PMd, SMA, cingulate motor areas) are likely to change their intracortical connectivity patterns, since their targets are destroyed (Eisner-Janowicz et al., 2008). If so, it follows that the brain with a focal injury is a very different system; it is not simply a normal system with a missing piece. If intracortical reorganization is a predictable process, as we think it is, then we may be able to begin to develop ways of enhancing adaptive connection patterns while suppressing maladaptive ones.

IMPLICATIONS OF PLASTICITY STUDIES FOR REHABILITATION

The significance of neuroplasticity for rehabilitation is that it provides a mechanistic rationale for understanding therapeutic interventions. Thus it may be possible to develop more effective recovery protocols if we can elucidate the effects of such interventions on physiological and anatomical plasticity in the injured brain. As demonstrated by the mapping studies after microinfarcts in nonhuman primates described above, it is clear that behavior is one of the most powerful modulators of postinjury recovery. Behavioral interventions to enhance recovery after stroke have been become increasingly popular, due to the success of such therapeutic interventions as constraint-induced movement therapy. Whether such behaviorally driven changes in motor performance are due to reestablishment of original motor programs in spared tissue, or due to compensatory use of unimpaired body parts, remains a controversial subject. Nonetheless, plastic changes must take place in the spared neuronal substrate, whether the improvement is due to true restoration of function or to compensation. Behavioral use clearly plays a role in the contralesional changes that take place in the uninjured cortex of rats following cortical infarction. Other studies have demonstrated that task-specific rehabilitative training is most effective in driving postinjury neuroanatomical changes. Thus it would appear that CNS injury produces an environment in which the neuronal network is particularly receptive to modulation by specific behavioral manipulations.

REFERENCES

Allard, T., Clark, S. A., Jenkins, W. M., & Merzenich, M. M. (1991). Reorganization of somatosensory area 3b representations in adult owl monkeys after digital syndactyly. *Journal of Neurophysiology, 66*(3), 1048–1058.

Altenmüller, E., & Jabusch, H.-C. (2010). Focal dystonia in musicians: Phenomenology, pathophysiology and triggering factors. *European Journal of Neurology, 17*(1), 31–36.

Aroniadou, V. A., & Keller, A. (1993). The patterns and synaptic properties of horizontal intracortical connections in the rat motor cortex. *Journal of Neurophysiology, 70*(4), 1553–1569.

Asanuma, H. (1975). Recent developments in the study of the columnar arrangement of neurons within the motor cortex. *Physiological Reviews, 55*(2), 143–156.

Barbay, S., Peden, E. K., Falchook, G., & Nudo, R. J. (1999). Sensitivity of neurons in somatosensory cortex (S1) to cutaneous stimulation of the hindlimb immediately following a sciatic nerve crush. *Somatosensensory and Motor Research, 16*(2), 103–114.

Biernaskie, J., Szymanska, A., Windle, V., & Corbett, D. (2005). Bi-hemispheric contribution to functional motor recovery of the affected forelimb following focal ischemic brain injury in rats. *European Journal of Neuroscience, 21*(4), 989–999.

Blake, D. T., Strata, F., Kempter, R., & Merzenich, M. M. (2005). Experience-dependent plasticity in S1 caused by noncoincident inputs. *Journal of Neurophysiology, 94*(3), 2239–2250.

Buonomano, D. V., & Merzenich, M. M. (1998). Cortical plasticity: From synapses to maps. *Annual Review of Neuroscience, 21*, 149–186.

Byl, N. N., Merzenich, M. M., & Jenkins, W. M. (1996). A primate genesis model of focal dystonia and repetitive strain injury: I. Learning-induced dedifferentiation of the representation of the hand in the primary somatosensory cortex in adult monkeys. *Neurology, 47*(2), 508–520.

Candia, V., Wienbruch, C., Elbert, T., Rockstroh, B., & Ray, W. (2003). Effective behavioral treatment of focal hand dystonia in musicians alters somatosensory cortical organization. *Proceedings of the National Academy of Sciences USA, 100*(13), 7942–7946.

Carmichael, S. T. (2003). Plasticity of cortical projections after stroke. *Neuroscientist, 9*(1), 64–75.

Churchill, J. D., Tharp, J. A., Wellman, C. L., Sengelaub, D. R., & Garraghty, P. E. (2004). Morphological correlates of injury-induced reorganization in primate somatosensory cortex. *BMC Neuroscience, 5*(1), 43.

Cirstea, M. C., & Levin, M. F. (2000). Compensatory strategies for reaching in stroke. *Brain, 123*(Pt. 5), 940–953.

Clark, S. A., Allard, T., Jenkins, W. M., & Merzenich, M. M. (1988). Receptive fields in the body-surface map in adult cortex defined by temporally correlated inputs. *Nature, 332*(6163), 444–445.

Dancause, N., Barbay, S., Frost, S. B., Plautz, E. J., Chen, D., Zoubina, E. V., et al. (2005). Extensive cortical rewiring after brain injury. *Journal of Neuroscience, 25*(44), 10167–10179.

Dancause, N., Duric, V., Barbay, S., Frost, S. B., Stylianou, A., & Nudo, R. J. (2008). An additional motor-related field in the lateral frontal cortex of squirrel monkeys. *Cerebral Cortex, 18*(12), 2719–2800.

Eisner-Janowicz, I., Barbay, S., Hoover, E., Stowe, A. M., Frost, S. B., Plautz, E. J., et al. (2008). Early and later changes in the distal forelimb representation of the supplementary motor area after injury to frontal motor areas in the squirrel monkey. *Journal of Neurophysiology, 100*(3), 1498–1512.

Elbert, T., Candia, V., Altenmüller, E., Rau, H., Sterr, A., Rockstroh, B., et al. (1998). Alteration of digital representations in somatosensory cortex in focal hand dystonia. *NeuroReport, 9*(16), 3571–3575.

Fetz, E. E., Cheney, P. D., & German, D. C. (1976). Corticomotoneuronal connections of precentral cells detected by postspike averages of EMG activity in behaving monkeys. *Brain Research, 114*(3), 505–510.

Friedman, R. M., Chen, L. M., & Roe, A. W. (2004). Modality maps within primate somatosensory cortex. *Proceedings of the National Academy of Sciences USA, 101*(34), 12724–12729.

Friel, K. M., Barbay, S., Frost, S. B., Plautz, E. J., Hutchinson, D. M., Stowe, A. M., et al. (2005). Dissociation of sensorimotor deficits after rostral versus caudal lesions in the primary motor cortex hand representation. *Journal of Neurophysiology, 94*(2), 1312–1324.

Fritsch, G., & Hitzig, E. (1870). Uber die elektrische Erregbarkeit des Grosshirns. *Archiv für Anatomie, Physiologie, und Wissenschaftliche Medizin, Leipzig, 37*, 300–332.

Frost, S. B., Barbay, S., Friel, K. M., Plautz, E. J., & Nudo, R. J. (2003). Reorganization of remote cortical regions after ischemic brain injury: A potential substrate for stroke recovery. *Journal of Neurophysiology, 89*(6), 3205–3214.

Garraghty, P. E., Arnold, L. L., Wellman, C. L., & Mowery, T. M. (2006). Receptor autoradiographic correlates of deafferentation-induced reorganization in adult primate somatosensory cortex. *Journal of Comparative Neurology, 497*(4), 636–645.

Glees, P., & Cole, J. (1950). Recovery of skilled motor functions after small repeated lesions of motor cortex in macaque. *Journal of Neurophysiology, 13*, 137–148.

Goldberger, M. E. (1972). Restitution of function in the CNS: The pathologic grasp in *Macaca mulatta. Experimental Brain Research, 15*(1), 79–96.

Hammond, G. (2002). Correlates of human handedness in primary motor cortex: A review and hypothesis. *Neuroscience and Biobehavioral Reviews, 26*(3), 285–292.

Heffner, R. S., & Masterton, R. B. (1983). The role of the corticospinal tract in the evolution of human digital dexterity. *Brain, Behavior and Evolution, 23*(3–4), 165–183.

Hess, G., & Donoghue, J. P. (1994). Long-term potentiation of horizontal connections provides a mechanism to reorganize cortical motor maps. *Journal of Neurophysiology, 71*(6), 2543–2547.

Hess, G., & Donoghue, J. P. (1996). Long-term depression of horizontal connections in rat motor cortex. *European Journal of Neuroscience, 8*(4), 658–665.

Hickmott, P. W., & Steen, P. A. (2005). Large-scale changes in dendritic structure during reorganization of adult somatosensory cortex. *Nature Neuroscience, 8*(2), 140–142.

Huntley, G. W., & Jones, E. G. (1991). Relationship of intrinsic connections to forelimb movement representations in monkey motor cortex: A correlative anatomic and physiological study. *Journal of Neurophysiology, 66*(2), 390–413.

Jackson, A., Mavoori, J., & Fetz, E. E. (2006). Long-term motor cortex plasticity induced by an electronic neural implant. *Nature, 444*(7115), 56–60.

Jackson, J. H. (1884). The Croonian Lectures on evolution and dissolution of the nervous system. *The British Medical Journal, 1*(1214), 660–663.

Jain, N., Qi, H.-X., Collins, C. E., & Kaas, J. H. (2008). Large-scale reorganization in the somatosensory cortex and thalamus after sensory loss in macaque monkeys. *Journal of Neuroscience, 28*(43), 11042–11060.

Jenkins, W. M., Merzenich, M. M., & Recanzone, G. (1990). Neocortical representational dynamics in adult primates: Implications for neuropsychology. *Neuropsychologia, 28*(6), 573–584.

Jones, E. G. (1993). GABAergic neurons and their role in cortical plasticity in primates. *Cerebral Cortex, 3*(5), 361–372.

Kleim, J. A., Barbay, S., Cooper, N. R., Hogg, T. M., Reidel, C. N., Remple, M. S., et al. (2002). Motor learning-dependent synaptogenesis is localized to functionally reorganized motor cortex. *Neurobiology of Learning and Memory, 77*(1), 63–77.

Kleim, J. A., Barbay, S., & Nudo, R. J. (1998). Functional reorganization of the rat motor cortex following motor skill learning. *Journal of Neurophysiology, 80*(6), 3321–3325.

Lashley, K. S. (1929). *Brain mechanisms and intelligence: A quantitative study of injuries to the brain.* Chicago: University of Chicago Press.

Lashley, K. S. (1930). Basic neural mechanisms in behavior. *Physiological Review, 37*, 1–24.

Lemon, R. N., & Griffiths, J. (2005). Comparing the function of the corticospinal system in different species: Organizational differences for motor specialization? *Muscle and Nerve, 32*(3), 261–279.

Liu, Y., & Rouiller, E. M. (1999). Mechanisms of recovery of dexterity following unilateral lesion of the sensorimotor cortex in adult monkeys. *Experimental Brain Research, 128*(1–2), 149–159.

Lowel, S., & Singer, W. (1992). Selection of intrinsic horizontal connections in the visual cortex by correlated neuronal activity. *Science, 255*(5041), 209–212.

Merzenich, M. M., Kaas, J. H., Wall, J., Nelson, R. J., Sur, M., & Felleman, D. (1983). Topographic reorganization of somatosensory cortical areas 3b and

1 in adult monkeys following restricted deafferentation. *Neuroscience, 8*(1), 33–55.

Monfils, M. H., Plautz, E. J., & Kleim, J. A. (2005). In search of the motor engram: Motor map plasticity as a mechanism for encoding motor experience. *Neuroscientist, 11*(5), 471–483.

Myers, W. A., Churchill, J. D., Muja, N., & Garraghty, P. E. (2000). Role of NMDA receptors in adult primate cortical somatosensory plasticity. *Journal of Comparative Neurology, 418*(4), 373–382.

Nudo, R. J., & Frost, S. B. (2007). The evolution of motor cortex and motor systems. In J. H. Kaas (Series Ed.) & T. Preuss (Vol. Ed.), *Evolution of nervous systems: A comprehensive reference. Vol. 3. Mammals.* Boston: Elsevier Academic Press.

Nudo, R. J., & Milliken, G. W. (1996). Reorganization of movement representations in primary motor cortex following focal ischemic infarcts in adult squirrel monkeys. *Journal of Neurophysiology, 75*(5), 2144–2149.

Nudo, R. J., Milliken, G. W., Jenkins, W. M., & Merzenich, M. M. (1996). Use-dependent alterations of movement representations in primary motor cortex of adult squirrel monkeys. *Journal of Neuroscience, 16*(2), 785–807.

Pascual-Leone, A., & Torres, F. (1993). Plasticity of the sensorimotor cortex representation of the reading finger in Braille readers. *Brain, 116*(Pt. 1), 39–52.

Penfield, W., & Rasmussen, T. (1950). *The cerebral cortex of man.* New York: Macmillan.

Plautz, E. J., Milliken, G. W., & Nudo, R. J. (2000). Effects of repetitive motor training on movement representations in adult squirrel monkeys: Role of use versus learning. *Neurobiology of Learning and Memory, 74*(1), 27–55.

Pons, T. P., Garraghty, P. E., Ommaya, A. K., Kaas, J. H., Taub, E., & Mishkin, M. (1991). Massive cortical reorganization after sensory deafferentation in adult macaques. *Science, 252*(5014), 1857–1860.

Rathelot, J. A., & Strick, P. L. (2006). Muscle representation in the macaque motor cortex: An anatomical perspective. *Proceedings of the National Academy of Sciences USA, 103*(21), 8257–8262.

Recanzone, G. H., Merzenich, M. M., & Schreiner, C. E. (1992). Changes in the distributed temporal response properties of SI cortical neurons reflect improvements in performance on a temporally based tactile discrimination task. *Journal of Neurophysiology, 67*(5), 1071–1091.

Schaechter, J. D., Moore, C. I., Connell, B. D., Rosen, B. R., & Dijkhuizen, R. M. (2006). Structural and functional plasticity in the somatosensory cortex of chronic stroke patients. *Brain, 129*(Pt. 10), 2722–2733.

Sherrington, C. (1912). On the instability of a cortical point. *Proceedings of the Royal Society of London, Series B, 85*, 250–277.

Stroemer, R. P., Kent, T. A., & Hulsebosch, C. E. (1995). Neocortical neural sprouting, synaptogenesis, and behavioral recovery after neocortical infarction in rats. *Stroke, 26*(11), 2135–2144.

Ungerleider, L. G., Doyon, J., & Karni, A. (2002). Imaging brain plasticity during motor skill learning. *Neurobiology of Learning and Memory, 78*(3), 553–564.

Wang, X., Merzenich, M. M., Sameshima, K., & Jenkins, W. M. (1995). Remodelling of hand representation in adult cortex determined by timing of tactile stimulation. *Nature, 378*(6552), 71–75.

Wellman, C. L., Arnold, L. L., Garman, E. E., & Garraghty, P. E. (2002). Acute reductions in GABAA receptor binding in layer IV of adult primate somatosensory cortex after peripheral nerve injury. *Brain Research, 954*(1), 68–72.

Whishaw, I. Q., Pellis, S. M., Gorny, B. P., & Pellis, V. C. (1991). The impairments in reaching and the movements of compensation in rats with motor cortex lesions: An endpoint, videorecording, and movement notation analysis. *Behavioural Brain Research, 42*(1), 77–91.

Woolsey, C. N., Settlage, P. H., Meyer, D. R., Sencer, W., Pinto Hamuy, T., & Travis, A. M. (1952). Patterns of localization in precentral and "supplementary" motor areas and their relation to the concept of a premotor area. *Research Publications of the Association for Research in Nervous and Mental Disease, 30*, 238–264.

Xerri, C., Merzenich, M. M., Peterson, B. E., & Jenkins, W. (1998). Plasticity of primary somatosensory cortex paralleling sensorimotor skill recovery from stroke in adult monkeys. *Journal of Neurophysiology, 79*(4), 2119–2148.

Zarzecki, P., Witte, S., Smits, E., Gordon, D. C., Kirchberger, P., & Rasmusson, D. D. (1993). Synaptic mechanisms of cortical representational plasticity: Somatosensory and corticocortical EPSPs in reorganized raccoon SI cortex. *Journal of Neurophysiology, 69*(5), 1422–1432.

CHAPTER 5

Cognitive Reserve

YAAKOV STERN

The idea of reserve against brain damage stems from the repeated observation that there does not appear to be a direct relationship between the degree of brain pathology or brain damage and the clinical manifestation of that damage. For example, Katzman et al. (1989) described 10 cases of cognitively normal elderly women who were discovered to have advanced Alzheimer's disease (AD) pathology in their brains at death. They speculated that these women did not express the clinical features of AD because their brains were larger than average, providing them with what these authors terms *brain reserve*. In more recent cohort studies, it has been estimated that approximately 25% of individuals who have postmortem neuropathological evidence of AD do not exhibit symptoms of dementia during their lives (Ince, 2001).

Brain reserve (Katzman, 1993) is an example of what might be called a "passive" model of reserve, in which reserve is derived from brain size or neuronal count. This and similar models are passive because reserve is defined in terms of the amount of brain damage that a person can sustain before reaching a threshold for clinical expression. The *threshold* model (Satz, 1993), one of the best-articulated passive models, revolves around the construct of *brain reserve capacity* (BRC). Although BRC is a hypothetical construct, concrete examples of BRC may include brain size or synapse count. The model recognizes that there are individual differences in BRC. It also presupposes that there is a critical threshold of BRC. Once BRC is depleted past this threshold, specific clinical or functional deficits emerge.

In contrast, the *cognitive reserve* (CR) model suggests that the brain actively attempts to cope with brain damage by using preexisting cognitive processing approaches or by enlisting compensatory approaches (Stern, 2002). According to this model, individuals with more CR will be more successful at coping with the same amount of brain damage. Thus the same amount of brain damage or pathology will have different effects on different people, even if BRC (e.g., brain size) is held constant. The concept of CR provides a ready explanation for why many studies have demonstrated that higher levels of intelligence and of educational and occupational attainment are good predictors of which individuals can sustain greater brain damage before demonstrating functional deficit. Rather than positing that these individuals' brains are grossly anatomically different from those of persons with less reserve (e.g., they have more synapses), the CR hypothesis posits that they process tasks in a manner that allows them to cope better with the brain damage. Brain reserve and CR concepts are not mutually exclusive, and it is likely that both are involved in providing reserve against brain damage.

I (Stern et al., 2005) have suggested that the neural implementation of CR may take two forms: neural reserve and neural compensation. *Neural reserve* refers to brain networks or cognitive paradigms that predate any type of brain damage and that are less susceptible to disruption, perhaps because they are more efficient or have greater capacity. This type of CR represents a normal process that is already in place in healthy individuals. Although healthy individuals may invoke these networks when coping with increased task demands, the networks may also help an individual cope with brain pathology. In imaging studies, networks underlying neural reserve should therefore be identical in healthy and impaired individuals, although they may be expressed to different degrees. *Neural compensation* refers to the process by which individuals suffering from brain pathology use brain structures or networks (and thus cognitive strategies) not normally used by individuals with intact brains, in order to compensate for brain damage. In imaging studies, neural compensation should translate into the impaired group's using brain areas of networks that are not used by the intact group. Thus the concepts of neural reserve and neural compensation are particularly important when researchers are attempting to formulate and interpret functional imaging studies that investigate CR.

MEASURES OF RESERVE

For advocates of the idea of brain reserve, anatomical measures such as brain volume, head circumference, synapse count, or dendritic branching are effective measures of reserve. Mounting evidence suggests that many of these measures are malleable over a person's lifetime and are influenced by life experience. Therefore, brain reserve may represent a summation of many aspects of life experience that are also thought to summate into CR.

Variables descriptive of lifetime experience are the most commonly used proxies for CR. These include measures of socioeconomic status, such as income or occupational attainment. Educational attainment has also been a widely used proxy for CR, probably because it is relatively easy to ascertain. Degree of literacy may be a better marker for CR than number of years of formal education, because it is a more direct measure of educational attainment (Manly, Schupf, Tang, & Stern, 2005; Manly, Touradji, Tang, & Stern, 2003). Finally, specific measured attributes have been used as indices of CR, including IQ and measures of various cognitive functions.

Education may also be a marker for innate intelligence, which may in turn be genetically based or a function of exposures. Some studies suggest that an estimate of IQ, or premorbid IQ, may actually be a more powerful measure of CR in some cases (Albert & Teresi, 1999; Alexander et al., 1997). Still, education and other life experiences probably impart CR over and above that obtained from innate intelligence. Studies have demonstrated separate or synergistic effects for higher educational and occupational attainment and leisure activities, suggesting that each of these life experiences contributes independently to CR (Evans et al., 1993; Mortel, Meyer, Herod, & Thornby, 1995; Rocca et al., 1990; Stern et al., 1994, 1995a). A prospective study showed that estimated IQ at age 53 was separately influenced by childhood cognition, educational attainment, and adult occupation (Richards & Sacker, 2003). These observations stress that CR is not fixed; at any point in one's lifetime, it results from a combination of exposures.

The simplest explanation for how CR forestalls the clinical effects of AD pathology does not posit that experiences associated with more CR have direct effects on brain reserve or the development of AD pathology. Rather, CR allows some people to cope better with the pathology and remain clinically more intact for longer periods of time. This has been the working assumption underlying the design and interpretation of many of my research group's studies. However, as mentioned above, many of the factors associated with CR may also have a direct impact on the brain itself. There is a demonstrated relationship between IQ and brain volume (Willerman, Schultz, Rutledge, & Bigler, 1991). Thus the child development literature suggests that intracranial brain volume and aspects of lifetime exposure are predictive of differential susceptibility to the effects of traumatic brain injury (Kesler, Adams, Blasey, & Bigler, 2003). Also, it is now clear that stimulating environments and exercise promote neurogenesis in the dentate gyrus of animals (Brown et al., 2003; van Praag, Shubert, Zhao, & Gage, 2005). In addition, there is evidence to suggest that environmental enrichment may act directly to prevent or slow the accumulation of AD pathology

(Lazarov et al., 2005). Thus a more complete accounting of CR will have to integrate these complex interactions among genetics, the environmental influences on brain reserve and pathology, and the ability to compensate actively for the effects of pathology.

EPIDEMIOLOGICAL EVIDENCE FOR CR

The concept of CR is relevant to any situation where the brain sustains injury. In addition, I argue that the concept of CR should be extended to encompass variation in healthy individuals' performance, particularly when they must perform at their maximum capacity. Nevertheless, many of the studies discussed in this chapter have been framed around AD, with the implicit assumption that the discussion has implications for brain damage in general. AD has some unique advantages for examining disease-induced changes in brain function. Its pathology affects cortical circuitry that subserves a wide range of cognitive functions, and because its pathology is more likely than conditions such as stroke to affect similar anatomical sites across subjects, it permits better generalization. AD is also slowly but inexorably progressive, providing a more sensitive indicator of the severity of brain insult required before cognitive networks change. On the other hand, the potential for adaptation of recovery may vary between slowly progressive and acute pathologies, so studies of AD may not always have direct implications for studies of other conditions.

Numerous studies have examined the relation between CR proxy variables and incident dementia. Parallel studies have often examined the relation between these variables and cognitive decline in normal aging. Several studies have reported no association between education and incident dementia (Chandra et al., 2001; Cobb, Wolf, Au, White, & D'Agostino, 1995; Graves et al., 1996; Hall, Gao, Unverzagt, & Hendrie, 2000; Paykel et al., 1994). However, lower rates of incident dementia in subjects with higher education have been reported in at least eight cohorts, in France (Letenneur, Commenges, Dartigues, & Barberger-Gateau, 1994), Sweden (Qiu, Backman, Winblad, Aguero-Torres, & Fratiglioni, 2001), Finland (Anttila et al., 2002), China (Zhang et al., 1990), and the United States (Evans et al., 1997; Stern et al., 1994; White et al., 1994; Evans et al., 1993). Similar associations emerged in a pooled analysis of four European population-based prospective studies of individuals 65 years and older (Launer et al., 1999).

There is also evidence for the role of education in age-related cognitive decline, with several studies of normal aging reporting slower cognitive and functional decline in individuals with higher educational attainment (Albert et al., 1995; Butler, Ashford, & Snowdon, 1996; Chodosh, Reuben, Albert, & Seeman, 2002; Christensen et al., 1997; Colsher & Wallace,

1991; Farmer, Kittner, Rae, Bartko, & Regier, 1995; Lyketsos, Chen, & Anthony, 1999; Snowdon, Ostwald, & Kane, 1989). These studies suggest that the same education-related factors that delay the onset of dementia also allow individuals to cope more effectively with the brain changes encountered in normal aging. In an ethnically diverse cohort of nondemented elders in New York City, increased literacy was also associated with slower decline in memory, executive function, and language skills (Manly et al., 2005).

Either no association or an equivocal association between occupation and incident AD was found in several population-based longitudinal studies (Anttila et al., 2002; Helmer et al., 2001; Jorm et al., 1998). In two other prospective studies, occupational position did not predict incident dementia (Paykel et al., 1994), or its predictive value might have been mediated by educational status (Evans et al., 1997). Nevertheless, several studies have noted a relationship between occupational attainment and incident dementia (Bickel & Cooper, 1994; Qiu et al., 2003; Schmand, Smit, Geerlings, & Lindeboom, 1997; Stern et al., 1994; White et al., 1994; Zhang, Li, & Zhang, 1999). As mentioned above, occupational attainment has often been noted to have independent effects or to interact with educational attainment.

Studies have also explored the relationship between leisure activities and incident dementia. A study from France reported that traveling, doing odd jobs, and knitting were associated with lower risk of incident dementia (Fabrigoule et al., 1995; Helmer et al., 1999). Community activities and gardening were also protective against incident dementia in China (Zhang et al., 1999). A longitudinal study in Sweden reported that having an extensive social network was protective against development of incident dementia (Fratiglioni, Wang, Ericsson, Maytan, & Winblad, 2000). The same research group later reported that engagement in mental, social, and productive activities was associated with decreased risk for incident dementia (Wang, Karp, Winblad, & Fratiglioni, 2002). Participation in a variety of leisure activities characterized as intellectual (e.g., reading, playing games, going to classes) or social (e.g., visiting with friends or relatives) was assessed in another population study of nondemented elderly persons in New York (Scarmeas, Levy, Tang, Manly, & Stern, 2001). During follow-up, subjects with high rates of leisure activity had 38% less risk of developing dementia. In another prospective study, frequency of participation in common cognitive activities (e.g., reading newspapers, magazines, books) was assessed at baseline for 801 elderly Catholic nuns, priests, and brothers without dementia (Wilson et al., 2002). Engagement in such cognitive activities was found to be associated with slower rates of cognitive decline. Finally, in another prospective cohort from New York, participation in leisure activities, particularly reading, playing board games or musical instruments, and dancing, was associated with a reduced risk for incident dementia (Verghese et al., 2003). Increased participation in cognitive activities was also associated with reduced rates of memory decline in this study.

A meta-analysis examined cohort studies of the effects of education, occupation, premorbid IQ, and mental activities on dementia risk (Valenzuela & Sachdev, 2005). A summary analysis was based on an integrated total of 29,279 individuals from 22 studies. The median follow-up was 7.1 years. The summary odds ratio of incident dementia for individuals with high brain reserve compared to low was 0.54 (95% confidence interval = 0.49–0.59, $p < .0001$)—a decreased risk of 46%. Of 33 data sets, 8 showed no significant effect, while the other 25 demonstrated a significant protective effect. The authors found a significant negative association between incident dementia risk (based on differential education) and the overall dementia rate for each cohort ($r = -.57$, $p = .04$), indicating that in these studies there was a lower overall risk of incident dementia in the cohort.

In contrast to the studies above, in which greater CR has been associated with better outcomes, a series of studies of patients with AD have suggested that those with higher CR have poorer outcomes. In a prospective study of patients matched for clinical severity of AD at baseline (Stern, Tang, Denaro, & Mayeux, 1995b), patients with greater education or occupational attainment died sooner than those with less attainment. Although at first these findings appear counterintuitive, they are consistent with the CR hypothesis. The hypothesis predicts that at any level of assessed clinical severity, the underlying pathology of AD will be more advanced in patients with CR than in those with CR. This should result in the clinical disease's emerging when pathology is more advanced, as suggested by the studies of incident AD reviewed above. This disparity in degree of pathology should be present at more advanced clinical stages of the disease as well. At some point, the greater degree of pathology in the high-CR patients should result in more rapid death. Although one study did not replicate this finding (Geerlings, Deeg, Schmand, Lindeboom, & Jonker, 1997), a follow-up study by the same group, using patients with more advanced dementia, did (Geerlings et al., 1999). Higher measured CR has also been associated with more rapid cognitive decline in patients with AD (Scarmeas, Albert, Manly, & Stern, 2006; Stern, Albert, Tang, & Tsai, 1999). Explanation of this finding is along similar lines. At some point, AD pathology must become too severe to support the processes that mediate CR. This point should arrive at an earlier stage of clinical severity in patients with higher CR, because the underlying AD pathology is more severe.

IMAGING STUDIES OF CR

Several imaging studies of CR in AD have used resting cerebral blood flow (CBF) as a surrogate for AD pathology (DeCarli et al., 1992; Friedland, Brun, & Bundinger, 1985; McGeer, McGeer, Harrop, Akiyama, & Kamo, 1990). Our original functional imaging study found that in patients matched for overall severity of dementia, the parietotemporal flow deficit was greater in those with more years of education (Stern, Alexander, Prohovnik, & Mayeux, 1992). This observation was confirmed in a later positron emission tomography (PET) study (Alexander et al., 1997). After clinical dementia severity was controlled, higher education was correlated with reduced cerebral metabolism in prefrontal, premotor, and left superior parietal association areas. The negative correlations are consistent with the CR model's prediction that at any given level of disease clinical severity, a subject with a higher level of CR should have greater AD pathology (i.e., lower CBF). These studies indicate that although pathology was more advanced in the patients with higher education, the clinical manifestations of the disease were comparable to those in patients with lower education and less pathology. Presumably the patients with more education had more CR. We made a similar observation for occupational attainment (Stern et al., 1995a), and later for leisure activities (Scarmeas et al., 2003). These findings were confirmed in a prospective study with subsequent neuropathological analysis. Education was found to modify the association between AD pathology and levels of cognitive function: For the same degree of brain pathology, there was better cognitive function with each year of education (Bennett et al., 2003).

In contrast to the resting studies, cognitive activation studies can be used to elucidate the nature of CR. The general logic behind this approach is that to the extent that CR reflects differences in how tasks are processed, functional imaging studies should be able to capture these differences. One approach to this problem is to identify patterns of task-related activation that differ between patients with AD and controls, and to determine whether they are compensatory. For example, in an early study (Stern et al., 2000), we tried to determine whether or not the pathology of AD alters the brain networks subserving performance on a memory task, while carefully controlling for task difficulty. $H_2[^{15}O]$ PET was used to measure regional CBF in patients and healthy elderly persons during the performance of a verbal recognition task. Task difficulty was matched across participants by adjusting the size of the list that each subject had to remember, so that each subject's recognition accuracy was 75%. In the healthy elders, a network of brain areas involving left anterior cingulate, anterior insula, and left basal ganglia was activated during task performance. Higher study list size (SLS) was associated with increased recruitment of this network, indicating that the network was associated with task performance and that subjects who could recruit it to a greater degree could perform the task better. Only three patients with AD expressed this network in a manner similar to that of the controls. This network may underlie neural reserve, in that it appears to be recruited to cope with the demands presented by the activation task, and differential recruitment of the network is directly related to the ability to perform the task. Individuals who are able to activate this network to a greater degree may have more reserve against brain damage. The remaining 11 patients with AD recruited a different network during task performance, consisting of left posterior temporal cortex, calcarine cortex, posterior cingulate, and the vermis. Again, in these patients, higher SLS was associated with increased activation of this network. We hypothesized that this alternate network may be used by most patients with AD to compensate for the effects of AD pathology. This is compatible with the concept of neural compensation, in which patients use brain networks not used by unaffected individuals to perform a task.

Whereas the criteria for neural compensation merely require that individuals with pathology use a brain network that is not used by unaffected individuals, one may further ask whether use of this alternate network is associated with better performance. For example, in several studies, some elders showed additional activation in areas contralateral to those activated by younger subjects; the elders who showed this additional activation performed better than those who did not, indicating that it was compensatory (Cabeza, Anderson, Locantore, & McIntosh, 2002; Rosen et al., 2002). Similarly, studies have shown that additional activation in patients with AD compared to controls is compensatory (Grady et al., 2003).

Other studies from my research group have taken a more direct approach to investigating brain networks associated with CR. One PET study identified brain areas whose activation during performance of a nonverbal memory task was correlated with an index of CR calculated from measures of education and literacy (Scarmeas et al., 2004). Such areas were identified in both healthy controls and patients with AD, suggesting that these areas may reflect the neural instantiation of CR. Interestingly, in some brain areas the directionality of the association between CR and cerebral activation differed in healthy controls and patients with AD. For example, some brain areas showed increased activation as a function of increased CR in the elderly controls and decreased activation in the patients. Given the assumption that individuals with higher measured CR should activate brain areas in a more adaptive way, these findings suggest that there has been some compensation for the effects of AD pathology in the patients, and that CR is mediated differently in the patients and controls. The changes in activation in the patients with AD are consistent with our definition of neural compensation. Similar observations have been noted in comparisons of young and elderly subjects (Stern et al., 2005).

In summary, the imaging evidence is beginning to provide support for the two hypothesized neural mechanisms underlying CR: neural reserve, which emphasizes preexisting differences in neural efficiency or capacity; and neural compensation, which reflects individual differences in the ability to develop new, compensatory responses to the disabling effects of pathology.

OTHER APPLICATIONS OF THE CR CONCEPT

The discussion of CR has focused on its application to aging in general and dementia in particular. However, it is equally applicable to any condition that has an impact on brain function. Thus it has been applied to the development of dementia in HIV (Farinpour et al., 2003), cognitive change in schizophrenia (Barnett, Salmond, Jones, & Sahakian, 2006), and recovery of function following either traumatic brain injury in adults (Kesler et al., 2003) or acquired brain injury in children (Dennis, Yeates, Taylor, & Fletcher, 2007).

More recently, there has been increasing interest in whether some experiences can impart CR. From the epidemiological data, we might expect that some combination of cognitively stimulating activities might promote CR and thus delay the effects of normal cognitive aging and AD. Unfortunately, the epidemiological data are not useful in specifying what types of experience would be ideal or what duration of exposure would be needed. However, it is clear that studies investigating this issue are forthcoming. We can therefore conceive of a time in the near future where we can actually promote CR to forestall the negative effects of later brain injury, and perhaps to hasten recovery from existing injury.

ACKNOWLEDGMENT

This work was supported by Grant No. RO1 AG26158 from the National Institute on Aging.

REFERENCES

Albert, M. S., Jones, K., Savage, C. R., Berkman, L., Seeman, T., Blazer, D., et al. (1995). Predictors of cognitive change in older persons: MacArthur studies of successful aging. *Psychology and Aging, 10*, 578–589.

Albert, S. M., & Teresi, J. A. (1999). Reading ability, education, and cognitive status assessment among older adults in Harlem, New York City. *American Journal of Public Health, 89*, 95–97.

Alexander, G. E., Furey, M. L., Grady, C. L., Pietrini, P., Mentis, M. J., & Schapiro, M. B. (1997). Association of premorbid function with cerebral metabolism in Alzheimer's disease: Implications for the reserve hypothesis. *American Journal of Psychiatry, 154*, 165–172.

Anttila, T., Helkala, E. L., Kivipelto, M., Hallikainen, M., Alhainen, K., Heinonen, H., et al. (2002). Midlife income, occupation, APOE status, and dementia: A population-based study. *Neurology, 59*, 887–893.

Barnett, J. H., Salmond, C. H., Jones, P. B., & Sahakian, B. J. (2006). Cognitive reserve in neuropsychiatry. *Psychological Medicine, 36*, 1053–1064.

Bennett, D. A., Wilson, R. S., Schneider, J. A., Evans, D. A., Mendes De Leon, C. F., Arnold, S. E., et al. (2003). Education modifies the relation of AD pathology to level of cognitive function in older persons. *Neurology, 60*(12), 1909–1915.

Bickel, H., & Cooper, B. (1994). Incidence and relative risk of dementia in an urban elderly population: Findings of a prospective field study. *Psychological Medicine, 24*, 179–192.

Brown, J., Cooper-Kuhn, C. M., Kemperman, G., van Praag, H., Winkler, J., & Gage, F. H. (2003). Enriched environment and physical activity stimulate hippocampal but not olfactory bulb neurogenesis. *European Journal of Neuroscience, 17*, 2042–2046.

Butler, S. M., Ashford, J. W., & Snowdon, D. A. (1996). Age, education, and changes in the Mini-Mental State Exam scores of older women: Findings from the Nun Study. *Journal of the American Geriatrics Society, 44*, 675–681.

Cabeza, R., Anderson, N. D., Locantore, J. K., & McIntosh, A. R. (2002). Aging gracefully: Compensatory brain activity in high-performing older adults. *NeuroImage, 17*, 1394–1402.

Chandra, V., Pandav, R., Dodge, H. H., Johnston, J. M., Belle, S. H., DeKosky, S. T., et al. (2001). Incidence of Alzheimer's disease in a rural community in India: The Indo-US study. *Neurology, 57*, 985–989.

Chodosh, J., Reuben, D. B., Albert, M. S., & Seeman, T. E. (2002). Predicting cognitive impairment in high-functioning community-dwelling older persons: MacArthur Studies of Successful Aging. *Journal of the American Geriatrics Society, 50*, 1051–1060.

Christensen, H., Korten, A. E., Jorm, A. F., Henderson, A. S., Jacomb, P. A., Rodgers, B., et al. (1997). Education and decline in cognitive performance: Compensatory but not protective. *International Journal of Geriatric Psychiatry, 12*, 323–330.

Cobb, J. L., Wolf, P. A., Au, R., White, R., & D'Agostino, R. B. (1995). The effect of education on the incidence of dementia and Alzheimer's disease in the Framingham Study. *Neurology, 45*, 1707–1712.

Colsher, P. L., & Wallace, R. B. (1991). Longitudinal application of cognitive function measures in a defined population of community-dwelling elders. *Annals of Epidemiology, 1*, 215–230.

DeCarli, C., Atack, J. R., Ball, M. J., Kay, J. A., Grady, C. L., Fewster, P., et al. (1992). Post-mortem regional neurofibrillary tangle densities but not senile plaque densities are related to regional cerebral metabolic rates for glucose during life in Alzheimer's disease patients. *Neurodegeneration, 1*, 113–121.

Dennis, M., Yeates, K. O., Taylor, H. G., & Fletcher, J. M. (2007). Reserve capacity in brain-injured children. In Y. Stern (Ed.), *Cognitve reserve: Theory and applications* (pp. 53–83). New York: Taylor & Francis.

Evans, D. A., Beckett, L. A., Albert, M. S., Hebert, L. E., Scherr, P. A., Funkenstein, H. H., et al. (1993). Level of education and change in cognitive function in a community population of older persons. *Annals of Epidemiology, 3*, 71–77.

Evans, D. A., Hebert, L. E., Beckett, L. A., Scherr, P. A., Albert, M. S., Chown, M. J., et al. (1997). Education and other measures of socioeconomic status and risk of incident Alzheimer disease in a defined population of older persons. *Archives of Neurology, 54*, 1399–1405.

Fabrigoule, C., Letenneur, L., Dartigues, J. F., Zarrouk, M., Commenges, D., & Barberger-Gateau, P. (1995). Social and leisure activities and risk of dementia: A prospective longitudinal study. *Journal of the American Geriatrics Society, 43*, 485–490.

Farinpour, R., Miller, E. N., Satz, P., Selnes, O. A., Cohen, B. A., Becker, J. T., et al. (2003). Psychosocial risk factors of HIV morbidity and mortality: Findings from the Multicenter AIDS Cohort Study (MACS). *Journal of Clinical and Experimental Neuropsychology, 25*, 654–670.

Farmer, M. E., Kittner, S. J., Rae, D. S., Bartko, J. J., & Regier, D. A. (1995). Education and change in cognitive function: The Epidemiologic Catchment Area study. *Annals of Epidemiology, 5*, 1–7.

Fratiglioni, L., Wang, H. X., Ericsson, K., Maytan, M., & Winblad, B. (2000). Influence of social network on occurrence of dementia: A community-based longitudinal study. *Lancet, 355*, 1315–1319.

Friedland, R. P., Brun, A., & Bundinger, T. F. (1985). Pathological and positron emission tomographic correlations in Alzheimer's disease. *Lancet, i*, 228.

Geerlings, M. I., Deeg, D. J. H., Penninx, B. W., Schmand, B., Jonker, C., Bouter, L. M., et al. (1999). Cognitive reserve and mortality in dementia: The role of cognition, functional ability and depression. *Psychological Medicine, 29*, 1219–1226.

Geerlings, M. I., Deeg, D. J. H., Schmand, B., Lindeboom, J., & Jonker, C. (1997). Increased risk of mortality in Alzheimer's disease patients with higher education?: A replication study. *Neurology, 49*, 798–802.

Grady, C. L., McIntosh, A. R., Beig, S., Keightley, M. L., Burian, H., & Black, S. E. (2003). Evidence from functional neuroimaging of a compensatory prefrontal network in Alzheimer's disease. *Journal of Neuroscience, 23*, 986–993.

Graves, A. B., Larson, E. B., Edland, S. D., Bowen, J. D., McCormick, W. C., McCurry, S. M., et al. (1996). Prevalence of dementia and its subtypes in the Japanese American population of King County, Washington state: The Kame Project. *American Journal of Epidemiology, 144*, 760–771.

Hall, K. S., Gao, S., Unverzagt, F. W., & Hendrie, H. C. (2000). Low education and childhood rural residence: Risk for Alzheimer's disease in African Americans. *Neurology, 54*, 95–99.

Helmer, C., Damon, D., Letenneur, L., Fabrigoule, C., Barberger-Gateau, P., Lafont, S., et al. (1999). Marital status and risk of Alzheimer's disease: A French population-based cohort study. *Neurology, 53*, 1953–1958.

Helmer, C., Letenneur, L., Rouch, I., Richard-Harston, S., Barberger-Gateau, P., Fabrigoule, C., et al. (2001). Occupation during life and risk of dementia in French elderly community residents. *Journal of Neurology, Neurosurgery and Psychiatry, 71*, 303–9.

Ince, P. G. (2001). Pathological correlates of late-onset dementia in a multicenter community-based population in England and Wales. *Lancet, 357*, 169–175.

Jorm, A. F., Rodgers, B., Henderson, A. S., Korten, A. E., Jacomb, P. A., Christensen, H., et al. (1998). Occupation type as a predictor of cognitive decline and dementia in old age. *Age and Ageing, 27*, 477–483.

Katzman, R. (1993). Education and the prevalence of dementia and Alzheimer's disease. *Neurology, 43*, 13–20.

Katzman, R., Aronson, M., Fuld, P., Kawas, C., Brown, T., Morgenstern, H., et al. (1989). Development of dementing illnesses in an 80-year-old volunteer cohort. *Annals of Neurology, 25*, 317–324.

Kesler, S. R., Adams, H. F., Blasey, C. M., & Bigler, E. D. (2003). Premorbid intellectual functioning, education, and brain size in traumatic brain injury: An investigation of the cognitive reserve hypothesis. *Applied Neuropsychology, 10*, 153–162.

Launer, L. J., Andersen, K., Dewey, M. E., Letenneur, L., Ott, A., Amaducci, L. A., et al. (1999). Rates and risk factors for dementia and Alzheimer's disease: Results from EURODEM pooled analyses. EURODEM Incidence Research Group and Work Groups. European Studies of Dementia. *Neurology, 52*, 78–84.

Lazarov, O., Robinson, J., Tang, Y. P., Hairston, I. S., Korade-Mirnics, Z., Lee, V. M., et al. (2005). Environmental enrichment reduces Abeta levels and amyloid deposition in transgenic mice. *Cell, 120*, 701–713.

Letenneur, L., Commenges, D., Dartigues, J. F., & Barberger-Gateau, P. (1994). Incidence of dementia and Alzheimer's disease in elderly community residents of south-western France. *International Journal of Epidemiology, 23*, 1256–1261.

Lyketsos, C. G., Chen, L.-S., & Anthony, J. C. (1999). Cognitive decline in adulthood: An 11.5-year follow-up of the Baltimore Epidemiologic Catchment Area study. *American Journal of Psychiatry, 156*, 58–65.

Manly, J. J., Schupf, N., Tang, M. X., & Stern, Y. (2005). Cognitive decline and literacy among ethnically diverse elders. *Journal of Geriatric Psychiatry and Neurology, 18*, 213–217.

Manly, J. J., Touradji, P., Tang, M.-X., & Stern, Y. (2003). Literacy and memory decline among ethnically diverse elders. *Journal of Clinical and Experimental Neuropsychology, 5*, 680–690.

McGeer, E. G., McGeer, P. L., Harrop, R., Akiyama, H., & Kamo, H. (1990). Correlations of regional postmortem enzyme activities with premortem local glucose metabolic rates in Alzheimer's disease. *Journal of Neuroscience Research, 27*, 612–619.

Mortel, K. F., Meyer, J. S., Herod, B., & Thornby, J. (1995). Education and occupation as risk factors for dementia of the Alzheimer and ischemic vascular types. *Dementia, 6*, 55–62.

Paykel, E. S., Brayne, C., Huppert, F. A., Gill, C., Barkley, C., Gehlhaar, E., et al. (1994). Incidence of dementia in a population older than 75 years in the United Kingdom. *Archives of General Psychiatry, 54*, 325–332.

Qiu, C., Backman, L., Winblad, B., Aguero-Torres, H., & Fratiglioni, L. (2001). The influence of education on clinically diagnosed dementia incidence and mortality data from the Kungsholmen Project. *Archives of Neurology, 58*, 2034–2039.

Qiu, C., Karp, A., von Strauss, E., Winblad, B., Fratiglioni, L., & Bellander, T.

(2003). Lifetime principal occupation and risk of Alzheimer's disease in the Kungsholmen Project. *American Journal of Industrial Medicine, 43*, 204–211.

Richards, M., & Sacker, A. (2003). Lifetime antecedents of cognitive reserve. *Journal of Clinical and Experimental Neuropsychology, 25*, 614–624.

Rocca, W. A., Bonaiuto, S., Lippi, A., Luciani, P., Turtu, F., Cavarzeran, F., et al. (1990). Prevalence of clinically diagnosed Alzheimer's disease and other dementing disorders: A door-to-door survey in Appignano, Macerata Province, Italy. *Neurology, 40*, 626–631.

Rosen, A. C., Prull, M. W., O'Hara, R., Race, E. A., Desmond, J. E., Glover, G. H., et al. (2002). Variable effects of aging on frontal lobe contributions to memory. *NeuroReport, 13*, 2425–8.

Satz, P. (1993). Brain reserve capacity on symptom onset after brain injury: A formulation and review of evidence for threshold theory. *Neuropsychology, 7*, 273–295.

Scarmeas, N., Albert, S. M., Manly, J. J., & Stern, Y. (2006). Education and rates of cognitive decline in incident Alzheimer's disease. *Journal of Neurology, Neurosurgery and Psychiatry, 77*, 308–316.

Scarmeas, N., Levy, G., Tang, M. X., Manly, J., & Stern, Y. (2001). Influence of leisure activity on the incidence of Alzheimer's disease. *Neurology, 57*, 2236–2242.

Scarmeas, N., Zarahn, E., Anderson, K. E., Habeck, C. G., Hilton, J., Flynn, J., et al. (2003). Association of life activities with cerebral blood flow in Alzheimer disease: Implications for the cognitive reserve hypothesis. *Archives of Neurology, 60*, 359–365.

Scarmeas, N., Zarahn, E., Anderson, K. E., Honig, L. S., Park, A., Hilton, J., et al. (2004). Cognitive reserve-mediated modulation of positron emission tomographic activations during memory tasks in Alzheimer disease. *Archives of Neurology, 61*, 73–78.

Schmand, B., Smit, J. H., Geerlings, M. I., & Lindeboom, J. (1997). The effects of intelligence and education on the development of dementia: A test of the brain reserve hypothesis. *Psychological Medicine, 27*, 1337–1344.

Snowdon, D. A., Ostwald, S. K., & Kane, R. L. (1989). Education, survival and independence in elderly Catholic sisters, 1936–1988. *American Journal of Epidemiology, 130*, 999–1012.

Stern, Y. (2002). What is cognitive reserve?: Theory and research application of the reserve concept. *Journal of the International Neuropsychological Society, 8*, 448–460.

Stern, Y., Albert, S., Tang, M. X., & Tsai, W. Y. (1999). Rate of memory decline in AD is related to education and occupation: Cognitive reserve? *Neurology, 53*, 1942–1957.

Stern, Y., Alexander, G. E., Prohovnik, I., & Mayeux, R. (1992). Inverse relationship between education and parietotemporal perfusion deficit in Alzheimer's disease. *Annals of Neurology, 32*, 371–375.

Stern, Y., Alexander, G. E., Prohovnik, I., Stricks, L., Link, B., Lennon, M. C., et al. (1995). Relationship between lifetime occupation and parietal flow: Implications for a reserve against Alzheimer's disease pathology. *Neurology, 45*, 55–60.

Stern, Y., Gurland, B., Tatemichi, T. K., Tang, M. X., Wilder, D., & Mayeux, R. (1994). Influence of education and occupation on the incidence of Alzheimer's disease. *Journal of the American Medical Association, 271*, 1004–1010.

Stern, Y., Habeck, C., Moeller, J., Scarmeas, N., Anderson, K. E., Hilton, H. J., et al. (2005). Brain networks associated with cognitive reserve in healthy young and old adults. *Cerebral Cortex, 15*, 394–402.

Stern, Y., Moeller, J. R., Anderson, K. E., Luber, B., Zubin, N., Dimauro, A., et al. (2000). Different brain networks mediate task performance in normal aging and AD: Defining compensation. *Neurology, 55*, 1291–1297.

Stern, Y., Tang, M. X., Denaro, J., & Mayeux, R. (1995b). Increased risk of mortality in Alzheimer's disease patients with more advanced educational and occupational attainment. *Annals of Neurology, 37*, 590–595.

Valenzuela, M. J., & Sachdev, P. (2005). Brain reserve and dementia: A systematic review. *Psychological Medicine, 35*, 1–14.

van Praag, H., Shubert, T., Zhao, C., & Gage, F. H. (2005). Exercise enhances learning and hippocampal neurogenesis in aged mice. *Journal of Neuroscience, 25*, 8680–8685.

Verghese, J., Lipton, R. B., Katz, M. J., Hall, C. B., Derby, C. A., Kuslansky, G., et al. (2003). Leisure activities and the risk of dementia in the elderly. *New England Journal of Medicine, 348*, 2508–2516.

Wang, H.-X., Karp, A., Winblad, B., & Fratiglioni, L. (2002). Late-life engagement in social and leisure activities is associated with a decreased risk of dementia: A longitudinal study from the Kungsholmen Project. *American Journal of Epidemiology, 155*, 1081–1087.

White, L., Katzman, R., Losonczy, K., Salive, M., Wallace, R., Berkman, L., et al. (1994). Association of education with incidence of cognitive impairment in three established populations for epidemiologic studies of the elderly. *Journal of Clinical Epidemiology, 47*, 363–374.

Willerman, L., Schultz, R., Rutledge, J. N., & Bigler, E. D. (1991). In vivo brain size and intelligence. *Intelligence, 15*, 223–228.

Wilson, R. S., Mendes De Leon, C. F., Barnes, L. L., Schneider, J. A., Bienias, J. L., Evans, D. A., et al. (2002). Participation in cognitively stimulating activities and risk of incident Alzheimer disease. *Journal of the American Medical Association, 287*, 742–748.

Zhang, M., Katzman, R., Salmon, D., Jin, H., Cai, G., Wang, Z., et al. (1990). The prevalence of dementia and Alzheimer's disease in Shanghai, China: Impact of age, gender and education. *Annals of Neurology, 27*, 428–437.

Zhang, X., Li, C., & Zhang, M. (1999). [Psychosocial risk factors of Alzheimer's disease]. *Zhonghua Yi Xue Za Zhi, 79*, 335–338.

CHAPTER 6

Practice-Related Changes in Brain Activity

SARAH A. RASKIN
GINGER N. MILLS
JULIANNE T. GARBARINO

The chapters of this volume by Jones (Chapter 3) and by Nudo and Bury (Chapter 4) have demonstrated the possibility of adult brain plasticity in nonhumans, primarily with regard to the motor and sensory cortices. Kolb, Cioe, and Williams (Chapter 2) demonstrate that the functional properties of neurons in the central nervous system (CNS) retain a significant degree of plasticity into adulthood. Neural representations can change in response to practice and experience, and these changes can occur at the synaptic level, as well as in cortical maps and neural networks. This chapter reviews the emerging research in recent years that has demonstrated the possibility of neuronal functional changes in response to experience in both nonhumans and humans. It is hoped that an understanding of changes that naturally take place through experience can help to inform strategies of rehabilitation.

There are, however, some difficulties with this literature. The theoretical understanding of these findings has been complicated by inconsistent findings. Some studies report increases in activation in response to experience; others report decreases in activity; and still others report functional reorganization of regional activations. In part, these diverse findings may represent different kinds of plasticity. For example, Kelly and Garavan (2005) suggest that increased neural efficiency (and reduced activation) occurs when practice leads to increased skill or reduced need for attention control areas to be active, whereas cortical functional reorganization reflects the development of a new strategy.

Furthermore, when considering only functional changes, some researchers have reported redistribution and others reorganization. Both redistribution and reorganization include both increases and decreases in activation. In redistribution, the activation may include the same areas, but changes occur in levels of activations within those areas. True reorganization, by contrast, is a change in the location of activations, reflecting a shift in the cognitive processes underlying task performance. So areas of reduced activity indicate less engagement of a particular cognitive process, and areas of increased activation indicate an engagement of an alternate system (Kelly & Garavan, 2005).

MOTOR LEARNING

Motor learning can be associated with an increase in synapses in the motor cortex. In a study conducted by Kleim and colleagues (Kleim, Lussnig, Schwartz, & Comery, 1996; Kleim et al., 1998), adult rats were trained to go through different obstacles. The animals were trained for three trials per day, and on each trial were required to go through 10 obstacles. The researchers measured changes in the amount of Fos protein as well as synapses in the motor cortex associated with motor learning. The results indicated that the trained animals had an increased number of synapses per neuron at later stages of training than that of the control animals. The researchers hypothesized that these changes in structure should indicate the synthesis or change in the presence of neuronal proteins. The results indicated just that: The animals in the experimental group had a higher percentage of Fos-positive cells. Thus the researchers suggest that Fos protein could be involved in skill acquisition. They also suggest that motor learning causes an increase in synapses in the motor cortex (Kleim et al., 1998).

Several studies have suggested that motor learning in nonhuman animals causes structural changes in the brain (e.g., Gilbert & Thach, 1997). This motor learning occurs through practice and is suggested to occur in the cerebellum. In an experiment run by Gilbert and Thach (1997), three monkeys were trained on a task, and recordings were taken from the cerebellar Purkinje cells. The monkeys were instructed over several months on a task that involved moving and turning a vertical handle in a specific way, and were rewarded after every three trials. The researchers measured changes in complex spikes (which are produced by single-climbing-fiber input) and simple spikes (which are produced by multiple parallel fibers) of the Purkinje cells. The results indicated a decrease in simple-spike frequency, despite the initial increase of complex-spike frequency and its return to baseline level in the trained monkeys. Thus the results are consistent with the hypothesis that motor learning occurs in the cerebellum through the changes in transmission strength of the parallel fiber synapses (Gilbert & Thach, 1997).

Similarly, Ojakangas and Ebner (1992) demonstrated changes in both complex-spike activity and simple-spike activity in the cerebellum in response to motor learning. Two monkeys were trained to do a task, and the recordings of 88 Purkinje cells were used to evaluate learning. The results indicated that in addition to changes in simple spike activity, a significant change in complex-spike activity was observed in 43% of the Purkinje cells. Thus the hypothesis that complex-spike and simple-spike activity changes play a role in learning in the cerebellum was supported (Kleim et al., 1996).

Applications to human motor plasticity have included complicated motor tasks, as indicated in studies of musicians (Krings et al., 2005). Pianists and nonmusicians underwent functional magnetic resonance imaging (fMRI). Both groups performed simple and complex movement sequences on a keyboard with the right hand; the sequences required different levels of ordinal complexity. The aim of this study was to characterize motor representations related to sequence complexity and to long-term motor practice. In nonmusicians, complex motor sequences showed higher fMRI activations of the presupplementary motor area (pre-SMA) and the rostral part of the dorsal premotor cortex (PMd) compared to simple motor sequences, whereas musicians showed no differential activations. These results may reflect the higher level of visual–motor integration required in the complex task in nonmusicians, whereas in musicians this rostral premotor network was employed during both tasks. Comparison of subject groups revealed increased activation in nonmusicians of a more caudal premotor network comprising the caudal part of the PMd and the SMA. This supports recent results suggesting a specialization within PMd. Furthermore, plasticity due to long-term practice appears to occur mainly in caudal motor areas that are directly related to motor execution. The slowly evolving changes in primary motor cortex during motor skill learning may extend to adjacent areas, leading to more effective motor representations in pianists. In a further study, Meister et al. (2005) found no significant behavioral differences in accuracy between musicians and nonmusicians on a simple piano sequence. However, whereas the nonmusicians had significantly greater activation of left PMd and bilateral pre-SMA in complex versus simple sequences, the musicians did not show any difference between the two types of sequences. The authors conclude that this is evidence for cortical reorganization due to long-term practicing.

Researchers have also looked at cortical changes associated with athletic practice and expertise. For example, a study that compared high jumpers who competed at a national level with novice high jumpers asked all participants to use internal imagery to visualize themselves doing a high jump (Olsson, Jonsson, Larsson, & Nyberg, 2008). The competitive high jumpers showed increased activation in left-lateralized motor areas, whereas the novices showed activation in visual and parietal areas. The finding that motor regions were activated during imagery was taken to suggest that competitive high jumpers have developed greater motor imagery ability.

PERCEPTUAL LEARNING

Perceptual learning occurs when experience shapes the way the cortex analyzes new sensory information. For example, Gilbert, Li, and Piech (2009) reported that even in adults, the visual cortex is capable of altering its functional properties as a result of experience with visual stimuli, and that these long-term changes play a role in functional recovery after damage to the CNS. In response to a retinal lesion, they found that long-term changes involve axonal sprouting and synaptogenesis. These results led the authors to speculate that adult neurons are dynamically tuned, changing their specificities with different sensory experiences. Thus the visual cortex retains the capacity for experience-dependent changes, or plasticity, of cortical function and cortical circuitry throughout life. These changes constitute the mechanism of perceptual learning in normal visual experience and in recovery of function after CNS damage (Kaas, 1991).

Such plasticity can be seen at multiple stages in the visual pathway, including in the primary visual cortex. The functional changes associated with perceptual learning involve both long-term modification of cortical circuits during the course of learning, and short-term dynamics in the functional properties of cortical neurons. These dynamics are subject to top-down influences of attention, expectation, and perceptual task. As a consequence, each cortical area is an adaptive processor, altering its function in accordance to immediate perceptual demands—even to the point of experimental rewiring, causing the auditory cortex to process visual information (Horng & Sur, 2006).

It has been shown that individuals who have practiced reading Braille show cortical plasticity, such that regions generally considered to be visual are recruited while reading. In one study, Burton et al. (2002) compared individuals with congenital blindness to persons with late-onset blindness. All subjects showed activation in visual cortex while reading; however, those with congenital blindness showed greater activation than those with late-onset blindness. In a further study, Burton, Snyder, Diamond, and Raichle (2003) used a verbal task with sighted individuals, persons with early-onset blindness, and persons with late-onset blindness. The task was one of generating verbs to nouns. Only the two groups of blind individuals showed activity in the occipital, temporal, and parietal components of visual cortex while performing this task.

These findings suggest that perceptual training may lead to improved functional performance as a result of neuroplastic changes (Karni & Bertini, 1997). Some studies of such training in humans have been conducted, such as tachistoscopic stimulation in people with partial cortical blindness (Pleger et al., 2003). Some authors have already suggested clinical applications of these findings, including treatment for children with ocular disorders, and retinal or cortical implants (Celesia, 2005).

WORKING MEMORY

One area that has been studied extensively for practice-related changes is working memory. Decreases in working memory activity after practice have been reported in a wide range of cognitive tasks, such as mirror reading, verb generation, delayed response tasks, and motor sequence learning (Van Raalten, Ramsey, Duyn, & Jasma, 2008). These findings have been interpreted in terms of reduced demands on domain-general cognitive control resources that support early learning or novel task performance (Van Raalten et al., 2008). It has also been shown that practice-induced activity decreases are closely related to one's capacity to concurrently perform an additional cognitive task, suggesting an increase in automatization. Better understanding of the mechanism behind automatization may help inform cognitive remediation strategies aimed at making effortful tasks more automatic (e.g., Raskin & Palmese, 2000).

One of the most common paradigms used to study practice changes in working memory is mirror reading. Typical studies provide daily practice at mirror reading for several weeks and measure changes in brain activation as a result of this practice (e.g., Ilg et al., 2008). In research using this paradigm, imaging techniques have provided evidence for practice-induced gray matter changes (Ilg et al., 2010). These authors report a shift of activation from right superior parietal to right dorsal occipital cortex, and a corresponding increase in gray matter after practice with mirror reading. Activation at the dorsal occipital cortex and bilateral parietal cortex (dorsal visual stream) was related to inverse text processing, whereas activation of areas at the inferior and ventral occipitotemporal cortex (ventral visual stream) was associated with decoding of mirrored words. The authors suggest that this indicates a dichotomy of content-related ("what") and process-related ("where") higher visual functions.

Van Raalten et al. (2008), using a modified Sternberg task, specifically examined the idea that practice should lead to automatization. In this case, practice reduced activation in the encoding network, identified as left dorsolateral prefrontal cortex and anterior cingulate cortex. However, response selection activity in these same regions did not show any effect of practice. The authors suggest that this counters the idea of a reduction in use of attention resources as a result of scaffolding task performance. They suggest instead that the data are most consistent with reduced working memory contributions.

Landau, Garavan, Schumacher, and D'Esposito (2007) used event-related fMRI to look more closely at different brain regions recruited for different components of working memory tasks. The delayed-recognition task involved encoding, maintenance, and retrieval of both objects and spatial materials, to permit the researchers to examine the influence of practice on different components of working memory. Decreases in activation were noted during encoding and retrieval, but not during maintenance. The authors suggest that the regions responsible for encoding and retrieval may have greater plasticity than those used for maintenance.

However, several studies have shown that practice-related changes in activation are not necessarily accompanied by changes in behavioral performance (Landau et al., 2007; Olesen, Westerberg, & Klingberg, 2004), indicating that it is not possible to determine a clear link between activation decreases and either faster reaction time or improved accuracy.

ENVIRONMENTS

Given findings of brain plasticity related to the richness of environments for rats, researchers have asked whether these findings can be applied to human environments. One study placed mentally ill persons living in a homeless shelter into either independent apartments or group homes. Each group home consisted of 6–10 people living in individual bedrooms but sharing facilities and taking over household management. Seidman et al. (2003) administered neuropsychological measures of cognitive function before and after an 18-month period. Participants in both groups demonstrated increased cognitive function on measures of delayed verbal memory, motor speed, and sequencing. Participants in independent apartments showed a decrease in executive function, while those in group homes showed a nonsignificant increase.

EFFECTS OF COGNITIVE EXPERIENCE IN HUMANS

Some of the most widely disseminated findings in experience-dependent plasticity in humans came from a series of studies by Maguire et al., involving London taxi drivers (Maguire, Woolett, & Spiers, 2006; Maguire et al., 2003). In these studies, the brains of taxi drivers—persons who have been thoroughly trained to navigate the streets of London—were imaged. The overall finding has been that the gray matter volume in the posterior hippocampus of London taxi drivers is greater than in age-matched controls, and that the size of the increase is correlated with length of taxi-driving experience. Their studies suggest that there is capacity for local plastic changes in the adult human brain in response to environmental stimulation, and specifically in the right posterior hippocampus, in relation to the representation of large-scale space.

Another well-disseminated example is the Nun Study, a longitudinal study of cognitive and brain changes associated with aging. Collecting data on older nuns at a convent in Minnesota, David Snowdon and his colleagues (e.g., Tyas, Snowdon, Desrosiers, Riley, & Markesbery, 2007) have documented early-life behaviors that affect later cognitive abilities. Nuns were separated into groups defined by performance on cognitive measures, activities of daily living, and self-report. Those nuns who progressed to mild cognitive impairment were those with the lowest levels of education, which suggested that education can protect against cognitive decline (see Stern, Chapter 5, this volume). In addition, those nuns with higher education lived longer than those with lower education. In further studies, it was shown that poor linguistic ability, as measured by autobiographies, was correlated with lower cognitive abilities and greater rates of Alzheimer's disease.

THERAPEUTIC APPLICATIONS

Psychotherapy

Recent research has given preliminary indications that brain changes occur during psychotherapy. Positron emission tomography (PET) scans, fMRI, and neuropsychological tests have been used to evaluate brain changes occurring during psychotherapy. The effects of psychotherapy on some parts of the brain are similar to the effects of medication, while in other parts they are not. Major depressive disorder (MDD), schizophrenia, and obsessive–compulsive disorder (OCD) are among the conditions affecting populations that have shown changes in the direction of normalization in brain glucose metabolic rates (Kumari & Cooke, 2006; Laatsch, Thulborn, Krisky, Shobat, & Sweeney, 2004).

The use of PET for comparison of groups receiving different treatments for depression (sometimes with a healthy control group) has been applied in a few studies, with differing results. For example, Goldapple et al. (2004) performed functional imaging studies to compare the effects of cognitive-behavioral therapy with those of paroxetine on individuals with major depression. Cognitive-behavioral treatment response was associated with increased activation in hippocampus and dorsal cingulate cortex, and decreased activation in dorsal, ventral, and medial frontal cortex. This pattern was distinct from that seen for paroxetine treatment, where prefrontal increases and hippocampal and subgenual cingulate decreases were seen. In contrast, Brody et al. (2001) compared interpersonal therapy to paroxetine treatment for individuals with MDD and found that both treatments led to a normalization of PET patterns in prefrontal cortex and temporal lobe, with no differences between the two treatments.

PET has been used in cases of OCD to try not only to determine patterns of change associated with treatments, but also to predict before treatment those subjects who are more likely to respond to one treatment versus another. For example, Brody et al. (1998) measured baseline and posttreatment activation in individuals with OCD, some of whom were treated with behavioral therapy and some with fluoxetine. They reported that those with low left orbitofrontal activation at baseline were most responsive to behavioral therapy, and that the left orbitofrontal activation normalized as a response to treatment. The opposite was true for fluoxetine treatment. This finding may be an important lesson for studies of cognitive remediation: Different treatments may be optimum for different brain dysfunctions within the same etiology.

Cognitive Rehabilitation

As has been discussed at various points in this book, cognitive rehabilitation can focus on restoring connections (direct restoration/restorative therapy) or on reorganizing and redistributing the cognitive workload (compensation strategy training; Raskin, 2010).

Two studies have looked at the effects of attention training on attention networks in the brain. Kim et al. (2009) used fMRI to examine performance on a visual–spatial attention task. Ten individuals with traumatic brain injury (TBI) who successfully completed attentional training underwent pretreatment and follow-up fMRI. Prior to treatment, fMRI analysis showed more activation in the frontal and temporoparietal lobes, as well as less activation in the anterior cingulate gyrus, SMA, and temporooccipital regions, compared to the healthy subjects. Following cognitive training, the patients' improved performance on attention tasks was accompanied by changes in attentional network activation: The activity of the frontal lobe decreased, whereas activation of the anterior cingulate cortices and precuneus increased.

Laatsch et al. (2004) used fMRI to demonstrate brain plasticity in response to cognitive rehabilitation in five individuals following mild TBI. The authors used neuropsychological tests and two fMRI activation tasks: visually guided saccades and a reading comprehension task. Cognitive rehabilitation was used to systematically address the identified deficits in visual scanning and language processing. As hypothesized, changes in the pattern and extent of activation within expected neuroanatomical areas occurred after cognitive rehabilitation. This study demonstrates how fMRI can illustrate the neurobiological mechanisms of recovery in individual subjects. The variability in subject responses to cognitive rehabilitation supports the notion of tailoring rehabilitation strategies to each subject in order to optimize recovery following brain injury.

In a series of case studies, Laatsch and Krisky (2006) used fMRI to examine activation patterns during presentation of a reading comprehension task in three adults with TBI. These subjects received cognitive rehabilitation therapy for visual processing and acquired reading deficits. fMRI and neuropsychological testing occurred before and after rehabilitation. The authors reported improvements in neuropsychological testing following cognitive rehabilitation, although the subjects with TBI were still demonstrated diffuse and variable activation patterns, compared to those of healthy adults.

Wayne Gordon and his colleagues have presented some preliminary data on computerized cognitive rehabilitation tasks specifically designed to take into account theories of plasticity. These preliminary data suggest that these techniques may be useful for improving attention and memory functions in both outpatients (Lebowitz et al., 2009) and inpatients (Dams-O'Connor, Lebowitz, Cantor, & Spina, 2009).

Similar results have been reported in research using cognitive remediation to treat cognitive deficits in people with schizophrenia (Wykes et al., 2002). This study used three groups: individuals with schizophrenia who received cognitive remediation, individuals with schizophrenia who received no cognitive intervention, and a group of healthy adults. All three groups were given a two-back task during fMRI and a battery of neuropsychological measures. The control group showed decreased activation, but the two patient groups showed an increase in activation over time. The patient group that received cognitive remediation had significantly increased brain activation in regions associated with working memory, particularly the frontocortical areas. More studies that directly measure brain changes following cognitive remediation are needed and might explain findings such as continued improvement after treatment is concluded (Raskin & Sohlberg, 2009).

CONCLUSIONS

Several morphometric studies have demonstrated both short- and long-term use-dependent changes in the cortex. Voxel-based morphometry has been used to study experience-related plasticity in response to explicit tasks such as spatial navigation (Maguire et al., 2003) or intensive studying (Draganski, Gaser, Kempermann, Kuhn, Winkler, et al., 2006), and implicit tasks including language skill learning (Mechelli, Crinion, Noppeney, O'Doherty, Ashburner, et al., 2004), musical training (Gaser & Schlaug, 2003), and juggling (Draganski, Gaser, Busch, Schuierer, Bogdahn, et al., 2004).

The question of the difference between pharmacotherapy and psychotherapy for psychological disorders and TBI still needs further investigation. Although brain imaging technology is more clearly revealing the effects that the two treatments do have on brain activity, and there is some evidence that certain symptoms respond better to one or the other, uncertainties still remain about the commonalities and differences between the pathways that drugs and psychotherapies take in effecting change. Future studies will need to look more closely at specific changes associated with specific treatment techniques.

Moreover, imaging studies must begin looking specifically at changes within individual groups to determine which treatments are most effective under which conditions. For example, an analysis of individual differences in people with TBI in a study of attention training indicated differences in treatment efficacy based on vigilance levels (Sohlberg et al., 2000). Finally, although changes noted in research using imaging techniques are suggestive of plastic changes in the brain, they must also be linked to improved function in daily life—the ultimate goal of all research in this area (Sohlberg & Raskin, 1996). The chapters that follow will take what is known about experience-based plasticity and apply it directly to rehabilitation of motor and cognitive functions.

REFERENCES

Brody, A., Saxena, S., Stoessel, P., Gillies, L., Fairbanks, L., Alborzian, S., et al. (2001). Regional brain metabolic changes in patients with major depression treated with either paroxetine or interpersonal therapy. *Archives of General Psychiatry, 58*, 631–640.

Brody, A. L., Saxena, S., Schwartz, J. M., Stoessel, P. W., Maidment, K., Phelps, M. E., et al. (1998). FDG-PET predictors of response to behavioral therapy and pharmacotherapy in obsessive compulsive disorder. *Psychiatry Research, 84*, 1–6.

Burton, H., Snyder, A., Conturo, T., Akbudak, E., Olinger, J., & Raichle, M. (2002). Adaptive changes in early and late blind: An fMRI study of Braille reading. *Journal of Neurophysiology, 87*, 589–607.

Burton, H., Snyder, A., Diamond, J., & Raichle, M. (2003). Adaptive changes in early and late blind: An fMRI study of verb generation to heard nouns. *Journal of Neurophysiology, 88*, 3359–3371.

Celesia, G. (2005). Visual plasticity and its clinical applications. *Journal of Physiological Anthropology and Applied Human Science*, 24, 23–27.

Dams-O'Connor, K., Lebowitz, M., Cantor, J., & Spina, L. (2009, October). *Feasibility of a computerized cognitive skill-building program in an inpatient TBI rehabilitation setting.* Poster presented at the American Congress of Rehabilitation Medicine, Denver, CO.

Dragonski, B., Gaser, C., Busch, V., Schuierer, O., Bogdahn, U., & May, A. (2004). Neuroplasticity: Changes in gray matter induced by training. *Nature, 427*, 311–312.

Dragonski, B., Gaser, C., Kempermann, G., Kuhn, H., Winkler, J., Büchel, C., & May, A. (2006). Temporal and spatial dynamics of brain structure changes during extensive learning. *Journal of Neuroscience, 26*, 6314–6317.

Gaser, C., & Schlaug, G. (2003). Gray matter differences between musicians and non-musicians. *Annual New York Academy, 999*, 514–517.

Gilbert, C. D., Li, W., & Piech, V. (2009). Perceptual learning and adult cortical plasticity. *Journal of Physiology, 29*(41), 12711–12716.

Gilbert, P., & Thach, W. T. (1977). Purkinje cell activity during motor learning. *Brain Research, 128*(2), 309–328.

Goldapple, K., Segal, Z., Garson, C., Lau, M., Beiling, P., Kennedy, S., et al. (2004). Modulation of cortical–limbic pathways in major depression: Treatment specific effects of cognitive behavior therapy. *Archives of General Psychiatry, 61*, 34–41.

Horng, S., & Sur, M. (2006). Visual activity and cortical rewiring: Activity dependent plasticity of cortical networks. *Progress in Brain Research, 157*, 3–11.

Ilg, R., Dauner, R., Wohlschlager, A., Liebau, Y., Zihl, J., & Muhlau, M. (2010, March 17). What and where in mirror reading. *Psychophysiology* [Epub ahead of print].

Ilg, R., Wohlschlager, A. M., Gaser, C., Liebau, Y., Dauner, R., et al. (2008). Gray matter increase induced by practice correlates with task-specific activation: A combined functional and morphometric magnetic resonance imaging study. *Journal of Neuroscience, 28*, 4210–4215.

Kaas, J. (1991). Plasticity in sensory and motor maps in adult mammals. *Annual Review of Neuroscience, 14*, 137–167.

Karni, A., & Bertini, G. (1997). Learning Perceptual Skills: Behavioral Probes into adult cortical plasticity. *Current Opinion in Neurobiology, 7*, 530–535.

Kelly, A., & Garavan, H. (2005). Human functional neuroimaging of brain changes associated with practice. *Cerebral Cortex, 15*, 1089–1102.

Kim, Y. H., Yoo, W. K., Ko, M. H., Park, C. H., Kim, S. T., & Na, D. L. (2009). Plasticity of the attentional network after brain injury and cognitive rehabilitation. *Neurorehabilitation and Neural Repair, 23*(5), 468–477.

Kleim, J. A., Lussnig, E., Schwartz, E. R., & Comery, T. A. (1996). Synaptogenesis and FOS expression in the motor cortex of the adult rat after motor skill learning. *Journal of Neuroscience, 16*(14), 4529–4535.

Kleim, J. A., Swain, R. A., Armstrong, K. A., Napper, R., Jones, T. A., & Greenough, W. T. (1998). Selective synaptic plasticity within the cerebellar cortex following complex motor skill learning. *Neurobiology of Learning and Memory, 69*(3), 274–289.

Krings, T., Topper, R., Foltys, H., Erberich, S., Sparing, R., & Willmes, K. (2000). Cortical activation patterns during complex motor tasks in piano players and control subjects: A functional magnetic resonance imaging study. *Neuroscience Letters, 278*, 189–193.

Kumari, V., & Cooke, M. (2006). Use of magnetic resonance imaging in tracking the course and treatment of schizophrenia. *Expert Review of Neurotherapy, 6*, 1005–1016.

Laatsch, L. K., & Krisky, C. M. (2006). Changes in fMRI activation following rehabilitation of reading and visual processing deficits in subjects with traumatic brain injury. *Brain Injury, 20*(13–14), 1367–1375.

Laatsch, L. K., Thulborn, K. R., Krisky, C. M., Shobat, D. M., & Sweeney, J. A. (2004). Investigating the neurobiological basis of cognitive rehabilitation therapy with fMRI. *Brain Injury, 18*(10), 957–974.

Landau, S., Garavan, H., Schumacher, E., & D'Esposito, M. (2007). Regional specificity and practice: Dynamic changes in object and spatial working memory. *Brain Research, 1180*, 78–89.

Lebowitz, M., Cantor, J., Dams-O'Connor, K., Ashman, T., Tsaousides, T., Gordon, W., et al. (2009, October). *Examining the usability of a computerized cognitive training program in people with traumatic brain injury (TBI): A pilot study.* Poster presented at the American Congress of Rehabilitation Medicine, Denver, CO.

Maguire, E., Spiers, H., Good, C., Hartley, T., Frackowiak, R., & Burgess, N. (2003). Navigation expertise and the human hippocampus: A structural brain imaging analysis. *Hippocampus, 13*, 250–259.

Maguire, E., Woolett, K., & Spiers, H. (2006). London taxi drivers and bus drivers: A structural MRI and neuropsychological analysis. *Hippocampus, 16*, 1091–1101.

Mechelli, A., Crinion, J., Noppeney, J., O'Doherty, J., Ashburner, J., Frackowiak,

R., & Price, C. (2004). Neurolinguistics: Structural plasticity in the bilingual brain. *Nature, 431*, 757.

Meister, I., Krings, T., Foltys, H., Boroojerdi, B., Muller, M., Topper, R., et al. (2005). Effects of long-term practice and task complexity in musicians and nonmusicians performing simple and complex motor tasks: Implications for cortical motor reorganization. *Human Brain Mapping, 25*, 345–352.

Ojakangas, C. L., & Ebner, T. J. (1992). Purkinje cell complex and simple spike changes during a voluntary arm movement learning task in the monkey [Abstract]. *Journal of Neurophysiology, 68*(6), 2222–2236.

Olesen, P., Westerberg, H., & Klingberg, T. (2004). Increased prefrontal and parietal activity after training of working memory. *Nature Neuroscience, 7*, 75–79.

Olsson, C.-J., Jonsson, B., Larsson, A., & Nyberg, L. (2005). Motor representation and practice affect brain systems underlying imagery: An fMRI study of internal imagery in novices and active high jumpers. *The Open Neuroimaging Journal, 2*, 5–13.

Palmese, C., & Raskin, S. (2000). The rehabilitation of attention in individuals with mild traumatic brain injury, using the APT-II programme. *Brain Injury, 14*, 535–548.

Pleger, B., Foerster, A., Widdig, W., Henschel, M., Nicolas, V., Jansen, A., et al. (2003). Functional magnetic resonance imaging mirrors recovery of visual perception after repetitive tachistoscopic stimulation in patients with partial cortical blindness. *Neuroscience Letters, 335*, 192–196.

Raskin, S. (2010). Current approaches to cognitive rehabilitation. In C. Armstrong & L. Morrow (Eds.), *Handbook of medical neuropsychology: Applications of cognitive neuroscience* (pp. 505–518). New York: Springer.

Raskin, S., & Sohlberg, M. (2009). Prospective memory intervention: A review and evaluation of a pilot restorative intervention. *Brain Impairment, 10*(1), 76–86.

Seidman, L., Schutt, R., Caplan, B., Tolomiczenko, G., Turner, W., & Goldfinger, S. (2003). The effects of housing interventions on neuropsychological functioning among homeless persons with mental illness. *Psychiatric Services, 54*, 905–908.

Sohlberg, M. M., McLaughlin, K. A., Pavese, A., Heidrich, A., & Posner, M. I. (2000). Evaluation of attention process training and brain injury education in persons with acquired brain injury. *Journal of Clinical and Experimental Neuropsychology, 22*(5), 656–676.

Sohlberg, M., & Raskin, S. (1996). Principles of generalization applied to attention and memory interventions. *Journal of Head Trauma Rehabilitation, 11*(2), 65–78.

Tyas, S., Snowdon, D., Desrosiers, M., Riley, K., & Markesbery, W. (2007). Healthy ageing in the Nun Study: Definition and neuropathologic correlates. *Age and Ageing, 36*(6), 650–655.

Van Raalten, T., Ramsey, N., Duyn, J., & Jasma, J. (2008). Practice induces function-specific changes in brain activity. *Plos One, 3*(10), e3270.

Wykes, T., Brammer, M., Mellers, J., Bray, P., Reeder, C., Williams, C., et al. (2002). Effects on the brain of a psychological treatment: Cognitive remediation therapy: functional magnetic resonance imaging in schizophrenia. *British Journal of Psychiatry, 181*, 144–152.

PART II

Interventions for Motor and Cognitive Deficits

CHAPTER 7

Activity-Based Interventions for Neurorehabilitation

DAVID M. MORRIS
C. SCOTT BICKEL

Injuries and diseases of the central nervous system (CNS) have a profound effect on the U.S. society. For example, stroke is the third leading cause of death after heart disease and cancer, and is a leading cause of serious longterm disability. Impaired movement is a major consequence of stroke; as a result, a large number of the more than 700,000 people in America sustaining a stroke each year have functional limitations and compromised quality of life (American Heart Association, 2000). The American Heart Association (2000) estimates the annual direct and indirect costs associated with stroke at $43.3 billion. Similarly, approximately 11,000 Americans sustain a spinal cord injury (SCI) each year (National Spinal Cord Injury Statistical Center, 2010). Nearly 200,000 people in the United States live with disability related to SCI (Berkowitz, O'Leary, Kruse, & Harvey, 1998). An analysis of medical and social costs by Berkowitz et al. (1998) suggested that SCI costs the nation an estimated $9.7 billion each year. Advances in medical care have dramatically reduced mortality in the acute phase of these injuries. However, with more individuals surviving, the number of persons living with disability due to neurological injury is rising. Consequently, the need for physical rehabilitation strategies to reduce the negative effects on neurological function is obvious.

A definition of *conventional physical rehabilitation* is difficult to formulate, because the treatments employed in clinical settings worldwide are diverse and are not connected by a single conceptual formulation. Conventional rehabilitation for neurological injuries has been described as consisting of two predominant philosophies: compensation or functional neurorecovery (Held, 2000; Shumway-Cook & Woollacott, 2001; Fisher & Sullivan, 2001). In a compensation-oriented approach, rehabilitation therapists do not (or minimally) incorporate patients' more affected extremities into therapeutic activities; instead, they encourage reliance on the less affected extremities for functional skills. One example of such an approach is teaching a patient recovering from stroke to tie his or her shoes with the less affected arm exclusively. Another is applying braces to the lower extremities of a person recovering from SCI and teaching him or her to walk using forearm crutches and a swing-through gait pattern. As a result of this approach, new movement patterns are used to compensate for those lost to injury. Functional neurorecovery incorporates activities with the more affected extremities to reestablish neural pathways affected by injury, and/or to recruit areas within the CNS that have been spared by the insult to assume control of extremity function. As a result, rehabilitation efforts attempt to help a patient "relearn" or "recover" movement patterns lost to the injury.

The preferred approach to rehabilitation has been a major topic of debate among neurorehabilitation professionals for many years. Although functional neurorecovery would seem to be the more desirable approach, clinicians are likely to embrace compensation in an effort to promote functional independence more quickly. Furthermore, the number of rehabilitation interventions shown to promote functional neurorecovery has been quite limited (Duncan, 1997, 2005). However, over the last decade, neurorehabilitation has been revolutionized by the introduction of activity-based therapies (ABTs). ABTs are standardized regimens based on functional neurorecovery principles from the fields of experimental psychology, exercise physiology, and neuroscience. Multiple factors have led to this paradigm shift in neurorehabilitation:

1. *A better understanding of the neuroplastic capabilities of the injured human CNS leading to a more optimistic view of the potential for functional neurorecovery.* Advances in neuroscience have led to a better understanding of how the CNS (somatosensory, auditory, and motor cortex, as well as the spinal cord) are reorganized after injury (see Kolb, Cioe, & Williams, Chapter 2; Jones, Chapter 3; and Nudo & Burg, Chapter 4,

this volume). This line of research suggests that the CNS can be modified long after the initial neurological insult, and in areas extending beyond the primary lesion. Convincing evidence indicates that a person's activity or lack of activity is largely responsible for these positive or negative neural plastic changes, respectively (see Chapter 4 in particular). These discoveries have led to suggestions that might reduce the negative impact on the CNS (e.g., a reduction in representation within the motor cortex) and promote positive CNS reorganization (e.g., recruitment of spared portions of the CNS to participate in the function of a more affected extremity). These neural-plasticity-enhancing strategies serve as fundamental principles for ABTs. Such principles are discussed extensively within this text.

2. *Improved technology for imaging the CNS has permitted examination of structural changes resulting from therapeutic interventions.* Various of imaging methods that have emerged in recent years allow detailed examination of the CNS in noninvasive ways. Some frequently used imaging procedures include functional magnetic resonance imaging (fMRI), neuroelectric source localization, positron emission tomography, and serial near-infrared spectroscopy. Within the last decade, the emergence of such technology has led to a dramatic increase in the use of CNS imaging as an outcome measure for rehabilitation research. Evidence of structural changes to the CNS, correlated with changes in behavioral measures, supports the effectiveness of the intervention approaches under study—including ABTs.

3. *An increase in randomized clinical trials (RCTs) to explore the effectiveness of emerging neurorehabilitation approaches.* To determine the number of RCT studies conducted up to 2003 for rehabilitation interventions, Johnston, Miklos, Michaliszyn, Ponce, and Gonzalez (2003) conducted an extensive MEDLINE search for rehabilitation-oriented medical subject headings for both relevant diagnostic groups and common types of interventions (excluding drug and mental health therapies). The results suggested that although progress has been made, many important areas of rehabilitation have received little attention by way of RCTs. Since the Johnston et al. article was published, two RCTs of neurorehabilitation have suggested that scientific efforts may be resulting in methodological advances in this area of research (Dobkin, 2006; Wolf, 2006).

The purpose of this chapter is to explore the recent paradigm shift in neurorehabilitation by using two ABTs as examples: Constraint-induced (CI) movement therapy for upper extremity (UE) use after stroke and locomotor training (LT) for functional gait restoration after SCI. For each approach, we explore its theoretical basis, the specific components of the intervention protocol, and evidence supporting its use as an effective rehabilitation intervention.

CI THERAPY FOR UE RECOVERY AFTER STROKE

Theoretical Basis

Learned Nonuse

CI therapy is derived from basic behavioral neuroscience research with primates by Edward Taub. When a single forelimb is deafferented in a monkey, the animal does not make use of it in the free-living situation (Knapp, Taub, & Berman, 1958, 1963). Several converging lines of evidence suggested that nonuse of a single deafferented limb is a learning phenomenon involving a conditioned suppression of movement (Knapp et al., 1958, 1963; Taub, 1976, 1977; Taub, Bacon, & Berman, 1965; Taub & Berman, 1963). The trauma induced by the deafferenting surgical procedure leads to a depression in all neural functions (sensory and motor)—a phenomenon commonly termed *neural shock*. In monkeys, the initial period of depressed functioning lasts from 2 to 6 months following forelimb deafferentation (Knapp et al., 1958, 1963; Taub, 1976, 1977; Taub et al., 1965; Taub & Berman, 1963). Thus, immediately after the operation, the monkeys cannot use a deafferented limb. An animal with one deafferented limb tries to use that extremity in the immediate postoperative situation, but it cannot. The monkey functions effectively in the laboratory environment on three limbs and is therefore positively reinforced for this pattern of behavior, which as a result is strengthened. Moreover, continued attempts to use the deafferented limb often lead to painful and otherwise aversive consequences, such as incoordination, falling, and loss of food objects. In general, a monkey fails in any attempts to use the deafferented limb functionally. These aversive consequences constitute punishment. Many learning experiments have demonstrated that punishment results in the suppression of behavior (Azrin & Holz, 1966; Catania, 1998; Estes, 1944). This response tendency persists, and consequently the monkeys never learn that several months after operation (after neural shock subsides), the limb has become potentially useful. In addition, after stroke (Liepert et al., 1998; Liepert, Bauder, Miltner, Taub, & Weiller, 2000) and presumably after extremity deafferentation, there is marked contraction in the size of the cortical representation of the limb; this is probably correlative with the report of patients with stroke that movement of the affected extremity is effortful.

These three processes (contraction of the cortical representation zone, effortful movement, and failure in attempts to use the deafferented limb) interact to produce a vicious downward spiral that results in a *learned nonuse* of the affected extremity, which is normally permanent (illustrated in Figure 7.1). However, a monkey with learned nonuse can be induced to use the deafferented extremity by restricting movement of the intact limb (Knapp et al., 1958, 1963; Taub, 1976, 1977, 1980; Taub et al., 1965;

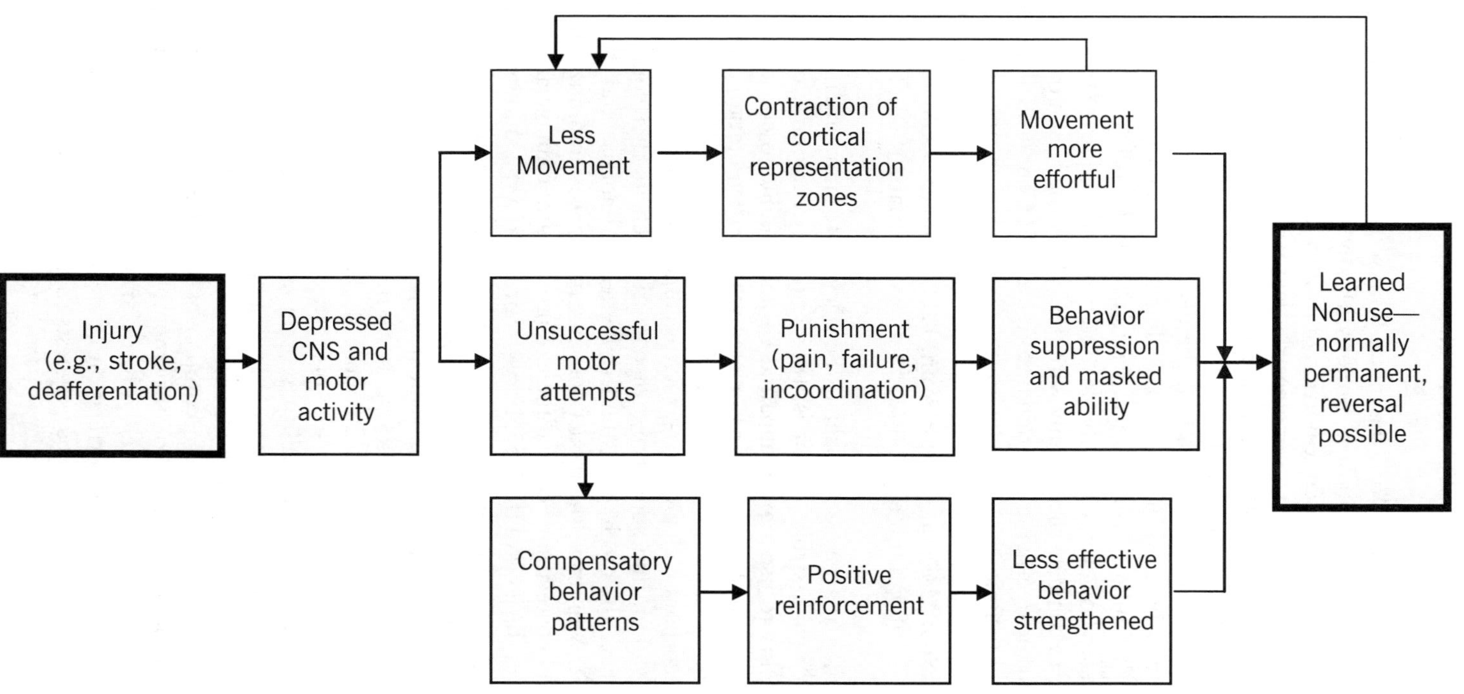

FIGURE 7.1. Schematic model for development of learned non-use.

Taub & Berman, 1963). With the intact limb restrained, the animal uses either the deafferented limb or it cannot with any degree of efficiency feed itself, walk, or carry out a large portion of its normal activities of daily life. This change in motivation overcomes the learned nonuse of the deafferented limb, and consequently the animal uses it. However, if the movement-restricting device is removed too soon after the early display of purposive movement, the newly learned use of the deafferented limb acquires little strength and is therefore quickly overwhelmed by the well-learned tendency not to use the limb. If the movement restriction device is left on for several days or longer, however, use of the deafferented limb acquires strength and is then able to compete successfully with the well-learned habit of nonuse of that limb in the free-living situation (see Figure 7.2). Conditioned responses and shaping techniques constitute another behavioral means of overcoming the inability to use a single deafferented limb in primates (Knapp et al., 1958, 1963; Morgan, 1974; Panyan, 1980; Skinner, 1938, 1968; Taub, 1976, 1977, 1980; Taub et al., 1965; Taub & Berman, 1963; Taub et al., 1994).

A similar analysis is thought to be relevant to human patients after brain injury (e.g., stroke). That is, the period of temporary, organically based inability to use a more impaired UE may be due to cortical mechanisms, rather than to processes associated with deafferentation at the level of the spinal cord. With respect to humans, the model of learned nonuse does not incorporate all modifiers, such as comorbidities, psychosocial support, motivation, and some types of cognitive deficits that could potentially influence the mechanisms underlying learned nonuse and those that overcome it. Moreover, the model does not in any way minimize the possible general correlation between the extent of neural damage after stroke (especially at the level of the medullary pyramids) and the amount of motor function that can be recovered through therapy on the more affected side. However, the fact that some survivors of stroke with a given extent and locus of lesions recover more movement than others having similar lesions do suggest that additional factors may be involved. One of these factors may be the operation of a learned-nonuse mechanism. Support for this view comes from the fact that a measure of learned nonuse developed by Mark and Taub (i.e., a measure of ability to use a more affected extremity when asked to do so in the laboratory minus a measure of actual amount of use of that extremity in the life situation) correlates ($r = .47$, $p < .0001$) with CI therapy outcome, whereas the component measures of this index correlate either not at all (initial laboratory motor function) or significantly but weakly (initial life situation use) with treatment outcome (Mark & Taub, 2004). The strength of the correlation of treatment outcome with a presumed measure of learned nonuse suggests that this measure is an index of a real entity.

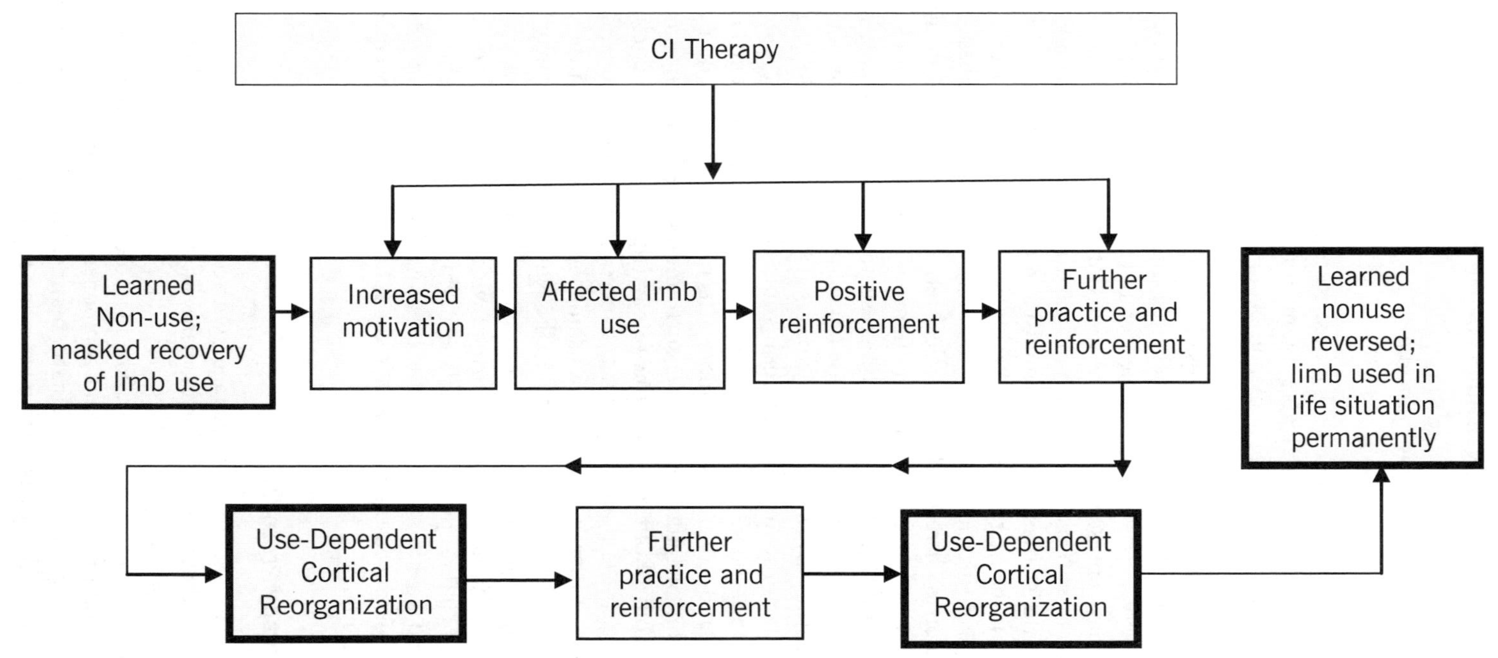

FIGURE 7.2. Schematic model of mechanism for overcoming learned non-use.

Use-Dependent Cortical Reorganization: A Linked but Independent Mechanism

Following the seminal work of Jenkins, Recanzone, Merzenich and colleagues on use dependent cortical reorganization in monkeys, imaging studies showed that the same phenomenon occurs in humans (Elbert, Pantev, Wienbruch, Rockstroh, & Taub, 1995; Elbert et al., 1997; Jenkins, Merzenich, Ochs, Allard, & Guic-Robles, 1990; Recanzone, Jenkins, & Merzenich, 1992; Recanzone, Merzenich, Jenkins, Grajski, & Dinise, 1992; Sterr et al., 1998). For example, Elbert et al. (1995) found that the cortical somatosensory representation of the digits of the left hand was larger in string players, who use their left hand for the dexterity-demanding task of fingering the strings, than in nonmusician controls. Moreover, the representation of the fingers of blind Braille readers, who use several fingers simultaneously to read, was enlarged (Sterr et al., 1998). These results, in conjunction with research on cortical reorganization in adult monkeys (Pons et al., 1991) and persons with phantom limb pain (Flor et al., 1995), suggest that the size of the cortical representation of a body part in adult humans depends on the amount of use of that part. The intracortical microstimulation study by Nudo and coworkers (reviewed by Nudo & Bury in Chapter 4) demonstrated that in adult squirrel monkeys that were surgically given an ischemic infarct in the cortical area controlling the movements of a hand, training of the more affected limb resulted in a cortical reorganization. Specifically, the area surrounding the infarct not normally involved in control of the hand came to participate in that function. These findings suggest the possibility that the increase in more affected arm use produced by CI therapy results in a use-dependent increase in the cortical representation of the more impaired UE, which provides the neural basis for a permanent increase in the use of that extremity.

This hypothesis has been confirmed with persons with chronic stroke who received CI therapy (discussed later in this chapter). These studies have demonstrated an alteration in brain organization or function associated with an ABT-induced improvement in the rehabilitation of movement after neurological injury in humans.

The CI Therapy Protocol

CI therapy is a "therapeutic package" with a number of different components. Some of these intervention elements have been employed in neurorehabilitation before, but usually as individual procedures and at a reduced intensity compared to CI therapy. The main novel feature of CI therapy is the combination of these treatment components and their application in a prescribed, integrated, and systematic manner to induce a patient to use a more impaired UE for many hours a day for a period of 2–3 consecutive weeks (depending on the severity of the initial deficit). CI therapy has evolved and undergone modification over the two decades of its existence. However, most of the original treatment elements remain part of the standard procedure. The present CI therapy protocol, as applied in research and clinical settings, consists of three main elements with multiple components and subcomponents under each (1) repetitive, task-oriented training of the more impaired UE for several hours a day for 10–15 consecutive weekdays (depending on the severity of the initial deficit); (2) applying a "transfer package" of adherence-enhancing behavioral methods designed to generalize gains made in the research laboratory or clinical setting to the patient's real world environment; and (3) constraining the patient to use the more impaired UE during waking hours over the course of treatment, sometimes by restraining the less impaired UE. The elements, components and subcomponents are described in the following sections (Mark & Taub, 2004; Morris, Crago, Pidikiti, & Taub, 1997; Morris, Taub, & Mark, 2006; Taub et al., 1993).

Repetitive, Task-Oriented Training

On each of the weekdays during the intervention period, participants receive training, under the supervision of an interventionist, for several hours each day. The original protocol called for 6 hours/day of this training. More recent studies indicate that a shorter daily training period (i.e., 3 hours/day) is as effective for higher-functioning patients (Dettmers et al., 2005; Sterr et al., 2002). Two distinct training procedures are employed as patients practice functional task activities: shaping and task practice. Shaping is a training method based on the principles of behavioral training (Morgan, 1974; Panyan, 1980; Skinner, 1938, 1968; Taub et al., 1994). In Shaping, a motor or behavioral objective is approached in small steps by "successive approximations"; for example, the task can be made more difficult in accordance with a participant's motor capabilities, or the requirement for speed of performance can be progressively increased. Each functional activity is practiced for a set of ten 30-second trials, and explicit feedback is provided regarding the participant's performance during each trial (Taub et al., 1994). Task practice is less structured; for example, the tasks are not set up to be carried out as individual trials of discrete movements. It involves functionally based activities performed continuously for a period of 15 to 20 minutes (e.g., wrapping a present, writing). In successive periods of task practice, the spatial requirements of the activities, or other parameters such as duration, can be changed to require more demanding control of limb segments for task completion. Global feedback about overall performance is provided at the end of the 15- to 20-minute period. A large bank of tasks has been created for each type of training procedure. The following are considered in selecting training tasks for each participant: (1) specific joint movements that exhibit the most pronounced deficits; (2) the joint movements that trainers believe have the greatest potential for improvement; and (3) the participant's preference among tasks that have similar potential for producing specific improvement. Frequent rest intervals are provided throughout the training day and intensity of training (i.e., the number of trials/hour [shaping] or the amount of time spent on each training procedure [task practice]) is recorded.

Adherence-Enhancing Behavioral Methods to Increase Transfer to the Life Situation

One of the overriding goals of CI therapy is to transfer gains made in the research or clinical setting into the participant's real-world environment (i.e., home, work/school and community settings). To achieve this goal, a set of techniques referred to as a "transfer package" is used to make the patient accountable for adherence to the requirements of the therapy. The participant must be actively engaged in and adherent to the intervention without constant supervision from an interventionist, especially in real-life situations where the interventionist is not present. Attention to adherence is directed toward using the more impaired UE during functional tasks, toward obtaining appropriate assistance from caregivers if present (i.e., assistance to prevent the participant from struggling excessively, but allowing him or her to try as many tasks independently as is feasible), and toward wearing the restraint as much as possible (when it is safe to do so).

Several individual intervention principles have been successfully applied to enhance adherence to exercise and physical-function oriented behaviors. Three are most relevant to and are utilized in the adherence-enhancing behavioral components of CI therapy: monitoring, problem solving, and behavioral contracting. All three have been used successfully, alone or in combination, to enhance adherence to physical activity in a variety of participant groups with a variety of physical conditions. These are essential aspects of the CI therapy approach. The full range of adherence-enhancing behavioral subcomponents currently employed in the CI therapy protocol includes daily administration of the Motor Activity Log (MAL), a structured interview that elicits information on how well and how often the more affected UE is used in 30 important activities of daily life (Taub et al., 1993; Uswatte, Taub, Morris, Barman, & Crago, 2006a; Uswatte, Taub, Morris, Vignolo, & McCulloch, 2005); a patient-kept home diary; problem solving; behavioral contracts with the patient and the caregiver independently; a daily schedule; home skill assignments and home practice. Each adherence-enhancing subcomponent is described in Table 7.1. Recent data from the UAB laboratory suggests that the transfer package may be the most important protocol component for inducing both behavioral and neural plastic changes following stroke (Gauthier et al., 2008). We believe

TABLE 7.1. Additional Techniques Employed in CI Therapy to Facilitate Transfer of Treatment Gains from the Therapeutic Setting to the Home

Technique	Description
Behavioral contract	At the outset of treatment, the therapist negotiates a contract with the participant and caregiver (if one is available) in which they agree that the participant will wear the restraint device whenever it is safe for up to 90% of waking hours and use his or her more impaired arm as much as possible outside the laboratory. Specific activities during which the participant can practice using the more impaired arm are discussed together and written down.
Daily home diary	During treatment, the participant catalogs how much he or she has worn the restraint device and used the more affected arm for the activities specified in the behavioral contract. The diary is kept for the part of the day spent outside the laboratory, and is reviewed each morning with the therapist.
Home practice exercises	During treatment, participants are asked to spend 15–30 minutes at home each day performing specific UE tasks repetitively with their more affected arm. The tasks typically employ materials that are commonly available (e.g., stacking Styrofoam cups). Toward the end of treatment, an individualized posttreatment home practice program is drawn up consisting of similar tasks. Participants are encouraged to do these tasks for 30 minutes daily after the 2-week treatment period.
Problem solving	During treatment and four weekly phone contacts following treatment, the therapist helps the participant to think through any barriers to using the more impaired arm. For example, if a patient is concerned about spilling liquid from a glass, the therapist may suggest only filling the glass halfway.
Home skill assignment	The Home skill assignment process encourages the participant to try activities of daily living (ADLs) that he or she may not otherwise have tried with the more impaired UE. The interventionist first reviews a list of common ADL carried out in the home. The tasks are categorized according to the rooms in which they are usually performed (e.g., kitchen, bathroom, bedroom, office). Starting on the second day of the intervention period, participants are asked to select 10 ADLs from the list; they agree to try these after they leave the laboratory/clinic and before they return for the next day of treatment. Tasks not on the list may be selected if desired by a participant. These tasks are to be carried out while wearing the mitt when doing so is possible and safe. The 10 items selected are recorded on an assignment sheet and given to each participant when he or she leaves the laboratory or clinic for the day. The goal is for approximately 30 minutes to be devoted to trying the specified ADLs at home each day. The Home skill assignment sheet is reviewed during the first part of the next treatment day and 10 additional ADL are selected for Home skill assignment for that evening. This process is repeated throughout the intervention.

(cont.)

TABLE 7.1. *(cont.)*

Technique	Description
Motor Activity Log (MAL) administration	The MAL is administered independently to the participant and an informant. MAL tasks include such activities as brushing teeth, buttoning a shirt or blouse, and eating with a fork or spoon. Information is gathered about more affected UE use prior to the participant's enrollment in the project, after the intervention, on each day of the intervention, weekly by phone for the 4 weeks after the end of treatment, and at several times during the 2-year follow-up period. Several studies concerning the clinimetric properties of the MAL have shown the measure to be reliable and valid. Moreover, the MAL does not produce a treatment effect when administered to persons receiving a placebo treatment at the same treatment schedule as those receiving CI therapy. Preliminary results from an ongoing experiment suggest that this self-monitoring instrument is a very important means of producing a transfer of improved performance from the laboratory/clinic to the life situation when used in conjunction with other aspects of the CI therapy package, particularly concentrated training.

that the use of adherence-enhancing strategies is the most often overlooked component of CI therapy therefore, interventionists wishing to employ CI therapy should further explore these strategies before using this ABT. The protocol article by Morris et al. (2006) may prove helpful for this purpose.

Constraining Use of the More Impaired UE

The most commonly applied treatment protocol in CI therapy is use of a restraint (either a sling or a protective safety mitt) on the less impaired UE to prevent participants from succumbing to the strong urge to use that UE during most or all functional activities, even when the interventionist is present. Over the last decade, the protective safety mitt (which eliminates the ability to use the fingers) has been preferred for restraint, as it prevents functional use of the less impaired UE for most purposes while still allowing protective extension of that UE in case of a loss of balance. When the mitt is employed, participants are taught to put it on and take it off independently, and decisions are made with the interventionist as to when its use is feasible and safe. The goal for mitt use is 90% of waking hours. This so called "forced use" is arguably the most visible element of the intervention to the rehabilitation community, and it is frequently and mistakenly described as synonymous with "CI therapy." However, Taub et al. (1998) has stated that "there is nothing talismanic about use of a sling, protective safety mitt or other constraining device on the less-affected UE," as long as the more-impaired UE is exclusively engaged in repeated practice. "Constraint," as used in the name of the therapy, is not intended to refer only to the application of a mitt or other physical restraint, but also to indicate a constraint of opportunity to use the less impaired UE for functional activities (Taub, Uswatte, & Pidikiti, 1999). As such, any strategy that encourages exclusive use of the more impaired UE is viewed as a constraining component of the treatment package. For example, shaping is meant to be considered as constituting a very important constraint on behavior: either a participant succeeds at a task, or he or she is not rewarded (e.g., by praise or knowledge of improvement).

Preliminary findings by Sterr and Freivogel (2004) indicated that a significant treatment effect was obtained when CI therapy was used without the physical restraint component. Swedish investigators also found that a CI therapy protocols could be employed without the use of a restraining mitt and that this protocol could yield similar results to CI therapy protocols employing the mitt (Brogårdh, Vestling, & Sjölund, 2009). In a 1-year follow-up investigation, both groups retained improvements equally (Brogårdh & Lexell, 2010) Likewise, the University of Alabama at Birmingham (UAB) laboratory has obtained similar findings with a small group of participants (n = 9) when a CI therapy protocol without physical restraint was employed (Morris et al., 1997; Taub et al., 1993; Uswatte et al., 2006a). However, our research suggested that this group experienced a larger decrement at the 2-year follow-up testing than groups where physical restraint was employed. If other treatment package elements developed in the UAB laboratory are not used, our clinical experience suggests that routine reminders not to use the less affected UE alone, without physical restraint, are not as effective as using the mitt. Consequently, we recommend using the mitt to minimize the need for the interventionist or caregiver to remind the participant to limit use of the less impaired UE during the intervention period.

Evidence Supporting the Effectiveness of CI Therapy

In the 1980s, Wolf and coworkers employed one of the two suggested techniques, restriction of the less affected extremity, to induce a significant remediation of motor impairment in patients with chronic stroke (Ostendorf & Wolf, 1981; Wolf, Lecraw, Barton, & Jann, 1989). While effective for this purpose, the effect size was quite small (d' = 0.2). Taub et al. (1993) expanded the protocol using two components—restriction and a variant of the shaping component (i.e., task practice of use of the more-impaired UE) in a small-sample pilot experiment. The participants were individuals with chronic stroke experienced from 1 to 18 years earlier. Patients with this degree of chronicity had traditionally been presumed to have reached a plateau in their motor recovery and were not expected to exhibit any further improvement for the rest of their lives even if therapy (of whatever type) was administered. Nine persons who met the initial study's inclusion criteria, including ability to extend at least 20° at the more impaired wrist and 10° at each of the more impaired finger joints, were assigned by a random process to either an experimental group ($n = 4$) or an attention-placebo control comparison group ($n = 5$). Patients in the experimental group signed a behavioral contract in which they agreed to wear a sling on their less-impaired UE for a target of 90% of waking hours for 14 days. On 10 of those days, the treatment subjects received 6 hours of supervised task practice using their more affected arm on a variety of tasks, interspersed with 1 hour of rest. Additional behavioral techniques were used that emphasized transfer of therapeutic gains in the laboratory to the life situation. Treatment efficacy was evaluated via two laboratory motor function tests and the MAL (Uswatte, Taub, Morris, Light, & Thompson, 2006b; Uswatte et al., 2005, 2006a). The MAL tracks arm use in a number of activities of daily living through a structured interview administered independently to patients and caregivers (Uswatte & Taub, 2002). The treatment group demonstrated a significant increase in motor ability, as measured by both laboratory motor tests (the Wolf Motor Function Test [WMFT; Morris, Uswatte, Crago, Cook, & Taub, 2001; Taub et al., 1993; Wolf et al., 2001, 2005] and the Arm Motor Ability Test [Kopp et al., 1997; McCulloch et al., 1988; Taub, Crago, & Uswatte, 1998]) over the treatment period, whereas the control patients showed no change or a decline in arm motor ability. The improvement on the WMFT was approximately eight times as great as in the work of Wolf et al. (1989). This presumably reflects the effect of expanding the protocol by adding practiced, repetitive movements to motor restriction of the unaffected limb. Indeed, subjects given intensive training only and no restraint exhibit 80% of the full treatment effect post-treatment (Morris, Crago, DeLuca, Pidikitti, & Taub, 1997; Taub, Crago, & Uswatte, 1998). On the MAL, the treatment group showed a very large increase in real-world arm use over the 2-week period and demonstrated a further small (but nonsignificant) increase in use when tested 2 years after treatment. Thus the improvement was long-term. The control patients exhibited no change or a decline in arm use over the same period.

These results have since been confirmed in an experiment from the UAB laboratory using less-affected UE restraint and training (by shaping) of the more-impaired UE instead of task practice, with a larger sample (20 subjects) and a credible placebo control group of equal size (Taub et al., 2006). As in other experiments, the treatment group demonstrated a significant increase in motor ability, as measured by a laboratory motor function test and a very large increase in real-world arm use over the intervention period. The control subjects did not show a significant improvement at the end of treatment. These studies from our laboratory have been replicated in published studies from four other laboratories (Dettmers et al., 2005; Kunkel et al., 1999; Miltner et al., 1999; Sterr et al., 2002).

To date, over 400 patients with chronic stroke have been treated in the UAB laboratory and its associated clinic. The mean effect size for increase of use of the more affected extremity in the life situation over all studies that have been conducted here has been 3.3. By convention, a large effect size is considered to be 0.8; thus the effect size for real-world use of the more affected arm is extremely large. The magnitude of the treatment effect is not correlated with the amount of time since stroke onset. The mean chronicity of deficits from stroke across all studies is 4.4 years; the patient whose time elapsed from stroke was longest (50 years) had a better-than-laboratory-average outcome. Treatment gain is also not correlated with age. Our oldest patient to date was 92 years at time of treatment, and his results were approximately as good as the laboratory average. We have had equivalent success with numerous patients in their 80s. This suggests that the plasticity of the nervous system remains throughout the lifespan and extends well into old age.

The largest controlled study of CI therapy to date was conducted by Wolf et al. (2005). The Extremity Constraint-Induced Therapy Evaluation (EXCITE) Trial was a prospective, single-blind, randomized, multisite clinical trial conducted at seven U.S. academic institutions. The EXCITE Trial enrolled 222 individuals who were in the subacute phase (3–9 months) of recovery from stroke and who had mild to moderate hemiparesis of the more-affected UE. In the study, 106 participants received CI therapy and 116 received usual and customary (and no CI therapy) only. From baseline to 12 months, the CI therapy group showed greater improvements than the control group in the WMFT performance time and functional ability scale as well as on the MAL Amount and Quality of Movement scales. The CI therapy group also experienced a significantly greater decrease in the self-perceived hand function difficulty portion of the Stroke Impact Scale at the 12-month follow-up. The investigators concluded that among participants who had had a stroke within the previous 3–9 months, CI therapy produced statistically significant and clinically relevant improvements in UE motor function that persisted for at least 2 years (Wolf et al., 2008, 2010).

The use of CI therapy has begun to spread. Numerous published studies using either the original technique used in the UAB laboratory or (in many cases) a variant of it. A 2009 Cochrane review included 19 studies including 619 participants (Sitori, Corbetta, Moja, & Gatti, 2009). These authors concluded that the approach was associated with a moderate reduction in disability but cited variable findings regarding retention of benefits. The originators of CI therapy state that the magnitude of the treatment effect has varied—in large part, it would seem, because of alterations in the protocol and outcome measures employed (Uswatte & Taub, 2005).

To date, at least 20 studies have explored neural plastic changes in humans, with hemiparesis due to stroke, who received the UE CI therapy protocol or a variant thereof. As such, CI therapy has been the most investigated neurorehabilitation approach with regard to its neurophysiological influence on the brain. Mark, Taub, and Morris (2006) published a review of these publications and noted that, without exception, these studies demonstrated positive neurophysiological changes that appeared to be related to participation in UE CI therapy. Various brain imaging techniques have been employed in these studies, including transcranial magnetic stimulation (TMS) (Liepert et al., 1998, 2000; Liepert, Haevernick, Weiller, & Barzel, 2006; Liepert, Hamzei, & Weiller, 2004; Liepert, Uhde, Graf, Leidner, & Weiller, 2001; Ro et al., 2006), neuroelectric source localization with electroencephalography (Kopp et al., 1999), single-photon emission computed tomography (Könönen et al., 2005), and fMRI (Dong, Dobkin, Cen, Wu, & Winstein, 2006; Gauthier et al., 2008; Greenberg et al., 2004; Johansen-Berg et al., 2002; Levy, Nichols, Schmalbrock, Keller, & Chakeres, 2001; Kim, Park, Ko, Jang, & Lee, 2004; Schaechter et al., 2002). In addition, four studies compared TMS with other physiological assessments (Hamzei, Leipert, Dettmers, Weiller, & Rijntjes, 2006; Park, Butler, Cavalheiro, Alberts, & Wolf, 2004; Wittenberg et al., 2003). All these studies either compared participants' pretreatment to posttreatment function or compared similar measures in intervention versus placebo control groups. Positive neurophysiological changes observed in these studies as resulting from participation in CI therapy can be summarized as including (1) an expansion of cortical representational zones for the more affected UE; (2) altered anatomical distribution of cortical activation with movements of the more affected hand; (3) altered cortical inhibition or excitation; and/or (4) altered regional cerebral blood flow in response to TMS over the motor cortex. In several of these studies, the positive changes in brain activity corresponded to real-world behavioral changes as assessed by the MAL. Interestingly, this relationship has not been as strong several months following the intervention. Specifically, the brain activation changes have appeared to normalize over this time period, while the MAL scores remain unchanged. Mark et al. (2006) suggest that the effect may be due to increased efficiency of the brain mechanisms involved in use of the more affected arm over time.

These studies represent ground-breaking work for exploring a direct link between a specific intervention protocol and neural plastic changes. However, the findings across the studies are inconsistent. This could be due to widespread inconsistency in the experimental methods used (e.g., participant criteria, brain imaging techniques employed, durations of follow-up testing). In addition, the sample sizes were generally small. Furthermore, none of the studies have directly compared the effects of CI therapy on brain reorganization to those of other recognized motor therapies. As such, this line of research could be greatly improved by using more uniform therapeutic and investigational techniques with larger participant groups and with standardized follow-up intervals. Despite some limitations, these studies have provided substantial evidence that for at least some patient populations with brain injury, UE CI therapy generally results in improved motor performance that is accompanied by changes in brain activity.

LOCOMOTOR TRAINING

Theoretical Basis

Locomotor training (LT), a physiologically based approach to gait rehabilitation, incorporates intrinsic mechanisms of the spinal cord that respond to specific afferent input in order to produce stepping motions (Barbeau, 2003; Barbeau & Blunt, 1991; Barbeau & Visintin, 2003; Behrman, Bowden, & Nair, 2006; Behrman & Harkema, 2000; Behrman et al., 2005; Beres-Jones & Harkema, 2004; Dietz, Colombo, & Jensen, 1994; Dietz, Colombo, Jensen, & Baumgartner, 1995; Dobkin, Harkema, Requejo, & Edgerton, 1995; Field-Fote, Lindley, & Sherman, 2005; Harkema et al., 1997; Stewart, Barbeau, & Gauthier, 1991; Visitin & Barbeau, 1989, 1994; Wernig, Muller, Nanassy, & Cagol, 1995). The approach developed from basic animal research demonstrating that cats with complete spinal cord transections were capable of responding to intensive walking training (Barbeau & Rossignol, 1987; de Leon, Hodgson, Roy, & Edgerton, 1998; Lovely, Gregor, Roy, & Edgerton, 1986). Despite the absence of supraspinal output, the cats were capable of generating stepping responses when provided with truncal support, manually assisted loading, and sensory signals initiated by a moving treadmill. This observation led to the belief that the spinal cord has an intrinsic capacity to integrate afferent input, interpret it, and respond with an appropriate motor output. This ability is believed to be possible through a network of spinal interneurons termed *central pattern generators* (CPGs) (Forssberg, 1979; Grillner, 1979, 1985; Pearson & Rossignol, 1991). The CPGs within an intact nervous system work in conjunction with afferent input and descending supraspinal ouput to control rhythmic movements (e.g., walking, swimming). Research with "spinalized" cats suggested that even in the absence of the descending supraspinal contributions, the cats were capable of learning a movement task when the CPGs were stimulated. However, training in this manner was task-specific. Cats trained either to stand or to step with their hindlimbs on a treadmill learned their respective task, but could not generalize that skill to other activities (Hodgson, Roy, de Leon, Dobkin, & Edgerton, 1994). This line of research suggested that the injured spinal cord is still capable of activity-dependent plasticity, and it serves as one prong of the scientific evidence supporting LT.

The second line of evidence driving LT comes from research exploring the specific afferent input to the neurological control of walking (Dietz & Duysens, 2000; Van de Crommert et al., 1998). These studies suggest that specific sensory cues are critical to the control of reciprocal stepping. For example, several lines of research indicate that proprioceptive input coming from a stretch to the hip flexor muscles is important for initiating the swing phase of gait (Sherrington, 1910). Therefore, sufficient hip extension in the terminal stance phase of the gait cycle is critical for effective reciprocal stepping. Also, extensor loads relayed by the Golgi tendon organs (Ib) in the ankle extensor muscles are believed to be important for stimulating appropriate muscle activation patterns needed during the stance-to-swing phase of gait (Dietz & Duysens, 2000; Van de Crommert, Mulder, Duysens, 1998). As such, the level of loading through the legs during gait is critical to reciprocal stepping. Therefore, guidelines for LT maximize loading the legs instead of the arms (i.e., as with using a walker) during gait training. Behrman and Harkema (2000, pp. 691–692), list the following the sensory cues as critical to inducing stepping:

> 1) generating stepping speeds approximating normal walking speeds (0.75–1.25 m/s); 2) providing the maximum sustainable load on the stance limb; 3) maintaining an upright and extended trunk and head; 4) approximating normal hip, knee, and ankle kinematics for walking; 5) synchronizing timing of extension of the hip in stance and unloading of the contralateral limb; 6) avoiding weight bearing on the arms and facilitating reciprocal arm swing; 7) facilitating symmetrical interlimb coordination; and 8) minimizing sensory stimulation that would conflict with sensory information associated with locomotion (e.g., stimulation of extensor afferents during swing and flexor afferents during stance).

Although it is critical for propulsion, reciprocal stepping alone is insufficient for controlled walking. Two additional mechanisms—balance (upright and dynamic equilibrium) and adaptability (the ability of the individual to respond to the demands of the environment and to meet personal behavioral goals)—are needed for functional walking behavior (Barbeau, 2003; Behrman et al., 2006; Forssberg, 1982). Research surrounding the control of balance and adaptability serves as the basis for LT intervention principles addressing the two additional mechanisms cited. Based on these findings, Behrman et al. (2005) have proposed a clinical decision-making algorithm that can be applied to LT for persons with incomplete SCI.

LT Protocols

LT protocols have been developed for persons with either complete or incomplete injuries of the spinal cord. For the purposes of this chapter, only LT protocols for persons with incomplete SCI are described. Specific guidelines for LT have been provided for two major categories of interventions: (1) body weight support treadmill training (BWSTT) and (2) progression to over-ground gait and balance skills. Subcomponents within each of these categories include specific guidelines for environmental adaptations (e.g., amount of weight bearing experienced by the participant, treadmill speed, equipment used, obstacles introduced), manual assistance provided (amount and location of facilitating input from trainers), and verbal cueing provided. In addition, over-ground training can be further subdivided into clinic and community gait and balance training components.

Body Weight Support Treadmill Training

A typical BWSTT protocol was the one used by Dobkin et al. (2003) during a multisite RCT of LT for persons with incomplete SCI. In this study, step training included a concentrated treatment session (approximately 1 hour in length) 3–5 days each week for a 12-week period. BWSTT was accomplished by using a parachute-type harness attached at the shoulders to an overhead lift. The apparatus was positioned over a treadmill and permitted adjustment of the amount of weight bearing experienced by the participant during step training. Each session began with a brief period of warm-up and stretching activities. The actual stepping bouts on the treadmill were tailored to each participant's endurance and gait capabilities. However, trainers worked toward a goal of 20 minutes of continuous stepping for each participant if this could be tolerated. During the stepping sessions, heart rate and blood pressure were monitored for safety. However, the primary purpose of the stepping was improving motor control as opposed to producing a specific aerobic conditioning effect, and activity intensity was not intended to produce more than minimal shortness of breath. A range of 20–50% of weight bearing was used during the initial treatment session, based on the participant's tolerance. The weight bearing was gradually increased in accordance to achieve maximum knee extension during stance without a buckling effect. Likewise, treadmill speed began with at least 1.6 mph but aimed to reach belt speeds of at least 2.0–2.5 mph. Participants received carefully prescribed verbal and physical assistance from the trainers during the training session. This input was directed at achieving optimal practice with trunk, hip, knee, and ankle control during the session. One trainer was placed next to each paretic leg to facilitate optimal movement by placing one hand above the popliteal fossa and the other above the heel. Another trainer stood behind the participant with hands placed on the participant's hips to facilitate optimal trunk extension, pelvic rotation, weight shift, and hip extension. Optimal hip extension was further enhanced passively by movement of the treadmill belt. Ankle–foot orthoses were not employed during the training. Instead, the ankle was supported manually by interventionists or by using a figure-of-eight wrap. The treadmill utilized did not have side railings because these might promote UE weight bearing during step training. Instead, participants were encouraged to use a reciprocal arm swing during step training, and this could be facilitated through use of poles held parallel to the floor by a trainer if needed. Pole assistance from the interventionist could be eventually replaced by an overhead suspension for the pole.

Over-Ground Training: Clinic

Over-ground training is begun when participants can support at least 80% of their weight and can generate appropriate stepping with at least one leg (Behrman & Harkema, 2000; Behrman et al., 2005). One of three methods can be used if a participant requires balance assistance to walk at "normal" speeds:

- *Method 1*: One trainer stands in front of and supports the participant by holding his or her hands. The trainer then walks backward and facilitates reciprocal arm swing while simultaneously providing the minimal amount of UE support required. Another trainer walks behind the participant to assist with pelvic rotation and hip extension as needed.
- *Method 2*: Two trainers (one in front and one behind the participant) provide assistance by means of a 4-foot pole on each side of the participant's body. The poles are held by the trainers at the level of the participant's greater trochanter. The participant holds onto the poles while the trainers move the poles forward and back in unison stepping of the legs. Since the trainers control the motion of the poles, UE weight bearing by the participant is minimized.
- *Method 3*: The participant uses an assistive device. Use of assistive devices may deviate from conventional methods to keep in line with LT training principles. For example, if a rolling walker is selected for training, the walker height is adjusted so that the walker handle achieves a level forearm with 90° of elbow flexion to minimize UE weight bearing and trunk flexion. This method may be selected if a participant is uncomfortable with the first two methods, if the availability of trainers is limited, or if the participant's locomotor skills require it. Since it does not allow reciprocal arm swing during gait, it is the least desirable method for over-ground training.

Regardless of the method selected, trainers gradually reduce their input as the participant demonstrates an improved gait pattern. Decision making algorithms guide the interventionist through the process of reducing assistance and increasing skill demands during over ground training. Interventionists interested in using this ABT are encouraged to refer to the article by Behrman et al. (2005) for more details about these decision-making algorithms.

Over-Ground Training: Community

As a patient's skill increases, a community locomotor decision-making algorithm guides over ground training in more challenging environments (Behrman et al., 2005). At this point of the training, balance and adaptability become particularly important. The participant's personal behavioral goals are also emphasized. For example, if outdoor activities are particularly important for a participant, the training may incorporate a variety of terrains (e.g., asphalt, grass, gravel) for skill practice.

Evidence Supporting the Effectiveness of LT

Hughes Barbeau and colleagues first described LT utilizing a body weight support system in conjunction with a treadmill in the late 1980s (Barbeau, Wainberg, & Finch, 1987). Their participants were supported in a harness over a treadmill, with a portion of their body weight supported through an overhead apparatus. The treadmill speed ranged from 0.26 to 1.5 meters per second, and the entire walking session lasted 1 hour. Seven subjects with SCI participated; they walked at full weight bearing when possible, or with 20% or 40% body weight supported by the system. The results of this preliminary study showed that self-selected maximum comfortable walking speed increased as a function of increasing body weight support (Barbeau et al., 1987). This study essentially established that the training was safe for humans with SCI and that progress could be made with ambulation.

Wernig and Müller (1992) conducted another study that utilized BWSTT in patients with SCI. Eight subjects with SCI, five of whom were classified as having complete motor SCI, were trained on the treadmill with a self-selected comfortable speed. The body weight support was initially set at 40% and gradually reduced to 0% throughout the course of the intervention. Training was conducted for 30–60 minutes daily, 5 days per week, for a period of 1.5 to 7 months. The subjects had variable locomotive capabilities prior to training, and all improved their gait speed on the treadmill with a concomitant decrease in body weight support (Wernig & Müller, 1992).

There were several other notable findings from the Wernig and Müller (1992) study. Four of the subjects they trained learned to ambulate over ground, despite the absence of voluntary limb movements in the resting position. This finding provides some evidence for the plasticity of the human spinal cord, perhaps illustrating the ability to learn tasks with minimal efferent signals from higher centers. The investigators believed that the primary manner in which locomotion was initiated was through assisted loading into passive hip extension, followed by a weight shift to unload the limb. In the same study, electromyographic (EMG) recordings were taken at rest, during attempted voluntary activity, and during gait. The EMG recordings demonstrated that during gait there were alternating muscle activity patterns within the flexors and extensors. These EMG data have since been replicated and studied in more depth by other investigators, further illustrating that the human spinal cord, when given the appropriate sensory inputs, can modulate motor output in a manner that can facilitate locomotion (Harkema et al., 1997; Maegele, Müller, Wernig, Edgerton, & Harkema, 2002).

Wernig et al. (1995) reported on 89 subjects with incomplete SCI who participated in LT over a period of several years. As of 1995, this was the largest report on patients who had participated in this type of training. The study reported on a group of subjects in the acute phase of recovery (injured for less than 20 weeks) and a group of subjects in the chronic phase of recovery (injured from 6 months to 18 years). The training was similar to that already reported. Body weight support was initially set at 40% and gradually reduced to 0% over a period of weeks of training. The treadmill speed was selected by each subject, and training was conducted for 30 minutes per day, 5 days per week. Over ground walking was initiated as soon as possible in all patients.

The acute group in the Wernig et al. (1995) study consisted of 45 subjects who received the LT and were compared against a group of 40 acute patients who had received conventional rehabilitation. The LT and conventional therapy groups were matched with regard to time since injury and had relatively similar levels of voluntary motor control. Prior to training, the acute LT group had 36 of 45 patients who were wheelchair-bound, however; by the end of the training, 92% (33) of them could independently ambulate at least 200 meters. In contrast, the acute conventional therapy group had approximately 50% of members walking in a similar manner. The authors noted that in this study there were no differences in the voluntary motor activity grades between groups, but there were differences in ambulatory ability, suggesting that the treadmill training was providing a stimulus capable of improving functional outcomes.

The chronic group in Wernig et al. (1995) study consisted of 44 subjects receiving LT. The investigators reported that nearly all of the subjects achieved some improvement in locomotor ability after training. Those subjects that could already ambulate independently could either walk faster or perform more complex walking patterns (e.g., maneuvering up or down stairs). Many subjects (75%) who were wheelchair-bound prior to training achieved the ability to walk either independently or with assistance after training. Additional reports from this study showed that the ability to ambulate was also maintained for 6 months after participants left the training program.

The studies cited above indicate that LT with the assistance of a body weight support system and treadmill could positively influence the ability to ambulate. However, one of the problems with the early studies was the lack of consistent training parameters and control groups. Behrman and Harkema (2000) expanded the evidence for LT with a series of case studies. These studies were important as the treadmill training and over ground training techniques were described in more detail. Behrman and Harkema described the treadmill training in terms of a team of therapists assisting each patient's legs and hips in an attempt to provide sensory feedback that would enhance neural output. These training principles were also utilized by Dobkin et al. (2003, 2006) in their RCT investigating the effects of BWSTT versus conventional training for walking during inpatient rehabilitation.

Behrman and Harkema (2000) described the effects of LT on four subjects, three with chronically incomplete SCI and one with chronically complete SCI. Each of the subjects with incomplete lesions improved their ability to step on the treadmill, one achieved the ability to ambulate over ground, and the other two improved. The individual with the complete lesion did not show signs of improvement in locomotor ability other than being able to tolerate upright standing for increased periods of time.

The largest controlled study to date was conducted by Dobkin et al. (2006). They conducted a single blind, multicenter RCT that compared BWSTT to over ground training for walking in patients with acute incomplete SCI. The study enrolled 146 subjects from six centers within 8 weeks of injury. Each group received 12 weeks of training, either BWSTT or a defined over-ground control of similar intensity. Results showed that post-training walking speeds were not different between groups, and that each group had an unusually high percentage of independent ambulators (92% of ASIA C or D).

A computer-controlled, driven gait orthosis called the Lokomat was developed to provide assisted LT in a less labor intensive manner. The Lokomat can be used along with BWSTT to provide critical sensory cues typically provided manually with other LT protocols. Wirz et al. (2005) reported improved overground walking in 20 participants with motor incomplete SCI who trained with the Lokomat and BWSTT 3–5 times each week for an 8-week period. A 2010 review of the effectiveness of robot-assisted gait training in persons with SCI examined two RCTs and 4 pre-experimental trials using the Lokomat or similar device (Swinnen, Duerinck, Baeyens, Meeusen, & Kerckhofs, 2010). While noting some improvements in body functions and activities, the authors believe the evidence to be inconclusive at this time and recommend further investigation.

Field-Fote and Roach (2010) examined the effects of using four variations of LT protocols with participants with minimal function due to chronic SCI. The participants were trained 5 days each week for a 12-week period with LT protocols that consisted of either a treadmill and manual assistance, treadmill and electrical stimulation, over-ground activities and electrical stimulation, or treadmill with robotic assistance. Outcome measures included over-ground walking speed and distance. All four training conditions significantly improved over-ground walking speed and distance. There were no significant differences in the improvements achieved between the treatment conditions for speed but the over-ground training with electrical stimulation was more effective for increasing walking distance. The findings of the Field-Fote and Roach (2010) study are consistent with conclusions drawn from a 2010 review article of 18 articles describing LT research, where the authors cited higher levels of independent walking with LT protocols including over-ground training compared with BWSTT only for persons with motor incomplete SCI (Wessels, Lucas, Eriks, & deGroot, 2010).

These studies represent classic examples of translational research. Basic scientists have known for years that animals with transected spinal cords could be taught to step on a treadmill or stand over ground. The animal research was then transferred to humans, first by Barbeau's group and then by many others, to see whether results done in quadrupeds could be translated to humans ambulating with two limbs. In doing so, the plasticity of the human spinal cord has been illustrated, and there is sufficient evidence to suggest that further studies on this intervention are warranted in this patient population.

CONCLUSION

In recent years, there has been a paradigm shift in neurorehabilitation to include activity-based intervention approaches that promote functional recovery instead of compensation. Driving forces behind this shift include an increased optimism regarding the potential of the CNS to experience positive changes after rehabilitation; multidisciplinary collaborations that facilitate a better understanding of the complex mechanisms underlying neural recovery; improved CNS imaging procedures; and an increasing number of multisite RCTs in rehabilitation research. Whereas this chapter has emphasized two interventions that directly influence motor impairment, similar ABTs have been proposed for cognitive and language restoration. Although those approaches show great promise for advancing outcomes in neurorehabilitation, several authorities advise the rehabilitation community to adopt these ABTs in the clinical setting with caution (Dobkin, 2006; Dromerick, Lum, & Hilder, 2006). They suggest that more development and research are needed before changes in clinical practice are warranted. Nevertheless, the ABT philosophy has made significant contributions to the advancement of neurorehabilitation, and it provides great promise for resolving many neurological deficits for which previously there was little hope of recovery.

REFERENCES

American Heart Association. (2000). *Heart and stroke statistical update.* Retrieved from *www.americanheart.org/statistics/stroke.htm.*

Azrin, N. H., & Holz, W. C. (1966). Punishment. In W. K. Honig (Ed.), *Operant behavior: Areas of research and application* (pp. 380–447). New York: Appleton-Century-Crofts.

Barbeau, H. (2003). Locomotor training in neurorehabilitation: Emerging rehabilitation concepts. *Neurorehabilitation and Neural Repair, 17,* 3–11.

Barbeau, H., & Blunt, R. (1991). A novel interactive locomotor approach using body weight support to retrain gait in spastic paretic subjects. In A. Wernig (Ed.), *Plasticity of motor neuronal connections* (pp. 461–474). New York: Elsevier.

Barbeau, H., & Rossignol, S. (1987). Recovery of locomotion after chronic spinalization in the adult cat. *Brain Research, 412,* 84–95.

Barbeau, H., Wainberg, M., & Finch, L. (1987). Description and application of a system for locomotor rehabilitation. *Medical and Biological Engineering and Computing, 25,* 341–344.

Barbeau, H., & Visintin, M. (2003). Optimal outcomes obtained with body-weight support combined with treadmill training in stroke subjects. *Archives of Physical Medicine and Rehabilitation, 84,* 1458–1465.

Behrman, A. L., Bowden, M. G., & Nair, P. M. (2006). Neuroplasticity after spinal cord injury and training: An emerging paradigm shift in rehabilitation and walking recovery. *Physical Therapy, 86,* 1406–1425.

Behrman, A. L., & Harkema, S. J. (2000). Locomotor training after human spinal cord injury: A series of case studies. *Physical Therapy, 80,* 688–700.

Behrman, A. L., Lawless-Dixon, A. R., Davis, S. B., Dowden, M. G., Nair, P., & Phadke, C. (2005). Locomotor training progression and outcomes after incomplete spinal cord injury. *Physical Therapy, 85,* 1356–1371.

Beres-Jones, J. A., & Harkema, S. J. (2004). The human spinal cord interprets velocity-dependent afferent input during stepping. *Brain, 127,* 2232–2246.

Berkowitz, M., O'Leary, P., Kruse D., & Harvey, C. (1998). *Spinal cord injury: An analysis of medical and social costs.* New York: Demos.

Brogårdh, C., & Lexell, J. (2010). A 1-year follow-up after shortened constraint-induced movement therapy with and without mitt poststroke. *Archives of Physical Medicine and Rehabilitation, 91,* 460–464.

Brogårdh, C., Vestling, M., & Sjölund, B. H. (2009). Shortened constraint-induced movement therapy in subacute stroke-no effect of using a restraint: A randomized controlled study with independent observers. *Rehabilitation Medicine, 41,* 231–236.

Catania, A. C. (1998). *Learning* (4th ed.). Upper Saddle River, NJ: Prentice Hall.

de Leon, R. D., Hodgson, J. A., Roy, R. R., & Edgerton, V. R. (1998). Locomotor capacity attributable to step training versus spontaneous recovery after spinalization in adult cats. *Neurophysiology, 79,* 1329–1340.

Dettmers, C., Teske, U., Hamzei, F., Uswatte, G., Taub, E., & Weiller, C. (2005). Distributed form of Constraint-Induced Movement therapy improves functional outcome and quality of life after stroke. *Archives Physical Medicine and Rehabilitation, 86*, 204–209.

Dietz, V., Colombo, G., & Jensen, L. (1994). Locomotor activity in spinal man. *Lancet, 344*, 1260–1263.

Dietz, V., Colombo, G., Jensen, L., & Baumgartner, L. (1995). Locomotor capacity of spinal cord in paraplegic patients. *Annals of Neurology, 37*, 574–582.

Dietz, V., & Duysens, J. (2000). Significance of load receptor input during locomotion: A review. *Gait and Posture, 11*, 102–110.

Dobkin, B. H., Apple, D., Barbeau, H., Basso, M., Berhman, A., & DeForge, D. (2003). Methods for a randomized trial of weight-supported treadmill training versus conventional training for walking during inpatient rehabilitation after traumatic spinal cord injury. *Neurorehabilitation and Neural Repair, 17*, 153–167.

Dobkin, B. H., Apple, D., Barbeau, H., Basso, M., Behrman, A., DeForge, D., et al. (2006). Weight-supported treadmill vs. overground training for walking after acute incomplete SCI. *Neurology, 66*, 484–493.

Dobkin, B. H., Harkema, S. J., Requejo, P. S., & Edgerton, V. R. (1995). Modulation of locomotor-like EMG activity in subjects with complete and incomplete spinal cord injury. *Neurologic Rehabilitation, 9*, 183–190.

Dong, Y., Dobkin, B. H., Cen, S. Y., Wu, A. D., & Winstein, C. J. (2006). Motor cortex activation during treatment may predict therapeutic gains in paretic hand function after stroke. *Stroke, 37*, 1552–1555.

Dromerick, A. W., Lum, P. S., & Hilder, J. (2006). Activity based therapies. *NeuroRx, 3*, 428–438.

Duncan, P. W. (1997). Synthesis of intervention trials to improve motor recovery following stroke. *Topics in Stroke Rehabilitation, 3*, 1–20.

Duncan, P. W., Zorowitz, R., Bates, B., Choi, J. Y., Glasberg, J. J., & Graham, G. D. (2005). Management of adult stroke rehabilitation care. *Stroke, 36*, 100–143.

Elbert, T., Pantev, C., Wienbruch, C., Rockstroh, B., & Taub, E. (1995). Increased use of the left hand in string players associated with increased cortical representation of the fingers. *Science, 220*, 21–23.

Elbert, T., Sterr, A., Flor, H., Rockstroh, B., Knecht, S., Pantev, C., et al. (1997). Input-increase and input-decrease types of cortical reorganization after upper extremity amputation in humans. *Experimental Brain Research, 117*, 161–164.

Estes, W. K. (1944). An experimental study of punishment. *Psychological Monographs, 57(Serial No. 263).*

Field-Fote, E. C., Lindley, S. D., & Sherman, A. L. (2005). Locomotor training approaches for individuals with spinal cord injury: A preliminary report of walking-related outcomes. *Neurologic Physical Therapy, 29*, 127–137.

Field-Fote, E. C., & Roach, K. E. (2010). Influence of a locomotor training approach on walking speed and distance in people with chronic spinal cord injury: A randomized clinical trial. *Physical Therapy, 91*, 48–60.

Fisher, B. E., & Sullivan, K. J. (2001). Activity-dependent factors affecting post-stroke functional outcomes. *Topics Stroke Rehabilitation, 8*, 31–44.

Flor, H., Elbert, T., Knecht, S., Wienbruch, C., Pantev, C., Birbaumer, N., et al.

(1995). Phantom limb pain as a perceptual correlate of massive reorganization in upper limb amputees. *Nature, 375*, 482–484.

Forssberg, H. (1979). Stumbling corrective reaction: A phase-dependent compensatory reaction during locomotion. *Neurophysioliology, 42*, 936–953.

Gauthier, L. V., Taub, E., Perkins, C., Ortmann, M., Mark, V. W., & Uswatte, G. (2008). Remodeling the brain: Plastic structural changes produced by different motor therapies after stroke. *Stroke, 39*, 1520–1525.

Greenberg, J. P., Butler, A. J., Sawaki, L., Schmalbrock, P., Mao, H., Nichols, D. S., et al. (2004). The effect of constraint-induced therapy for stroke on functional MRI motor maps. *Society for Neuroscience Abstracts, 30*, 431–437.

Grillner, S. (1979). Interaction between central and peripheral mechanisms in the control of locomotion. *Progress in Brain Research, 50*, 227–235.

Grillner, S. (1985). Neurobiological bases of rhythmic motor acts in vertebrates. *Science, 228*, 143–149.

Hamzei, F., Liepert, J., Dettmers, C., Weiller, C., & Rijntjes, M. (2006). Two different reorganization patterns after rehabilitative therapy: An exploratory study with fMRI and TMS. *NeuroImage, 31*, 710–720.

Harkema, S. J., Hurley, S. L., Patel, U. K., Reguejo, P. S., Dobkin, B. H., & Edgerton, V. R. (1997). Human lumbosacral spinal cord interprets loading during stepping. *Neurophysiology, 77*, 797–811.

Held, J. (2000). Recovery of function after brain damage: Theoretical implications for therapeutic intervention. In J. Carr & R. Shepherd (Eds.), *Movement science: Foundations for physical therapy in rehabilitation.* Gaithersburg, MD: Aspen.

Hilder, J. M. (2005). What is next for locomotor-based studies? *Rehabilitation Research Development, 42*, 10–16.

Hodgson, J. A., Roy, R. R., de Leon, R., Dobkin, B., & Edgerton V. R. (1994). Can the mammalian lumbar spinal cord learn a motor task? *Medicine Science Sports and Exercise, 26*, 1491–1497.

Jenkins, W., Merzenich, M., Ochs, M., Allard, T., & Guic-Robles, E. (1990). Functional reorganization of primary somatosensory cortex in adult owl monkeys after behaviorally controlled tactile stimulation. *Journal of Neurophysiology, 63*, 82–104.

Johansen-Berg, H., Dawes, H., Guy, C., Smith, S. M., Wade, D. T., & Matthews, P. M. (2002). Correlation between motor improvements and altered fMRI activity after rehabilitative therapy. *Brain, 125*, 2731–3742.

Johnston, M. V., Miklos, C., Michaliszyn, D., Ponce, M., & Gonzalez, S. (2003). Clinical trials in rehabilitation: An overview of the scientific literature [Abstract]. *American Journal of Physical Medicine and Rehabilitation, 82*, 10.

Kim, Y. H., Park, J. W., Ko, M. H., Jang, S. H., & Lee, P. K. (2004). Plastic changes of motor network after constraint-induced movement therapy. *Yonsei Medical Journal, 45*, 241–246.

Knapp, H. D., Taub, E., & Berman, A. J. (1958). Effects of deafferentation on a conditioned avoidance response. *Science, 128*, 842–843.

Knapp, H. D., Taub, E., & Berman, A. J. (1963). Movement in monkeys with deafferented limbs. *Experimental Neurology, 7*, 305–315.

Könönen, M., Kuikka, J. T., Husso-Saastamoinen, M., Vanninen, E., Vanninen,

R., Soimakallio, S., et al. (2005). Increased perfusion in motor areas after constraint-induced movement therapy in chronic stroke: A single-photon emission computerized tomography study. *Cerebral Blood Flow and Metabolism, 25*, 1668–1674.

Kopp, B., Kunkel, A., Flor, H., Platz, T., Rose, U., Mauritz, K.-H., et al. (1997). The Arm Motor Ability Test (AMAT): Reliability, validity, and sensitivity to change of an instrument for assessing ADL disability. *Archives of Physical Medicine and Rehabilitation, 78*, 615–620.

Kopp, B., Kunkel, A., Muhlnickel, W., Villringer, K., Taub, E., & Flor, H. (1999). Plasticity in the motor system correlated with therapy-induced improvement of movement after stroke. *NeuroReport, 10*, 807–810.

Kunkel, A., Kopp, B., Muller, G., Villringer, K., Villringer, A., Taub, E., et al. (1999). Constraint-induced movement therapy: A powerful new technique to induce motor recovery in chronic stroke patients. *Archives of Physical Medicine and Rehabilitation, 80*, 624–628.

Levy, C. E., Nichols, D. S., Schmalbrock, P. M., Keller, P., & Chakeres, D. W. (2001). Functional MRI evidence of cortical reorganization in upper-limb stroke hemiplegia treated with constraint-induced movement therapy. *American Physical Medicine and Rehabilitation, 80*, 4–12.

Liepert, J., Bauder, H., Miltner, W., Taub, E., & Weiller, C. (2000). Treatment induced cortical reorganization after stroke in humans. *Stroke, 31*, 1210–1216.

Liepert, J., Haevernick, K., Weiller, C., & Barzel, A. (2006). The surround inhibition determines therapy-induced cortical reorganization. *NeuroImage, 32*, 1216–1220.

Liepert, J., Hamzei, F., & Weiller, C. (2004). Lesion-induced and training-induced brain reorganization. *Restorative Neurology and Neuroscience, 22*, 269–277.

Liepert, J., Miltner, W., Bauder, H., Sommer, M. Dettermers, C., Taub, E., et al. (1998). Motor cortex plasticity during constraint-induced movement therapy in stroke patients. *Neuroscience Letters, 250*, 5–8.

Liepert, J., Uhde, I., Graf, S., Leidner, O., & Weiller, C. (2001). Motor cortex plasticity during forced-use therapy in stroke patients: A preliminary study. *Neurology, 248*, 315–321.

Lovely, R. G., Gregor, R. J., Roy, R. R., & Edgerton, V. R. (1986). Effects of training on the recovery of full-weight-bearing stepping in the adult spinal cat. *Experimental Neurology, 92*, 421–435.

Maegele, M., Müller, S., Wernig, A., Edgerton, V. R., & Harkema, S. J. (2002). Recruitment of spinal motor pools during voluntary movements versus stepping after human spinal cord injury. *Neurotrauma, 19*, 1217–1229.

Mark, V. W., & Taub, E. (2004). Constraint-induced movement therapy for chronic stroke hemiparesis and other disability. *Restorative Neurology and Neuroscience, 22*, 317–336.

Mark, V. W., Taub, E., & Morris, D. M. (2006). Neural plasticity and constraint-induced movement therapy. *Europa Medicophysica, 42*, 269–284.

McCulloch, K., Cook, E., III, Fleming, W., Novack, T., Nepomeceno, C. S., &

Taub, E. (1988). A reliable test of upper extremity ADL function [abstract]. *Archives of Physical Medicine and Rehabilitation, 69*, 755.

Miltner, W., Bauder, H., Sommer, M., Dettmers, C., & Taub, E. (1999). Effects of Constraint-induced movement therapy on chronic stroke patients: A replication. *Stroke, 30*, 586–592.

Morgan, W. (1974). The shaping game: A teaching technique. *Behavior Therapy, 5*, 271–272.

Morris, D. M., Crago, J., DeLuca, S., Pidikiti, R., & Taub, E. (1997). Constraint-induced (CI) movement therapy for motor recovery after stroke. *NeuroRehabilitation, 9*, 29–43.

Morris, D. M., Taub, E., & Mark, V. W. (2006). Constraint-induced movement therapy: Characterizing the intervention protocol. *Europa Mediphysica, 42*, 257–268.

Morris, D. M., Uswatte, G., Crago, J. E., Cook, E. W., & Taub, E. (2001). The reliability of the Wolf Motor Function Test for assessing upper extremity function after stroke. *Archives of Physical Medicine and Rehabilitation, 82*, 750–755.

National Spinal Cord Injury Statistical Center. (2010). *Facts and figures at a glance.* Retrieved from *www.nscisc.uab.edu.*

Ostendorf, C. G., & Wolf, S. L. (1981). Effect of forced use of the upper extremity of a hemiplegic patient on changes in function. *Physical Therapy, 61*, 1022–1028.

Panyan, M. (1980). *How to use shaping.* Lawrence, KS: H & H Enterprises.

Park, S. W., Butler, A. J., Cavalheiro, V., Alberts, J. L., & Wolf, S. L. (2004). Changes in serial optical topography and TMS during task performance after constraint-induced movement therapy in stroke: A case study. *Neurorehabil Neural Repair, 18*, 95–105.

Pearson, L. G., & Rossignol, S. (1991). Fictive motor patterns in chronic spinal cats. *Journal of Neurophysiology, 66*, 1874–1887.

Pons, T. P., Garraghty, P. E., Ommaya, A. K., Kaas, J. H., Taub, E., & Mishkin, M. (1991). Massive cortical reorganization after sensory differentiation in adult macaques. *Science, 252*, 1857–1860.

Recanzone, G., Jenkins, W., & Merzenich, M. (1992). Progressive improvement in discriminative abilities in adult owl monkeys performing a tactile frequency descrimination task. *Journal of Neurophysiology, 67*, 1015–1030.

Recanzone, G., Merzenich, M., Jenkins, W., Grajski, A., & Dinise, H. (1992). Topographic reorganization of the hand representation in area 3b of owl monkeys trained in a frequency descrimination task. *Journal of Neurophysiology, 67*, 1031–1056.

Ro, T., Noser, E., Boake, C., Johnson, R., Gaber, M., Speroni, A., et al. (2006). Functional reorganization and recovery after constraint-induced movement therapy in subacute stroke: Case reports. *Neurocase, 12*, 50–60.

Schaechter, J. D., Kraft, E., Hilliard, T. S., Dijkhuizen, R. M., Benner, T., Finklestein, S. P., et al. (2002). Motor recovery and cortical reorganization after constraint-induced movement therapy in stroke patients: A preliminary study. *Neurorehabilitation Neural Repair, 16*, 326–338.

Sherrington, C. S. (1910). Flexion-reflex of the limb, crossed extension-reflex, and reflex stepping and standing. *Physiology, 40*, 28–121.

Shumway-Cook, A., & Woollacott, M. (2001). *Motor control: Theory and practical applications*. Philadelphia: Lippincott.

Skinner, B. F. (1938). *The behavior of organisms*. New York: Appleton-Century-Crofts.

Skinner, B. F. (1968). *The technology of teaching*. New York: Appleton-Century-Crofts.

Sterr, A., Elbert, T., Berthold, I., Kölbel, S., Rockstroh, B., & Taub, E. (2002). CI therapy in chronic hemiparesis: The more the better? *Archives of Physical Medicine and Rehabilitation, 83*, 1374–1377.

Sterr, A., & Freivogel, S. (2004). Intensive training in chronic upper limb hemiparesis does not increase spasticity or synergies. *Neurology, 63*, 2176–2177.

Sterr, A., Mueller, M., Elbert, T., Rockstroh, B., Pantev, C., & Taub, E. (1998). Changed perceptions in Braille readers. *Nature, 391*, 134–135.

Stewart, J. E., Barbeau, H., & Gauthier, S. (1991). Modulation of locomotor patterns and spasticity with clonidine in spinal cord injured patients. *Canadian Neurological Sciences, 18*, 321–332.

Swinnen, E., Duerinck, S., Baeyens, J. P., Meeusen, R., & Kerckhofs, E. (2010). Effectiveness of robot-assisted gait training in persons with spinal cord injury: A systematic review. *Rehabilitation Medicine, 42*, 520–526.

Taub, E. (1976). Motor behavior following deafferentation in the developing and motorically mature monkey. In R. Herman, S. Grillner, H. J. Ralson, P. S. G. Stein, & D. Stuart (Eds.), *Neural control of locomotion* (pp. 675–705). New York: Plenum Press.

Taub, E. (1977). Movement in nonhuman primates deprived of somatosensory feedback. *Exercise and Sports Science Reviews, 4*, 335–374.

Taub, E. (1980). Somatosensory deafferentation research with monkeys: implications for rehabilitation medicine. In L. Ince (Ed.), *Behavioral psychology in rehabilitation medicine* (pp. 371–401). Baltimore: Williams & Wilkins.

Taub, E., Bacon, R., & Berman, A. J. (1965). The acquisition of a trace-conditioned avoidance response after deafferentation of the responding limb. *Journal of Comparative and Physiological Psychology, 58*, 275–279.

Taub, E., & Berman, A. J. (1963). Avoidance conditioning in the absence of relevant proprioception and exteroceptive feedback. *Journal of Comparative and Physiological Psychology, 56*, 1012–1016.

Taub, E., Burgio, L., Miller, N. E., Cook, E., III, Groomes, T., DeLuca, S., et al. (1994). An operant approach to overcoming learned nonuse after CNS damage in monkeys and man: The role of shaping. *Journal of the Experimental Analysis of Behavior, 61*, 281–293.

Taub, E., Crago, J. E., & Uswatte, G. (1998). Constraint-induced movement therapy: A new approach to treatment in physical rehabilitation. *Rehabilitation Psychology, 43*, 152–170.

Taub, E., Miller, N. E., Novack, T., Cook, E., III, Fleming, W., Nepomeceno, C. S., et al. (1993). Technique to improve chronic motor deficit after stroke. *Archives of Physical Medicine and Rehabilitation, 74*, 347–354.

Taub, E., Uswatte, G., King, D. K., Morris, D. M., Crago, J. E., & Chatterjee, A. (2006). A placebo controlled trial of Constraint-Induced Movement therapy for upper extremity after stroke. *Stroke, 37*, 1045–1049.

Taub, E., Uswatte, G., & Pidikiti, R. (1999). Constraint-induced movement therapy: A new family of techniques with broad application to physical rehabilitation—A clinical review. *Rehabilitation Research and Development, 36*, 237–251.

Uswatte, G., & Taub, E. (2002). Constraint-induced movement therapy: New approaches to outcome measurement in rehabilitation. In D. Stuss, G. Winocur, & I. H. Robertson (Eds.), *Cognitive neurorehabilitation: A comprehensive approach*. Cambridge: University Press.

Uswatte, G., & Taub, E. (2005). Implications of the learned nonuse formulation for measuring rehabilitation outcomes: Lessons from constraint-induced movement therapy. *Rehabilitation Psychology, 50*, 34–42.

Uswatte, G., Taub, E., Morris, D., Barman, J., & Crago, J. (2006a). Contribution of the shaping and restraint components of Constraint-induced movement therapy to treatment outcome. *NeuroRehabilitation, 21*, 147–156.

Uswatte, G., Taub, E., Morris, D., Light, K., & Thompson, P. (2006b). The Motor Activity Log-28: A method for assessing daily use of the hemiparetic arm after stroke. *Neurology, 67*, 1189–1194.

Uswatte, G., Taub, E., Morris, D., Vignolo, M., & McCulloch, K. (2005). Reliability and validity of the upper-extremity Motor Activity Log-14 for measuring real-world arm use. *Stroke, 36*, 2493–2496.

Van de Crommert, H. W., Mulder, T., & Duysens, J. (1998). Neural control of locomotion: Sensory control of the central pattern generator and its relation to treadmill training. *Gait and Posture, 7*, 251–263.

Visintin, M., & Barbeau, H. (1989). The effects of body weight support on the locomotor pattern of spastic paretic patients. *Canadian Neurological Sciences, 16*, 315–325.

Visintin, M., & Barbeau, H. (1994). The effects of parallel bars, body weight support and speed on the modulation of the locomotor pattern of spastic paretic gait: A preliminary communication. *Paraplegia, 32*, 540–553.

Wernig, A., & Müller, S. (1992). Laufband locomotion with body weight support improved walking in persons with severe spinal cord injuries. *Paraplegia, 30*, 229–238.

Wernig, A., Müller, S., Nanassy, A., & Cagol, E. (1995). Laufband therapy based on "rules of spinal locomotion" is effective in spinal cord injured persons. *European Neuroscience*, 7823–7829. (Erratum in European Journal of Neuroscience, 7, 1429.)

Wessels M., Lucas, C., Eriks, I., deGroot, S. (2010). Body weight-supported gait training for restoration of walking in people with an incomplete spinal cord injury: A systematic review. *Rehabilitation Medicine, 42*, 513–519.

Wirz, M., Zemon, D. H., Rupp, R., Scheel, A., Colombo, G., Dietz, V., et al. (2005). Effectiveness of automated locomotor training in patients with chronic incomplete spinal cord injury: A multicenter trial. *Archives of Physical Medicine and Rehabilitation, 86*, 672–680.

Wittenberg, G. F., Chen, R., Ishii, K., Bushara, K. O., Taub, E., Gerber, L. H., et al. (2003). Constraint-induced therapy in stroke: Magnetic-stimulation motor maps and cerebral activation. *Neurorehabilitation and Neural Repair, 17*, 48–57.

Wolf, S. L., Catlin, P. A., Ellis, M., Archer, A. L., Morgan, B., & Piacentino, A. (2001). Assessing the Wolf Motor Function Test as outcome measure for research in patients after stroke. *Stroke, 32*, 1635–1639.

Wolf, S. L., Lecraw, D. E., Barton, L., & Jann, B. (1989). Forced use of hemiplegic upper extremities to reverse the effect of learned nonuse among chronic stroke and head-injured patients. *Experimental Neurology, 104*, 125–132.

Wolf, S. L., Thompson, P. A., Morris, D. M., Rose, D. K., Winstein, C. J., Taub, E., et al. (2005). The EXCITE Trial: Attributes of the Wolf Motor Function Test in patients with subacute stroke. *Neurorehabilitation and Neural Repair, 19*, 194–205.

Wolf, S. L., Thompson, P. A., Winstein, C., Miller, J. P., Blanton, S. R., Nichols-Larsen, D. S., et al. (2010). The EXCITE stroke trial: Comparing early and delayed constraint induced movement therapy. *Stroke, 41*, 2309–2315.

Wolf, S. L., Winstein, C., Miller, J. P., Taub, E., Uswatte, G., Morris, D. M., et al. (2006). Effect of constraint-induced movement therapy on upper extremity function 3 to 9 months after stroke. The EXCITE randomized clinical trial. *American Medical Association, 296*, 2095–2104.

Wolf, S. L., Winstein, C., Miller, J. P., Thompson, P. A., Taub, E., Uswatte, G., et al. (2008). Retention of upper limb function in stroke survivors who have received constraint-induced movement therapy: The EXCITE randomized trial. *Lancet Neurology, 7*, 33–40.

CHAPTER 8

Malleability and Plasticity in the Neural Systems for Reading and Dyslexia

BENNETT A. SHAYWITZ
SALLY E. SHAYWITZ

Developmental dyslexia is characterized by unexpected difficulty in reading in children or adults who otherwise possess the intelligence and motivation considered necessary for accurate and fluent reading (Lyon, Shaywitz, & Shaywitz, 2003). *Unexpected* here means that these children (or adults) appear to have all of the factors (intelligence, motivation, exposure to reasonable reading instruction) needed to be good readers, but that they nevertheless continue to struggle with reading (S. Shaywitz, 1998). Recent evidence provides empirical support for defining dyslexia as *unexpected* difficulty in reading. Using data from the Connecticut Longitudinal Study, we (Ferrer, Shaywitz, Holahan, Marchione, & Shaywitz, 2010) demonstrated that in typical readers, reading and IQ development are dynamically linked over time. Not only do reading and IQ track together over time, they also influence one another. Such mutual interrelationships are not perceptible in dyslexic readers, suggesting that reading and cognition develop more independently in these individuals (Figure 8.1). These findings provide the first empirical demonstration of a coupling between cognition and reading in typical readers, confirming the general public perception that people who are good readers are likely to be very intelligent, and, conversely, that people who struggle to read may be less intelligent. Because these new data also demonstrate a developmental uncoupling between cognition and reading in dyslexic readers they indicate that dyslexia is a special case violating the assumption that reading and IQ are always linked. In other words, they confirm that in dyslexia, one can be highly intelligent and still struggle to read.

Our findings of an uncoupling between IQ and reading in dyslexia, and the influence of this uncoupling on the developmental trajectory of reading, provide evidence to support the conceptual basis of dyslexia as an unexpected difficulty in reading in individuals who otherwise have the intelligence and motivation to learn to read. Based on dynamic models, the uncoupling of reading and cognition observed demonstrate that in the special case of dyslexia, a child or adult can be both bright and accomplished, along with having a much lower reading level than would be expected for a person with his or her intelligence, education, or professional status. They

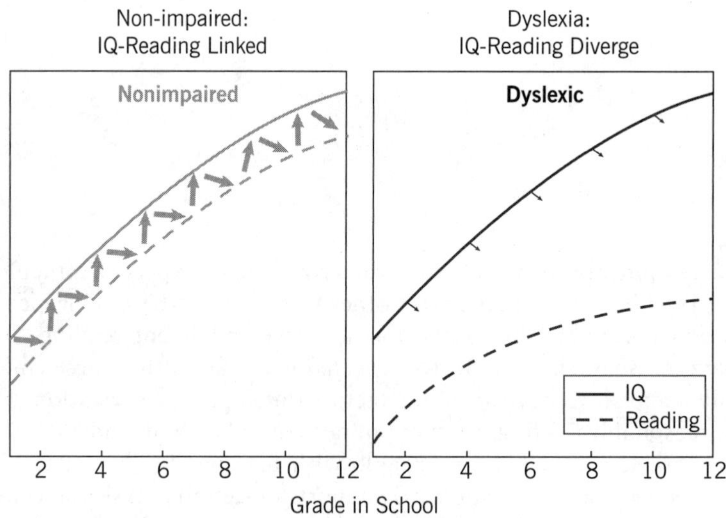

FIGURE 8.1. Uncoupling of reading and IQ over time: Empirical evidence for a definition of dyslexia. The left panel shows that in typical readers, reading and IQ development are dynamically linked over time. In contrast, the right panel shows that in dyslexic readers, reading and IQ development are dissociated; in other words, a person can be highly intelligent and still struggle with reading. Data from Ferrer et al. (2010).

also demonstrate that in dyslexia, the reading difficulty is unexpected for an *individual's* level of intelligence or education; that is, the difficulty is defined as a disparity existing *within* the individual. The implication is that for a person with dyslexia, the appropriate comparison is between the person's ability and his or her reading. Thus, in dyslexia, a highly intelligent person may read at a level above average but below that expected, based on his or her intelligence, education, or accomplishments. These new findings provide an explanation for the "unexpected" nature of developmental dyslexia, and provide the long-sought empirical evidence for the seeming paradox involving cognition and reading in individuals with developmental dyslexia.

Dyslexia (or specific reading disability) is the most common and most carefully studied of the learning disabilities, affecting 80% of all individuals identified as having such disabilities. This chapter reviews recent advances in our knowledge of the epidemiology, etiology, cognitive influences, and neurobiology of reading and dyslexia in children and adults, with an emphasis on plasticity and malleability of the neural systems serving reading.

Historically, dyslexia in adults was first noted in the latter half of the 19th century, and developmental dyslexia in children was first reported by Morgan (1896). Our understanding of the neural systems for reading began when Dejerine (1891) suggested that a portion of the posterior brain region is critical for reading. Another posterior brain region—this one more ventral, in the occipitotemporal area—was also described by Dejerine (1892) as critical in reading.

EPIDEMIOLOGY

Recent epidemiological data indicate that, like hypertension and obesity, dyslexia fits a dimensional model. In other words, within the population, reading ability and disability occur along a continuum, with reading disability representing the lower tail of a normal distribution of reading ability (S. Shaywitz, Escobar, Shaywitz, Fletcher, & Makuch, 1992). Dyslexia is perhaps the most common neurobehavioral disorder affecting children, with prevalence rates ranging from 5% to 17.5% (Interagency Committee on Learning Disabilities, 1987; S. Shaywitz, 1998). Longitudinal studies, both prospective (Francis, Shaywitz, Steubing, Shaywitz, & Fletcher, 1996; B. Shaywitz et al., 1995) and retrospective (Bruck & Treiman, 1992; Felton, Naylor, & Wood, 1990), indicate that dyslexia is a persistent, chronic condition; it does not represent a transient "developmental lag" (Figure 8.2). Over time, poor readers and good readers tend to maintain their relative positions along the spectrum of reading ability.

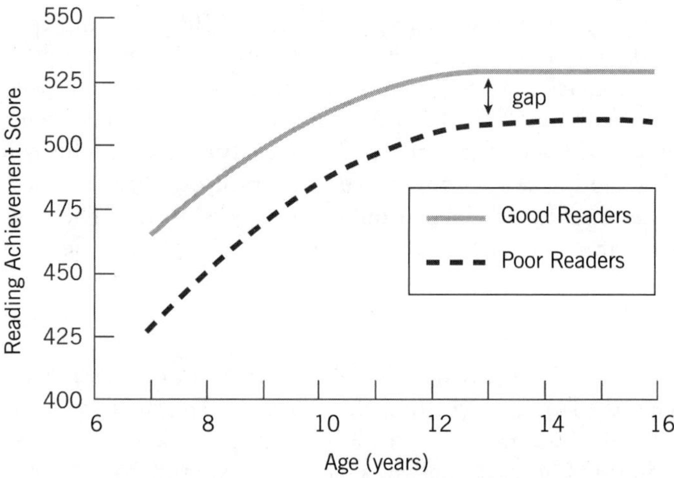

FIGURE 8.2. Trajectory of reading skills over time in nonimpaired and dyslexic readers. Numbers on the ordinate are Rasch scores (*W* scores) from the Woodcock–Johnson reading test (Woodcock & Johnson, 1989), and numbers on the abscissa are ages in years. Both dyslexic and nonimpaired readers improve their reading scores as they get older, but the gap between the dyslexic and nonimpaired readers remains. Dyslexia is a deficit, not a developmental lag. Adapted from S. Shaywitz (2003). Copyright 2003 by S. Shaywitz. Adapted by permission.

ETIOLOGY

Dyslexia is both familial and heritable (Pennington & Gilger, 1996). Family history is one of the most important risk factors: From 23% to as many as 65% of children who have a parent with dyslexia are reported to have the disorder (S. Shaywitz, 2003). A rate among siblings of affected persons of approximately 40%, and a rate among parents ranging from 27% to 49% (Pennington & Gilger, 1996), provide opportunities for early identification of affected siblings and often for delayed but helpful identification of affected adults.

Given that dyslexia is familial and heritable, initial hopes that dyslexia would be explained by a one or just a few genes have been disappointing. Thus, along with genome-wide association studies (GWAS) of a great many other common disorders and diseases, GWAS of dyslexia have so far identified genetic variants that account for only a very small percentage of the risk—in this case, less than 1% (Meaburn, Harlaar, Craig, Schalkwyk, & Plomin, 2008). Current evidence suggests "that common diseases involve thousands of genes and proteins interacting on complex pathways" (Duncan, 2009), and that, similar to experience with other complex disorders (e.g., heart disease, diabetes), it is unlikely that a single gene or even a few genes will identify people with dyslexia. Rather, dyslexia is best explained by *multiple* genes, each contributing a *small* amount of the variance. Thus current evidence suggests that the etiology of dyslexia is best conceptualized within a multifactorial model, with multiple genetic and environmental risk and protective factors leading to the disorder.

COGNITIVE INFLUENCES

The Phonological Theory of Developmental Dyslexia

Among investigators in the field, there is now a strong consensus supporting the phonological theory of developmental dyslexia. According to this theory, speech is natural and inherent, while reading is acquired and must be taught. To read, the beginning reader must recognize that the letters and letter strings (the *orthography*) represent the sounds of spoken language. In order to read, a child has to develop the insight that spoken words can be pulled apart into the elemental particles of speech (*phonemes*), and that the letters in a written word represent these sounds (S. Shaywitz, 2003); such awareness is largely missing in dyslexic children and adults (Bruck, 1998; Fletcher et al., 1994; Liberman & Shankweiler, 1991; Shankweiler, Liberman, Mark, Fowler, & Fischer, 1979; S. Shaywitz, 2003; Torgesen & Wagner, 1995; Wagner & Torgesen, 1987). Results from large and well-studied populations with reading disability confirm that in young school-age children (Fletcher et al., 1994; Stanovich & Siegel, 1994) as well as in adolescents (S. Shaywitz et al., 1999), a deficit in phonology represents the most robust and specific correlate of reading disability (Morris et al., 1998; Ramus et al., 2003). Such findings form the basis for the most successful and most firmly evidence-based interventions designed to improve reading (National Reading Panel, 2000).

Implications of the Phonological Model

Reading comprises two main processes—decoding and comprehension (Gough & Tunmer, 1986). In dyslexia, a deficit at the level of the phonological module impairs the ability to segment a spoken word into its underlying phonological elements and then to link the letters to their corresponding sounds. As a result, the reader experiences difficulty first in decoding the word, and then in identifying it. The phonological deficit is domain-specific; that is, it is independent of other (nonphonological) abilities. In particular, the higher-order cognitive and linguistic functions involved in comprehension, such as general intelligence/reasoning, vocabulary (Share & Stanovich, 1995), and syntax (Shankweiler et al., 1995), are generally intact. This pattern—a deficit in phonological analysis contrasted with intact higher-order cognitive abilities—offers an explanation for the paradox of otherwise intelligent, often gifted people who experience great difficulty in reading (S. Shaywitz, 1996, 2003).

According to the model, a circumscribed deficit in a lower-order linguistic function (phonology) blocks access to higher-order processes and to the ability to draw meaning from text. The problem is that the affected reader cannot use his or her higher-order linguistic skills to access the meaning until the printed word has first been decoded and identified. Suppose, for example, that Mary knows the precise meaning of the spoken word *apparition*; however, she will not be able to use her knowledge of the meaning of the word until she can decode and identify the printed word on the page, and it will appear that she does not know the word's meaning.

NEUROBIOLOGICAL STUDIES OF DYSLEXIA

To a large degree, these advances in understanding the cognitive basis of dyslexia have informed and facilitated studies examining the neurobiological underpinnings of reading and dyslexia. Thus a range of neurobiological investigations using postmortem brain specimens (Galaburda, Sherman, Rosen, Aboitiz, & Geschwind, 1985), brain morphometry (Brown et al., 2001; Eliez et al., 2000), and diffusion tensor imaging (Klingberg et al., 2000) suggests that there are differences in the temporo-parieto-occipital brain regions between dyslexic and nonimpaired readers. By far, the most consistent and replicable data have come from studies using functional magnetic resonance imaging (fMRI), and we focus on such studies in the remainder of this chapter.

FMRI IN STUDIES OF READING AND DYSLEXIA

General Considerations

fMRI has proven to be a powerful tool for understanding the brain's organization for reading and dyslexia, and promises to supplant other methods for its ability to map the brain's response to specific cognitive stimuli. Since it is noninvasive and safe, it can be used repeatedly—properties that make it ideal for studying humans, especially children. In principle, the signal used to construct magnetic resonance images changes by a small amount (typically on the order of 1–5%), in regions that are activated by a stimulus or task. The increase in signal results from the combined effects of increases in the tissue blood flow, volume, and oxygenation, though the precise contribution of each of these is still somewhat uncertain. Image intensity increases when deoxygenated blood is replaced by oxygenated blood. A variety of methods can be used to record the changes that occur, but one preferred approach makes use of ultrafast imaging, such as echo planar imaging, in which complete images are acquired in times substantially shorter than a second. Echo planar imaging can provide images at a rate fast enough to capture the time course of the hemodynamic response to neural activation and to permit a wide variety of imaging paradigms over large volumes of the brain. Details of fMRI are reviewed elsewhere (Anderson & Gore, 1997; Frackowiak et al., 2004; Jezzard, Matthews, & Smith, 2001).

Identification and Localization of Specific Systems and Their Differences in Good and Poor Readers

We (B. Shaywitz et al., 2002) used fMRI to study 144 right-handed children: 70 dyslexic (DYS) readers (21 girls, 49 boys, ages 7–18 years, mean age = 13.3 years) and 74 nonimpaired (NI) readers (31 girls, 43 boys, ages 7–17 years, mean age = 10.9 years) as they read pseudowords and real words. This study was designed to minimize some of the problems encountered in previous studies, and thus we examined a large sample, particularly for a functional imaging study; we included a broad age range and studied both boys and girls. We found significant differences in brain activation patterns during phonological analysis between the NI and DYS children. Specifically, the NI children demonstrated significantly greater activation than did the DYS children in predominantly left-hemisphere sites (including the inferior frontal, superior temporal, parietotemporal, and middle temporal–middle occipital gyri) and a few right-hemisphere sites (including an anterior site around the inferior frontal gyrus and two posterior sites—one in the parietotemporal region, the other in the occipitotemporal region) (Plate 8.1). These data converge with reports from many investigators using functional brain imaging, which show a failure of left-hemisphere posterior brain systems to function properly during reading (Bradley & Bryant, 1983; Helenius, Tarkiainen, Cornelissen, Hansen, & Salmelin, 1999; Horwitz, Rumsey, & Donohue, 1998; Paulesu et al., 2001; Rumsey et al., 1992; Salmelin, Service, Kiesila, Uutela, & Salonen, 1996; Seki et al., 2001; B. Shaywitz et al., 2002; S. Shaywitz et al., 2003; Temple et al., 2000), as well as during nonreading visual processing tasks (Demb, Boynton, & Heeger, 1998; Eden et al., 1996). These findings indicate that dyslexia is characterized by an inefficient functioning of posterior reading systems—a phenomenon that, as illustrated in Plate 8.2, has been termed the *neural signature of dyslexia*. The consistency of the functional brain imaging in dyslexia has been critical in making a heretofore hidden disability visible.

Compensatory Systems in Dyslexic Readers

Our study in children also allowed for the examination of compensatory systems that dyslexic readers develop. Two kinds of information were helpful in examining this issue. One involved the relationship between brain activation and age. During the most difficult and specific phonological task (nonword rhyming), *older* compared to younger DYS readers engaged the left and right inferior frontal gyrus; in contrast, few differences emerged between older and younger NI readers. Another clue to compensatory systems comes from the findings of the relationship between reading skill and brain activation, where a significant positive correlation was noted between reading skill and activation in the left occipitotemporal word form area. We also found a *negative* correlation between brain activation and reading skill in the *right* occipitotemporal region; that is, the poorer the reader, the greater the activation in the right occipitotemporal region. Thus compensatory systems seem to involve areas around the inferior frontal gyrus in both hemispheres, and perhaps the right-hemisphere homologue of the left occipitotemporal word form area as well (Plate 8.3).

Development of Reading Systems in Dyslexia

Although converging evidence points to three important neural systems for reading, few studies have examined age-related changes in these systems in either typical readers or dyslexic children. In a recent report (B. Shaywitz et al., 2007), we used fMRI to study age-related changes in reading in a cross-sectional study of 232 right-handed children 7–18 years of age (113 dyslexic readers and 119 nonimpaired readers) as they read pseudowords. Our findings indicated that the neural systems for reading that develop with age in nonimpaired readers differ from those in dyslexic readers.

The most significant contrasts were found in those systems within the left occipitotemporal area. Here, older compared to younger nonimpaired readers demonstrated an increased engagement of the left anterior lateral occipitotemporal region. In contrast, older compared to younger dyslexic readers demonstrated an increase in activation in the left posterior medial occipitotemporal region. These findings indicate that the systems for reading that develop with age in dyslexic readers differ from those in nonimpaired readers, primarily in being localized to a more posterior and medial, rather than a more anterior and lateral, occipitotemporal region. Interestingly, this difference in activation patterns between the two groups of readers has parallels to reported brain activation differences observed during reading of two Japanese writing systems, *kana* and *kanji*. For example, left anterior lateral occipitotemporal activation, similar to that seen in nonimpaired readers, occurs during the reading of *kana* (Nakamura, Dehaene, Jobert, Le Bihan, & Kouider, 2005). *Kana* script employs symbols that are linked to the sound or phoneme (as in English and other alphabetic scripts). In *kana* and in alphabetic scripts, children initially learn to read words by learning how letters and sounds are linked; over time, these linkages are integrated and permanently instantiated as a word form. Knowledge of how letters and sounds are linked allows a reader to sound out and read new words.

Considerable research supports the notion that the anterior lateral occipitotemporal system—a region that Cohen and Dehaene have termed the *visual word form area* (Cohen et al., 2000; Dehaene, Cohen, Sigman, & Vinckier, 2005; Dehaene et al., 2001; McCandliss, Cohen, & Dehaene, 2003)—is associated with the ability to read words fluently, the hallmark of a skilled reader. Just how this area functions to integrate phonology (sounds) and orthography (print) is as yet unknown. Current studies are now focusing on whether visual word recognition takes place serially, in a step-by-step approach (Dehaene et al., 2005; Vinckier et al., 2007), or whether the left anterior lateral occipitotemporal system functions as an interface between bottom-up visual form information and top-down semantic and phonological properties in a more dynamic integrative process (McCrory, Mechelli, Frith, & Price, 2005; Price et al., 2003). Studies using functional imaging combined with sophisticated task presentations may help to resolve this question (Devlin, Jamison, Gonnerman, & Matthews, 2006).

In contrast, posterior medial occipitotemporal activation, comparable to that observed in dyslexic readers, has been noted during reading of *kanji* script (Nakamura et al., 2005). Consideration of the mechanisms used for reading *kanji* compared to *kana* provide insights into potentially different mechanisms that develop with age in dyslexic versus nonimpaired readers. *Kanji* script uses ideographs, and each character must be memorized, suggesting that the posterior medial occipitotemporal region functions as part of a memory-based system. We suppose that as dyslexic children mature, this posterior medial system supports memorization rather than the progressive sound–symbol linkages observed in nonimpaired readers. And there is evidence that dyslexic readers are not able to make good use of sound–symbol linkages as they mature; instead, they come to rely on memorized words. For example, phonological deficits continue to characterize struggling readers even as they enter adolescence and adult life (Bruck & Treiman, 1992; S. Shaywitz et al., 1999), and (as described in the next section) persistently poor adult readers read words by memorization so that they are able to read familiar words but have difficulty reading unfamiliar words (S. Shaywitz, 2003).

Thus our findings support and now extend previous findings to indicate that the system responsible for the integration of letters and sounds, the anterior lateral occipitotemporal system, is the neural circuit that develops with age in nonimpaired readers. Conversely, dyslexic readers, who struggle to read new or unfamiliar words, come to rely on an alternative system—the posterior medial occipitotemporal system, which functions via memory networks.

Types of Reading Disability

Using data from participants in a longitudinal epidemiological study, we (S. Shaywitz et al., 2003) examined the neural systems for reading in two groups of young adults who were poor readers as children—a group with relatively good compensated and a group with persistent reading difficulties—and compared them to nonimpaired readers. In addition, we wanted to determine whether there were any factors distinguishing the good compensators from the persistently poor readers that might account for their different outcomes. To this end, we took advantage of the availability of a cohort participating in the Connecticut Longitudinal Study: a representative sample of individuals (now young adults) who have been prospectively followed since 1983 when they were age 5 years, and who have had their reading performance assessed yearly throughout their primary and secondary schooling (B. Shaywitz, Fletcher, Holahan, & Shaywitz, 1992; S. Shaywitz et al., 1999; S. Shaywitz, Shaywitz, Fletcher, & Escobar, 1990).

Three groups of young adults, ages 18.5–22.5 years, were created. First, persistently poor readers (PPR, $n = 24$) met criteria for poor reading in grade 2 or 4 and again in grade 9 or 10. Second, accuracy- (but not fluency-) improved (compensated) readers (AIR, $n = 19$) satisfied criteria for poor reading in grade 2 or 4 but not in grade 9 or 10. Finally, nonimpaired (NI) readers ($n = 27$) were selected on the basis of not meeting the criteria for poor reading in any of the grades (2–10); having a reading standard score over 94 (above the 40th percentile), to prevent overlap with the PPR and AIR groups; and having an average Full Scale IQ lower than 130, to avoid a supernormal control group. Findings during pseudoword rhyming in both groups of poor readers (AIR, PPR) were similar to those observed in previous studies; that is, these groups showed a relative underactivation in posterior neural systems located in the superior temporal and the occipitotemporal regions. But when participants were reading real words, the findings were quite surprising: Brain activation patterns in the AIR and PPR groups diverged. As they had for pseudoword reading, AIR participants demonstrated relative underactivation in left posterior regions, compared to NI readers. By contrast, during real-word reading the PPR subjects activated posterior systems; thus there was comparable activation in the NI and PPR groups in the posterior reading systems. These findings were both new and unexpected. Despite the significantly better reading performance in the NI group than in the PPR group on every reading task administered, left posterior reading systems were activated during reading real words in both these groups.

We hypothesized that the PPR participants were reading real words very differently from the NI readers—that is, reading the very simple real words primarily by memory. Support for this belief came from the PPR group's performance on a real-word (in contrast to the nonword) pronunciation task: They were accurate while reading high-frequency words, but far less accurate when reading low-frequency and unfamiliar words. Further support for this hypothesis comes from a functional connectivity analysis. This strategy involves examining a *seed voxel* (in this case, a voxel in the left occipitotemporal region) and determining those regions most functionally related to the seed voxel (McIntosh, Bookstein, Haxby, & Grady, 1996; McIntosh, Nyberg, Bookstein, & Tulving, 1997). We hypothesized that in NI readers the occipitotemporal region processes print in a linguistically structured manner and should interact with other areas implicated in orthographic and phonological processing. We further hypothesized that in PPR individuals the occipitotemporal area serves as a visually based memory system and should interact with other areas implicated in memory retrieval.

Results indicated that the NI readers demonstrated connectivity between the left occipitotemporal seed region and the left inferior frontal gyrus, a traditional language region. In contrast, the PPR subjects demonstrated functional connectivity between the seed region and right prefrontal areas often associated with working memory and memory retrieval (Fletcher, Frith, & Rugg, 1997; MacLeod, Buckner, Miezin, Petersen, & Raichle, 1998)—a finding consistent with the hypothesis that in PPR individuals the occipitotemporal area functions as a component of a memory network. This finding, together with the more recent data on the development of reading systems described in the preceding section, amplify the importance of memory systems in dyslexic readers.

PLASTICITY OF NEURAL SYSTEMS FOR READING

Studies of Plasticity of Language Systems after Brain Injury

A number of studies have used fMRI to examine the development of neural systems for language and reading after brain injury in children. For example, Fair, Brown, Petersen, and Schlaggar (2006) examined the neuroanatomical pattern of brain activation in a boy who had suffered a perinatal stroke affecting his left middle cerebral artery. He was studied via fMRI at ages 9 and 13 years while doing tasks that required him to generate words to both visual and auditory stimuli. For the most part, his brain activation was similar to that observed in a large number of nonimpaired children. Other studies have examined neural plasticity in children who have undergone temporal lobe resection for intractable epilepsy. Noppeney, Price, Duncan, and Koepp (2005) examined sentence reading in children following left anterior temporal lobe resection and found similarities in activation in the two groups in the left hemisphere, but also differences in the right. In both the children with temporal lobe resection and control children, reading ability predicted activations in *left* middle temporal regions. By contrast, in patients but not controls, reading ability predicted activation in the *right* inferior frontal region, right hippocampus, and right inferior temporal region. Berl et al. (2005) used fMRI to determine asymmetry of activation during silent reading to study 50 children and adults after surgery for intractable epilepsy. Patients with left-hemisphere seizure foci were more likely to exhibit atypical language representation than either controls or children with right-hemisphere seizure foci were. Liegeois et al. (2004) studied 10 children with epilepsy primarily originating in the left hemisphere. Brain imaging showed bilateral or right language lateralization in 5 of 10 children, leading the authors to conclude that it is difficult to predict language reorganization.

Thus the results from studies of individuals with brain injury are difficult to interpret. More consistent reports have emerged from studies using fMRI before and after a reading intervention and are discussed next.

Effects of Reading Interventions on Neural Systems for Reading

Given the converging evidence for a disruption of posterior reading systems in dyslexia, an obvious question relates to the plasticity of these neural systems—that is, whether they are malleable and can be changed by an effective reading intervention. We (B. Shaywitz et al., 2004) hypothesized that the provision of an evidence-based, phonologically mediated reading intervention would improve reading fluency and the development of the neural systems serving skilled reading. The experimental intervention was structured to help children gain phonological knowledge (develop an awareness of the internal structure of spoken words) and, at the same time, develop their understanding of how the orthography represents the phonology.

Seventy seven right-handed children, ages 6.1–9.4 years, were recruited for three experimental groups: experimental intervention (EI, n = 37); community intervention (CI, n = 12); and a community control (CC) group of nonimpaired readers (n = 28). Children in the CI group met criteria for reading disability and received a variety of interventions commonly provided within the schools; however, specific, systematic, explicit phonologically based interventions comparable to the experimental intervention were not used in any of the reading programs that were provided to this group. The experimental intervention provided second- and third-grade poor readers with 50 minutes of daily individual tutoring that was explicitly and systematically focused on helping children understand the alphabetic principle (how letters and combinations of letters represent the small segments of speech known as phonemes), and that provided many opportunities to practice applying the letter–sound linkages taught. Children were imaged on three occasions: preintervention, immediately postintervention, and 1 year after the intervention was complete.

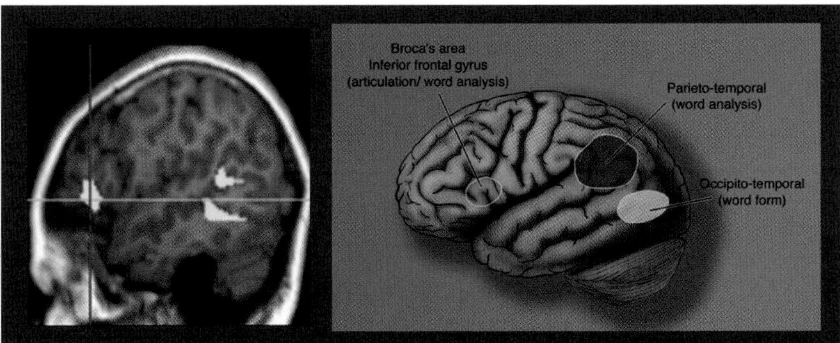

PLATE 8.1. Three neural systems for reading are illustrated for the surface of the left hemisphere. The left figure is a composite fMRI depiction of 74 typical readers contrasted with 70 dyslexic readers; regions more active in typical than in dyslexic readers are shown as yellow. The right figure is a schematic view. Both images show three systems for reading: an anterior system in the region of the inferior frontal gyrus (Broca's area), which is believed to serve articulation and word analysis; and two posterior systems—one in the parietotemporal region, which is believed to serve word analysis, and a second in the occipitotemporal region (the word form area), which is believed to serve the rapid, automatic, fluent identification of words. Adapted from S. Shaywitz (2003). Copyright 2003 by S. Shaywitz. Adapted by permission.

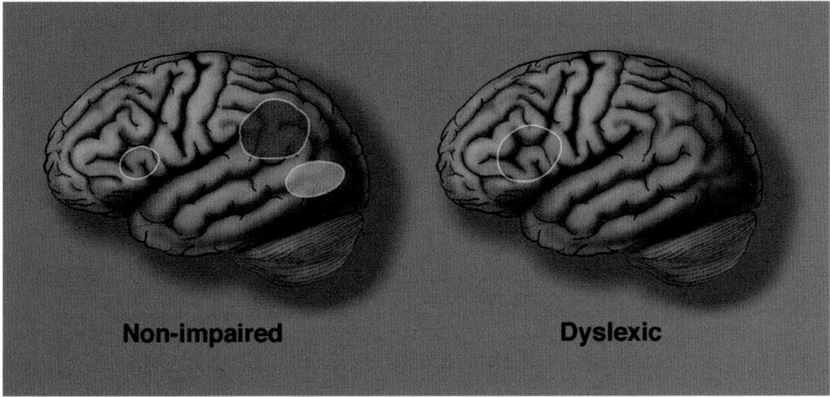

PLATE 8.2. A neural signature for dyslexia is illustrated in this schematic view of left-hemisphere brain systems in nonimpaired (left) and dyslexic (right) readers. In typical readers, the three systems provided in Plate 8.1 are shown. In dyslexic readers, the anterior system is slightly overactivated, compared with that of typical readers; in contrast, the two posterior systems are underactivated. This pattern of underactivation in left posterior reading systems is referred to as the *neural signature for dyslexia*. Adapted from S. Shaywitz (2003). Copyright 2003 by S. Shaywitz. Adapted by permission.

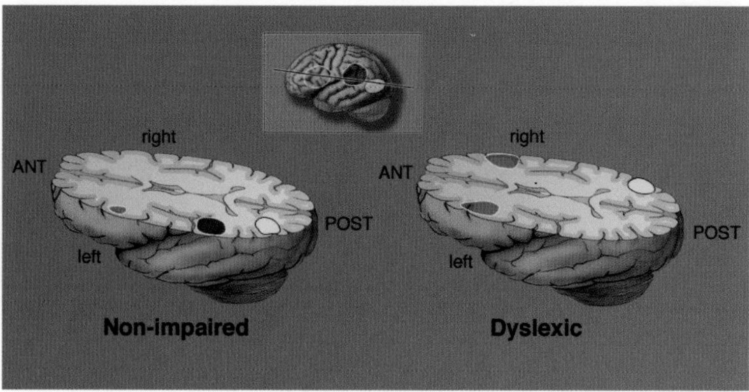

PLATE 8.3. Compensatory neural systems and the neural basis for the requirement for extended time for dyslexic students on high-stakes testing. Each image is a cutaway view of the brain showing the left and right hemispheres. Typical readers activate three left-hemisphere neural systems for reading: an anterior system and two posterior systems. Dyslexic readers have inefficient functioning in the left-hemisphere posterior neural systems for reading, but compensate by developing anterior systems in the left and right hemispheres and the posterior homologue of the visual word form area in the right hemisphere. Adapted from S. Shaywitz (2003). Copyright 2003 by S. Shaywitz. Adapted by permission.

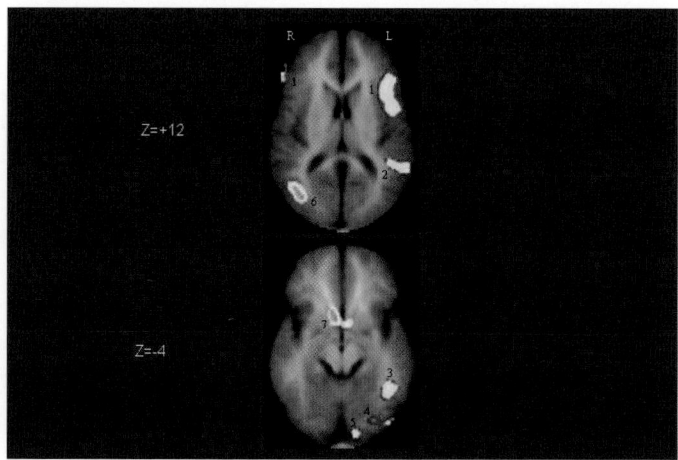

PLATE 8.4. Composite maps indicating the difference in activation between year 3 and year 1 in the experimental intervention (EI) study group (n = 25). Red-yellow indicates brain regions that were more active (p = .05) in the third year; blue-purple indicates brain regions that were more active (p = .05) in the first year. The slice locations are z = 12 and z = −4 in Talairach space. Brain regions (Talairach x, y, z, coordinates in parentheses) more active in the third year than in the first were (1) bilateral inferior frontal gyri (±41, 23, 12); (2) the left superior temporal sulcus (+51, −42, +12); (3) the occipitotemporal region involving the posterior aspects of the middle and inferior temporal gyri and the anterior aspect of the middle occipital gyrus (+42, −49, −4); (4) the inferior occipital gyrus (+34, −71, −4), and (5) the lingual gyrus (+13, −88, −4). The brain region more active in the first year than in the third year were (6) the right middle tempora l gyrus (−35, −69, +12) and (7) the caudate nucleus (−7, +10, −4). Figure from B. Shaywitz et al. (2004). Copyright 2004 by the Society of Biological Psychiatry. Reprinted by permission.

Children in the EI group improved their reading accuracy, reading fluency, and reading comprehension, though they did not improve so much that they were reading as well as the control children, and a gap in reading between the dyslexic and control children still remained. Compared to the CI group, both the CC and EI groups demonstrated increased activation in left-hemisphere regions, including the inferior frontal gyrus and the posterior aspect of the middle temporal gyrus. One year after the experimental intervention had ended (Plate 8.4), compared to their preintervention images, the EI children were activating bilateral inferior frontal gyri; the left superior temporal sulcus; the occipitotemporal region involving the posterior aspects of the middle and inferior temporal gyri and the anterior aspect of the middle occipital gyrus; the inferior occipital gyrus; and the lingual gyrus.

These findings indicate that the nature of the remedial educational intervention is critical to successful outcomes in children with reading disabilities, and that the use of an evidence-based reading intervention facilitates the development of those fast-paced neural systems that underlie skilled reading. Our findings indicate that a phonologically based reading intervention leads to the development of neural systems in both anterior (inferior frontal gyrus) and posterior (middle temporal gyrus) brain regions.

Other investigators, too, have found that an effective reading intervention influences neural systems in very much the same fashion. Two studies from the same investigative group have used fMRI to examine the effects of a commercial reading program (Fast ForWord) on both adults and children with dyslexia. The first study examined three adults with dyslexia who received Fast ForWord training during a task requiring that subjects respond to a high-pitched stimulus. Following 33 training days, two of the three subjects demonstrated greater activation in the left prefrontal cortex after training than before training, and these two adults also showed improvement on both rapid auditory processing and auditory language comprehension after training; the one adult who did not show a change in fMRI after training failed to show behavioral changes (Temple et al., 2000). In another study, immediate short-term improvement in reading accuracy and brain activation changes were observed in 20 children with dyslexia—changes that included the areas observed in our study, as well as areas in the right hemisphere and cingulate cortex (Temple et al., 2003).

Richards et al. (2000) used proton magnetic resonance spectroscopy to measure brain lactate concentrations at two time points, 1 year apart, in eight dyslexic and seven control boys before and after 3 weeks of a phonologically based reading intervention. Measuring lactate is a direct measure of brain metabolism, with lower levels reflecting more efficient metabolism. Before treatment, the dyslexic boys demonstrated increased lactate concentration (compared to controls) in the left anterior quadrant during a phonological task. After treatment, brain lactate concentrations were no different in the dyslexic and control boys, and the dyslexic boys' reading improved after treatment, reflecting an improvement in the efficiency of brain function after the intervention. This same investigative group reported fMRI changes in areas similar to those reported here following 28 hours of an intensive phonological and morphological reading intervention (Aylward et al., 2003).

Simos et al. (2002) used magnetoencephalography (MEG) in eight children with dyslexia and eight controls before and after 8 weeks of a phonologically based reading intervention. Prior to intervention, the dyslexic readers demonstrated little or no activation of the posterior portion of the superior temporal gyrus. After intervention, reading improved and activation increased in the left superior temporal gyrus. Using a phonologically based intervention consisting of 3-hour daily sessions for 8 weeks, Eden et al. (2004) compared 9 adults (age 40) who had been diagnosed with dyslexia as children to 10 adults who did not receive the intervention. Although real-word reading did not improve, tests of phonemic awareness did improve, and posterior brain systems in the left hemisphere (as well as right-hemisphere homologues) increased in activation compared to the preintervention imaging.

These findings after a reading intervention suggest plasticity of the neural systems for reading in children. They parallel those observed after a variety of therapies in individuals with stroke (Carey et al., 2002) and after surgical removal of a hemisphere in a child with Rasmussen's syndrome (Hertz-Pennier et al., 2002). Importantly, the effects of the experimental intervention—both in promoting skilled reading and in activating the occipitotemporal word form area shown to be critical for skilled reading (B. Shaywitz et al., 2002, 2007)—are similar to the co-occurrence of visual–spatial proficiency and cortical specialization reported in adults. Thus Gauthier et al. (2000) have demonstrated a progressive increase in activation of the right-hemisphere fusiform face area and right lateral occipital cortex with increasing proficiency in identifying novel face-like stimuli they called "Greebles." The findings described here suggest that, as in recognition of Greebles, an intervention that improved proficiency in reading was the most important element in functional reorganization of the neural systems for reading.

Interventions in Acquired Alexia

Studies of acquired alexia also demonstrate the utility of brain imaging in aiding intervention. For example, Leff, Spitsyna, Plant, and Wise (2006) used structural brain imaging to differentiate two groups of adults who had suffered posterior cerebral artery thrombosis: one group with hemianopic alexia, the other with pure alexia. Hemianopic alexia impairs text reading more than single-word reading, because in reading text from left to right, readers must be able to make use of visual information to the right of fixation. In contrast, pure alexia results from damage to the visual word form area (discussed earlier). Those with hemianopic alexia respond to interventions focusing on visual field restoration or ocular–motor rehabilitation. Those with damage to the visual word form area require substantially different interventions—for example, interventions focused on attempting to improve word form identification. Such an intervention was described by Beeson, Magloire, and Robey (2005), who reported on a 59-year-old man who developed sudden onset of alexia after a stroke in the distribution of the left posterior cerebral artery. MRI indicated damage to the left occipitotemporal word form area affecting reading fluency. Intervention focused on multiple oral readings, similar to those used to improve fluency in children. The intervention resulted in an improved reading rate. Cases of acquired pure alexia are much less frequently observed in children (reviewed in Paquier, DeSmet, Marien, Poznanski, & VanBogaert, 2006, and Fiori et al., 2006). Fiori et al. (2006) used fMRI to study a 9-year-old who had suffered brain injury after an anesthetic accident at age 6 years, which required subtotal resection of the left temporal lobe. By age 9 his aphasia had improved, but he still exhibited severe difficulties in reading and writing. fMRI imaging during reading of familiar compared to unfamiliar words demonstrated activation of posterior reading systems, particularly the left occipitotemporal word form area, with familiar words. On the basis of the fMRI, an intervention program focusing on sight words and syllabic units of words was instituted, with subsequent improvement in reading accuracy (though not in fluency). We suppose that the boy had learned to read by using the posterior medial portion of the word form area that appears to support memory systems in reading.

CONCLUSIONS AND FUTURE DIRECTIONS

Within the last two decades, overwhelming evidence from many laboratories has converged to indicate the cognitive basis for dyslexia: Dyslexia represents a disorder within the language system, and more specifically within a particular subcomponent of that system, phonological processing. Recent advances in imaging technology and the development of tasks that sharply isolate the subcomponent processes of reading now allow the localization of phonological processing in the brain; as a result, they provide for the first time the possibility of elucidating a biological signature for reading and reading disability. Converging evidence from a number of laboratories using functional brain imaging indicates a disruption of left hemisphere posterior neural systems while children and adults with dyslexia are performing reading tasks, with an additional suggestion for an associated increased reliance on ancillary systems (e.g., in the frontal lobes and right-hemisphere posterior circuits).

Extended longitudinal studies provide an increasingly appreciated paradigm for the study of the development of neural systems for reading and dyslexia. As noted above, data from the Connecticut Longitudinal Study have been helpful in demonstrating two types of reading disability. Studies are currently underway to further examine the development of reading systems in this group as they enter mature adulthood.

At yet another, more practical level, brain imaging studies offer the possibility of using biological metrics for diagnosing individuals with dyslexia, as well as for evaluating the effects of specific reading interventions not only on groups of children but on individual children. Currently, diagnosis of young adults and of adults who have compensated to some degree for their dyslexia is often difficult. When brain imaging is perfected to allow reliable measures in *individual* subjects with dyslexia, it will be useful, for example, to demonstrate that such individuals have a disruption in the word form area. Furthermore, it is often very difficult to predict dyslexia in preschool children. Here, structural brain imaging may be very helpful in indicating whether a preschool child is at high risk for the development of dyslexia.

Brain imaging may also prove helpful in intervention studies. Thus it may be possible to obtain results of the effects of various interventions with fewer subjects than are currently needed in intervention studies relying only on behavioral measures.

Finally, newer studies demonstrate the importance of fMRI in studies of self-regulation and plasticity. These studies implicitly recognize three distinct but not necessarily incompatible theories of brain development (Johnson, 2001, 2007): a maturational theory (related to newly emerging brain functions associated with specific neuroanatomical development); a skill learning theory (i.e., the development of expertise, similar to the development of face recognition by the fusiform face area); and an interactive specialization theory (wherein certain brain regions are biased toward particular stimuli, and as these stimuli are encountered, the brain systems become attuned to the stimuli and more specialized). Weiskopf et al. (2004) review studies that demonstrate the possibility of physiological self-regulation of the blood-oxygen-level-dependent signal related to neuronal activity and that offer the possibility of using fMRI in biofeedback, paralleling studies using electroencephalographic biofeedback. To demonstrate the utility of such an approach, deCharms et al. (2005) used real-time fMRI to guide training for reduction of chronic pain. Both normal subjects and individuals with chronic pain were able to learn to control activation in the anterior cingulate cortex, an area believed to be involved in pain perception. In addition to biofeedback studies, newer studies using repetitive transcranial magnetic stimulation have been used to modify neural systems (Tegenthoff et al., 2005). We anticipate that in the not too distant future, these newer techniques will be brought to bear on dyslexia—probably first in adults, but eventually in children.

ACKNOWLEDGMENTS

The work described in this chapter was supported by Grant Nos. P50 HD25802, RO1 HD046171, and R01 HD057655 from the National Institute of Child Health and Human Development to Sally E. Shaywitz and Bennett A. Shaywitz, as well as by grants from Eli Lilly Ltd. And the Yale Center for Dyslexia and Creativity. Portions of this chapter are based on S. Shaywitz and Shaywitz (2008) and on S. Shaywitz and Shaywitz (in press).

REFERENCES

Anderson, A., & Gore, J. (1997). The physical basis of neuroimaging techniques. *Child and Adolescent Psychiatric Clinics of North America*, *6*, 213–264.

Aylward, E., Richards, T., Berninger, V., Nagy, W., Field, K., Grimme, A., et al. (2003). Instructional treatment associated with changes in brain activation in children with dyslexia. *Neurology*, *61*, 212–219.

Beeson, P., Magloire, J., & Robey, R. (2005). Letter-by-letter reading: Natural recovery and response to treatment. *Behavioral Neurology*, *16*, 191–202.

Berl, M., Balsamo, L., Xu, B., Moore, E., Weinstein, S., Conry, J., et al. (2005). Seizure focus affects regional language networks assessed by fMRI. *Neurology*, *65*, 1604–1611.

Bradley, L., & Bryant, P. E. (1983). Categorizing sounds and learning to read—a causal connection. *Nature*, *301*, 419–421.

Brown, W. E., Eliez, S., Menon, V., Rumsey, J. M., White, C. D., & Reiss, A. L. (2001). Preliminary evidence of widespread morphological variations of the brain in dyslexia. *Neurology*, *56*(6), 781–783.

Bruck, M. (1998). Outcomes of adults with childhood histories of dyslexia. In C. Hulme & R. Joshi (Eds.), *Cognitive and linguistic bases of reading, writing, and spelling* (pp. 179–200). Mahwah, NJ: Erlbaum.

Bruck, M., & Treiman, R. (1992). Learning to pronounce words: The limitations of analogies. *Reading Research Quarterly*, *27*, 375–388.

Carey, J., Kimberley, T., Lewis, S., Auerbach, E., Dorsey, L., Rundquist, P., et al. (2002). Analysis of fMRI and finger tracking training in subjects with chronic stroke. *Brain*, *125*, 773–788.

Cohen, L., Dehaene, S., Naccache, L., Lehericy, S., Dehaene-Lambertz, G., Henaff, M., et al. (2000). The visual word form area: Spatial and temporal characterization of an initial stage of reading in normal subjects and posterior split-brain patients. *Brain*, *123*, 291–307.

deCharms, C. R., Maeda, F., Glover, G. H., Ludlow, D., Pauly, J. M., Soneji, D., et al. (2005). Control over brain activation and pain learned by using real-time functional MRI. *Proceedings of the National Academy of Sciences USA*, *102*(51), 18626–18631.

Dehaene, S., Cohen, L., Sigman, M., & Vinckier, F. (2005). The neural code for written words: A proposal. *Trends in Cognitive Sciences*, *9*(7), 335–341.

Dehaene, S., Naccache, L., Cohen, L., Le Bihan, D., Mangin, J., Poline, J., et al. (2001). Cerebral mechanisms of word masking and unconscious repetition priming. *Nature Neuroscience*, *4*, 752–758.

Dejerine, J. (1891). Sur un cas de cécité verbale avec agraphie, suivi d'autopsie. *Comptes Rendus de la Société de Biologie*, *43*, 197–201.

Dejerine, J. (1892). Contribution a l'étude anatomo-pathologique et clinique des differentes variétés de cecite verbale. *Mémoires de la Société de Biologie*, *4*, 61–90.

Demb, J., Boynton, G., & Heeger, D. (1998). Functional magnetic resonance imaging of early visual pathways in dyslexia. *Journal of Neuroscience*, *18*, 6939–6951.

Devlin, J., Jamison, H., Gonnerman, L., & Matthews, P. (2006). The role of the posterior fusiform gyrus in reading. *Journal of Cognitive Neuroscience*, *18*(6), 911–922.

Duncan, D. (2009, August 24). Scientist at work: Eric Schadt, enlisting computers to unravel the true complexity of disease. *The New York Times*, p. D3.

Eden, G., Jones, K., Cappell, K., Gareau, L., Wood, F., Zeffiro, T., et al. (2004). Neural changes following remediation in adult developmental dyslexia. *Neuron*, *44*(3), 411–422.

Eden, G., VanMeter, J. W., Rumsey, J. M., Maisog, J. M., Woods, R. P., & Zeffiro, T. A. (1996). Abnormal processing of visual motion in dyslexia revealed by functional brain imaging. *Nature*, *382*, 66–69.

Eliez, S., Rumsey, J. M., Giedd, J. N., Schmitt, J. E., Patwardhan, A. J., & Reiss, A. L. (2000). Morphological alteration of temporal lobe gray matter in dyslexia: An MRI study. *Journal of Child Psychology and Psychiatry*, *41*(5), 637–644.

Fair, D. A., Brown, T. T., Petersen, S. E., & Schlaggar, B. L. (2006). fMRI reveals novel functional neuroanatomy in a child with perinatal stroke. *Neurology*, *67*, 2246–2249.

Felton, R. H., Naylor, C. E., & Wood, F. B. (1990). Neuropsychological profile of adult dyslexics. *Brain and Language*, *39*, 485–497.

Ferrer, E., Shaywitz, B. A., Holahan, J. M., Marchione, K., & Shaywitz, S. E. (2010). Uncoupling of reading and IQ over time: Empirical evidence for a definition of dyslexia. *Psychological Science*, *21*(1) 93–101.

Fiori, A., Huber, W., Dietrich, T., Schnitker, R., Shah, J., Herpertz-Dahlmann, B., et al. (2006). Acquired dyslexia after stroke in the prereading stage: A single case treatment study with fMRI. *Neurocase*, *12*, 252–262.

Fletcher, J., Shaywitz, S., Shankweiler, D., Katz, L., Liberman, I., Stuebing, K., et al. (1994). Cognitive profiles of reading disability: Comparisons of discrepancy and low achievement definitions. *Journal of Educational Psychology*, *86*(1), 6–23.

Fletcher, P., Frith, C., & Rugg, M. (1997). The functional anatomy of episodic memory. *Trends in Neurosciences*, *20*, 213–218.

Frackowiak, R., Friston, K., Frith, C., Dolan, R., Price, C., Zeki, S., et al. (2004). *Human brain function* (2nd ed.). Amsterdam: Elsevier Academic Press.

Francis, D., Shaywitz, S., Steubing, K., Shaywitz, B., & Fletcher, J. (1996). Developmental lag versus deficit models of reading disability: A longitudinal, individual growth curves analysis. *Journal of Educational Psychology*, *88*, 3–17.

Galaburda, A. M., Sherman, G. F., Rosen, G. D., Aboitiz, F., & Geschwind, N. (1985). Developmental dyslexia: Four consecutive patients with cortical anomalies. *Annals of Neurology*, *18*(2), 222–233.

Gauthier, I., Tarr, M., Moylan, J., Skudlarski, P., Gore, J. C., & Anderson, A. (2000). The fusiform "face area" is part of a network that processes faces at the individual level. *Journal of Cognitive Neuroscience*, *123*, 495–504.

Gough, P. B., & Tunmer, W. E. (1986). Decoding, reading, and reading disability. *Remedial and Special Education*, *7*, 6–10.

Helenius, P., Tarkiainen, A., Cornelissen, P., Hansen, P. C., & Salmelin, R. (1999). Dissociation of normal feature analysis and deficient processing of letter-strings in dyslexic adults. *Cerebral Cortex*, *4*, 476–483.

Hertz-Pennier, L., Chiron, C., Jambaque, I., Renaux-Kieffer, V., Van de Moortele, P., Delalande, O., et al. (2002). Late plasticity for language in a child's non-dominant hemisphere: A pre- and post-surgery fMRI study. *Brain*, *125*, 361–372.

Horwitz, B., Rumsey, J. M., & Donohue, B. C. (1998). Functional connectivity of the angular gyrus in normal reading and dyslexia. *Proceedings of the National Academy of Sciences USA*, *95*, 8939–8944.

Interagency Committee on Learning Disabilities. (1987). *Learning disabilities: A report to the U.S. Congress.* Washington, DC: U.S. Government Printing Office.

Jezzard, P., Matthews, P., & Smith, S. (2001). *Functional MRI: An introduction to methods.* Oxford: Oxford University Press.

Johnson, M. H. (2001). Functional brain development in humans. *Nature Reviews Neuroscience*, *2*, 475–483.

Johnson, M. H. (2007). Developing a social brain. *Acta Paediatrica*, *96*, 3–5.

Klingberg, T., Hedehus, M., Temple, E., Salz, T., Gabrieli, J., Moseley, M., et al. (2000). Microstructure of temporo-parietal white matter as a basis for reading ability: Evidence from diffusion tensor magnetic resonance imaging. *Neuron*, *25*, 493–500.

Leff, A., Spitsyna, G., Plant, G., & Wise, R. (2006). Structural anatomy of pure and hemianopic alexia. *Journal of Neurology, Neurosurgery and Psychiatry*, *77*, 1004–1007.

Liberman, I., & Shankweiler, D. (1991). *Phonology and beginning reading: A tutorial.* Hillsdale, NJ: Erlbaum.

Liegeois, F., Connelly, A., Cross, J. H., Boyd, S., Gadian, D., Vargha-Khadem, F., et al. (2004). Language reorganization in children with early-onset lesions of the left hemisphere: An fMRI study. *Brain*, *127*, 1229–1236.

Lyon, G., Shaywitz, S., & Shaywitz, B. (2003). A definition of dyslexia. *Annals of Dyslexia*, *53*, 1–14.

MacLeod, A., Buckner, R., Miezin, F., Petersen, S., & Raichle, M. (1998). Right anterior prefrontal cortex activation during semantic monitoring and working memory. *NeuroImage*, *7*, 41–48.

McCandliss, B., Cohen, L., & Dehaene, S. (2003). The visual word form area: Expertise in reading in the fusiform gyrus. *Trends in Cognitive Sciences*, *7*(7), 293–299.

McCrory, E., Mechelli, A., Frith, U., & Price, C. (2005). More than words: A common neural basis for reading and naming deficits in developmental dyslexia? *Brain, 128*(2), 261–267.

McIntosh, A., Bookstein, F., Haxby, J., & Grady, C. (1996). Spatial pattern analysis of functional brain images using partial least squares. *NeuroImage, 3*, 143–157.

McIntosh, A., Nyberg, L., Bookstein, F., & Tulving, E. (1997). Differential functional connectivity of prefrontal and medial temporal cortices during episodic memory retrieval. *Human Brain Mapping, 5*, 323–327.

Meaburn, E., Harlaar, N., Craig, I., Schalkwyk, L., & Plomin, R. (2008). Quantitative trait locus association scan of early reading disability and ability using pooled DNA and 100K SNP microarrays in a sample of 5760 children. *Molecular Psychiatry, 13*, 729–740.

Morgan, W. P. (1896). A case of congenital word blindness. *British Medical Journal*, 1378.

Morris, R., Stuebing, K., Fletcher, J., Shaywitz, S., Lyon, G., Shankweiler, D., et al. (1998). Subtypes of reading disability: Coherent variability around a phonological core. *Journal of Educational Psychology, 90*, 347–373.

Nakamura, K., Dehaene, S., Jobert, A., Le Bihan, D., & Kouider, S. (2005). Subliminal convergence of *kanji* and *kana* words: Further evidence for functional parcellation of the posterior temporal cortex in visual word perception. *Journal of Cognitive Neuroscience, 17*(6), 954–968.

National Reading Panel. (2000). *Teaching children to read: An evidence based assessment of the scientific research literature on reading and its implications for reading instruction* (NIH Publication No. 00-4754). Washington, DC: U.S. Department of Health and Human Services, Public Health Service, National Institutes of Health, National Institute of Child Health and Human Development.

Noppeney, U., Price, C. J., Duncan, J. S., & Koepp, M. J. (2005). Reading skills after left anterior temporal lobe resection: An fMRI study. *Brain, 128*, 1377–1385.

Paquier, P., DeSmet, H., Marien, P., Poznanski, N., & VanBogaert, P. (2006). Acquired alexia with agraphia syndrome in childhood. *Journal of Child Neurology, 21*(4), 324–330.

Paulesu, E., Demonet, J.-F., Fazio, F., McCrory, E., Chanoine, V., Brunswick, N., et al. (2001). Dyslexia—Cultural diversity and biological unity. *Science, 291*, 2165–2167.

Pennington, B., & Gilger, J. (1996). How is dyslexia transmitted?: Neural, cognitive, and genetic mechanism. In C. H. Chase, G. D. Rosen, & G. F. Sherman (Eds.), *Developmental dyslexia* (pp. 41–61). Baltimore: York Press.

Price, C., Gorno-Tempini, M., Graham, K., Biggio, N., Mechelli, A., Patterson, K., et al. (2003). Normal and pathological reading: converging data from lesion and imaging studies. *NeuroImage, 20*, S30–S41.

Ramus, F., Rosen, S., Dakin, S., Day, B., Castellote, J., White, S., et al. (2003). Theories of developmental dyslexia: Insights from a multiple case study of dyslexic adults. *Brain, 126*, 841–865.

Richards, T., Corina, D., Serafini, S., Steury, K., Echelard, D., Dager, S., et al. (2000). Effects of a phonologically driven treatment for dyslexia on lactate levels measured by proton MRI spectroscopic imaging. *American Journal of Neuroradiology*, *21*, 916–922.

Rumsey, J. M., Andreason, P., Zametkin, A. J., Aquino, T., King, C., Hamburber, S. D., et al. (1992). Failure to activate the left temporoparietal cortex in dyslexia. *Archives of Neurology*, *49*, 527–534.

Salmelin, R., Service, E., Kiesila, P., Uutela, K., & Salonen, O. (1996). Impaired visual word processing in dyslexia revealed with magnetoencephalography. *Annals of Neurology*, *40*, 157–162.

Seki, A., Koeda, T., Sugihara, S., Kamba, M., Hirata, Y., Ogawa, T., et al. (2001). A functional magnetic resonance imaging study during reading in Japanese dyslexic children. *Brain and Development*, *23*, 312–316.

Shankweiler, D., Crain, S., Katz, L., Fowler, A. E., Liberman, A. M., Brady, S. A., et al. (1995). Cognitive profiles of reading-disabled children: Comparison of language skills in phonology, morphology, and syntax. *Psychological Science*, *6*(3), 149–156.

Shankweiler, D., Liberman, I. Y., Mark, L. S., Fowler, C. A., & Fischer, F. W. (1979). The speech code and learning to read. *Journal of Experimental Psychology: Human Learning and Memory*, *5*(6), 531–545.

Share, D. L., & Stanovich, K. E. (1995). Cognitive processes in early reading development: Accommodating individual differences into a model of acquisition. *Issues in Education: Contributions from Educational Psychology*, *1*(1), 1–57.

Shaywitz, B., Fletcher, J. M., Holahan, J. M., & Shaywitz, S. E. (1992). Discrepancy compared to low achievement definitions of reading disability: Results from the Connecticut Longitudinal Study. *Journal of Learning Disabilities*, *25*(10), 639–648.

Shaywitz, B., Holford, T., Holahan, J., Fletcher, J., Stuebing, K., Francis, D., et al. (1995). A Matthew effect for IQ but not for reading: Results from a longitudinal study. *Reading Research Quarterly*, *30*(4), 894–906.

Shaywitz, B., Shaywitz, S., Blachman, B., Pugh, K., Fulbright, R., Skudlarski, P., et al. (2004). Development of left occipito-temporal systems for skilled reading in children after a phonologically-based intervention. *Biological Psychiatry*, *55*, 926–933.

Shaywitz, B., Shaywitz, S., Pugh, K., Mencl, W., Fulbright, R., Skudlarski, P., et al. (2002). Disruption of posterior brain systems for reading in children with developmental dyslexia. *Biological Psychiatry*, *52*(2), 101–110.

Shaywitz, B., Skudlarski, P., Holahan, J., Marchione, K., Constable, R., Fulbright, R., et al. (2007). Age-related changes in reading systems of dyslexic children. *Annals of Neurology*, *61*, 363–370.

Shaywitz, S. (1996). Dyslexia. *Scientific American*, *275*(5), 98–104.

Shaywitz, S. (1998). Current concepts: Dyslexia. *New England Journal of Medicine*, *338*(5), 307–312.

Shaywitz, S. (2003). *Overcoming dyslexia: A new and complete science-based program for reading problems at any level*. New York: Knopf.

Shaywitz, S., Escobar, M., Shaywitz, B., Fletcher, J., & Makuch, R. (1992). Evidence that dyslexia may represent the lower tail of a normal distribution of reading ability. *New England Journal of Medicine*, *326*(3), 145–150.

Shaywitz, S., Fletcher, J., Holahan, J., Shneider, A., Marchione, K., Stuebing, K., et al. (1999). Persistence of dyslexia: The Connecticut Longitudinal Study at adolescence. *Pediatrics, 104*(6), 1351–1359.

Shaywitz, S., Morris, R., & Shaywitz, B. (2008). The Education of dyslexic children from childhood to young adulthood. *Annual Review of Psychology, 59*, 451–475.

Shaywitz, S., & Shaywitz, B. (2008). Paying attention to reading: The neurobiology of reading and dyslexia. *Development and Psychopathology, 20*, 1329–1349.

Shaywitz, S., & Shaywitz, B. (in press). Dyslexia. In K. F. Swaiman, S. Ashwal, D. M. Ferriero, & N. F. Schor (Eds.), *Pediatric neurology: Principles and practice* (5th ed.). Philadelphia: Elsevier.

Shaywitz, S., Shaywitz, B., Fletcher, J., & Escobar, M. (1990). Prevalence of reading disability in boys and girls: Results of the Connecticut Longitudinal Study. *Journal of the American Medical Association, 264*(8), 998–1002.

Shaywitz, S., Shaywitz, B., Fulbright, R., Skudlarski, P., Mencl, W., Constable, R., et al. (2003). Neural systems for compensation and persistence: Young adult outcome of childhood reading disability. *Biological Psychiatry, 54*(1), 25–33.

Simos, P., Fletcher, J., Foorman, B., Francis, D., Castillo, E., Davis, R., et al. (2002). Brain activation profiles during the early stages of reading acquisition. *Journal of Child Neurology, 17*(3), 159–163.

Stanovich, K., & Siegel, L. (1994). Phenotypic performance profile of children with reading disabilities: A regression-based test of the phonological-core variable-difference model. *Journal of Educational Psychology, 86*(1), 24–53.

Talairach, J., & Tournoux, P. (1988). *Coplanar stereotaxic atlas of the human brain: Three-dimensional proportional system. An approach to cerebral imaging.* New York: Thieme Medical.

Tegenthoff, M., Ragert, P., Peger, B., Schwenkreis, P., Forster, A.-F., Nicolas, V., et al. (2005). Improvement of tactile discrimination performance and enlargement of cortical somatosensory maps after 5 Hz rTMS. *PLoS Biology, 3*(11), e362.

Temple, E., Deutsch, G., Poldrack, R., Miller, S., Tallal, P., Merzenich, M., et al. (2003). Neural deficits in children with dyslexia ameliorated by behavioral remediation: Evidence from fMRI. *Proceedings of the National Academy of Sciences USA, 100*(5), 2860–2865.

Temple, E., Poldrack, R., Protopapas, A., Nagarajan, S., Salz, T., Tallal, P., et al. (2000). Disruption of the neural response to rapid acoustic stimuli in dyslexia: Evidence from functional MRI. *Proceedings of the National Academy of Sciences USA, 97*, 13907–13912.

Torgesen, J., & Wagner, R. (1995, May 11). *Alternative diagnostic approaches for specific developmental reading disabilities.* Paper presented at the National Research Council's Board on Testing and Assessment, Workshop on IQ Testing and Educational Decision Making, Washington, DC.

Vinckier, F., Dehaene, S., Jobert, A., Dubus, J., Sigman, M., & Cohen, L. (2007). Hierarchical coding of letter strings in the ventral stream: Dissecting the inner organization of the visual word form system. *Neuron, 55*(1), 143–156.

Wagner, R., & Torgesen, J. (1987). The nature of phonological processes and its causal role in the acquisition of reading skills. *Psychological Bulletin*, *101*, 192–212.

Weiskopf, N., Scharnowski, F., Veit, R., Goebel, R., Birbaumer, N., & Mathiak, K. (2004). Self-regulation of local brain activity using real-time functional magnetic resonance imaging (fMRI). *Journal of Physiology—Paris*, *98*, 357–373.

Woodcock, R., & Johnson, M. (1989). *Woodcock–Johnson Psycho-Educational Battery—Revised (WJ-R)*. Allen, TX: Developmental Learning Materials.

CHAPTER 9

Neuroplasticity and Rehabilitation of Attention in Children

JENNIFER A. ENGLE
KIMBERLY A. KERNS

> If I have ever made any valuable discoveries, it has been owing more to patient attention, than to any other talent.
>
> —ISAAC NEWTON

Although there is controversy over what specific aspects of cognitive functions compose the concept of *attention*, there is general agreement that attention can be divided into several components, each of which is associated with an underlying neural system (Kerns & Mateer, 1996; Sohlberg & Mateer, 2001b). These systems, which are complex, highly integrated, and slow to develop, are especially vulnerable to dysfunction associated with developmental disorders or damage from acquired brain injury.

Dysfunction of attention can have far-reaching impact. Intact attention is vital for the utilization of higher-level functions. For example, impaired attention may lead to difficulty in learning new information, and therefore may present as memory problems. In addition, if information is not attended to, that information cannot be used to help solve problems and guide appropriate behavior. Children who cannot pay attention in class will be disadvantaged in academic situations, which could potentially show a "snowball effect," as basic skills required for later learning are not acquired. Peer socialization may also be affected by impaired attention, as attention is necessary in order to navigate complex social situations successfully.

Adults with attention and other cognitive deficits may be reintegrated into their home and work lives with external supports and training in key specific skills, such as driving, vocational, and adaptive living skills (see Park & Ingles, 2001, for a review). Reacquisition of these important specific, functional skills allows an individual to live with a maximal amount of independence. A retrained skill typically relies on intact brain systems; that is, the skill is rerouted through new neural mechanisms. Generalization to untrained skills is not expected.

Children with attention and other cognitive deficits, however, must function in the dynamic environment of school, where the ability to learn is more important than acquisition of specific skills. Therefore, children have the most to benefit from an approach that directly improves the function of the networks underlying attention. Increased neural plasticity (especially in younger children) also makes children especially suited to benefiting from this approach. This chapter examines direct approaches to attention rehabilitation in children, focusing on plasticity of neural systems in the developing brain.

BRAIN DAMAGE/DYSFUNCTION IN CHILDREN

Three groups of children have been the primary foci of research in attention rehabilitation: (1) children with acquired brain injury; (2) children with attention deficits, including attention-deficit/hyperactivity disorder (ADHD); and (3) children who have received cancer treatment affecting the central nervous system (CNS), or whose cancer directly affects the CNS. Recently, some work has also been done on children with reading disabilities, children with Fetal Alcohol Spectrum Disorders, and on typically developing preschoolers. This section examines epidemiology, pathophysiology, and associated behavioral, cognitive, and socioemotional problems for each of the three main groups typically studied.

Acquired Brain Injury

Acquired brain injury is a serious public health concern for children. Traumatic brain injury (TBI) is the most frequent cause of death and new disabilities in childhood (Luerssen, 1991). Less common forms of acquired brain injury include stroke, anoxia, infection, chemical poisoning, and tumor.

In the pediatric population, stroke can be classified as perinatal (28 weeks' gestation to 1 month of age) or childhood (1 month of age to 18 years). Perinatal stroke is estimated to occur in approximately 1 in 4,000 live births. Perinatal strokes typically involve occlusion of the middle cerebral artery due to thromoboembolism from a cranial vessel, the heart, or the placenta (Lynch & Nelson, 2001). Childhood strokes are less common, with an estimated incidence rate ranging from 1.3 to 13 per 100,000 children per year. More than half of these children will suffer permanent motor or cognitive disability, and 5–20% will not survive. The most common causes of childhood strokes are cardiac disorders, blood disorders, vasculopathies, and viral infections (Lynch, 2004). Max et al. (2002) found that strokes involving the frequently affected dopamine-rich ventral posterior putamen were associated with the development of postinjury ADHD or traits of ADHD. The clinical profile of children with ADHD following stroke was similar to the predominantly inattentive type of ADHD, rather than the more common combined type, which includes aspects of impulsivity and hyperactivity (Max et al., 2005).

Estimates of TBI incidence vary widely, due to differences in injury definitions, criteria for diagnosis, and sources of data. Across research studies, Kraus (1995) found an annual incidence rate of 180 per 100,000 children (from birth to age 14) admitted to hospital with medical diagnoses of brain injury. This number was averaged across studies from three countries and six U.S. states. A more recent analysis examined data from the Centers for Disease Control and Prevention in three representative states and summarized TBI-related deaths, hospitalizations, and emergency department visits for children from birth to age 14, between 1995 and 2001 (Langlois, Rutland-Brown, & Thomas, 2005). This study found much lower hospitalization rates than previously documented, presumably due to changes in hospital admission practices (i.e., more individuals are now served in an outpatient setting). Per 100,000 children from birth to age 14, the average annual death rate from TBI was 4.5, hospitalizations were 63, and emergency department visits were 731. When the data were examined by age, the highest rates in each category were in the birth-to-4 age group. In addition, for this youngest age group, rates for hospitalizations and deaths were significantly higher for blacks than for whites. Causes of injury also varied by age. Infants were most likely to be injured by falls or child abuse. As children become more mobile in the preschool years, they were more at risk for pedestrian accidents and falls. School-age children were most likely to be injured by sporting, cycling, pedestrian, and motor vehicle accidents (Anderson, Northam, Hendy, & Wrennall, 2001; Langlois et al., 2005). Finally, studies consistently show differences in epidemiology by gender: Males are at greater risk than females, with ratios varying between 1.6:1 and 2.8:1 (Kraus & Chu, 2005).

Penetrating brain injuries are relatively rare in children, accounting for only about 10% of TBIs (Anderson et al., 2001). Such injuries may result from the penetration of skull fragments into the brain or from the penetration of a foreign object. Damage from a penetrating head injury tends to be localized, frequently leading to specific neurological deficits and/or post-traumatic epilepsy.

In the more common closed head injury, there are typically multiple sites of injury, as well as diffuse axonal damage caused by the stretching and tearing of the long axonal fibers that connect the brainstem to the cortex. Due to the structure of the brain and skull, areas most vulnerable to injury include the orbitofrontal regions and the temporal lobes (Anderson et al., 2001). Following the initial damage from injury, further damage may occur secondary to *excitotoxicity* (high levels of excitatory amino acids immediately following injury). Excitotoxicity may disrupt cell function and lead to cell death. Damage to blood vessels, increase in fluid in the brain, or failure of autoregulatory mechanisms of cerebral blood flow may lead to the formation of hematomas, cerebral edema, or raised intracranial pressure, resulting in decreased consciousness and risk of death (Anderson et al., 2001).

As the causes of brain injury frequently differ between children and adults, differences in pathophysiology and functional outcome can also be expected. However, it is also important to recognize that even the seemingly same injury can manifest quite different results in children and adults, due to physical differences in CNS development, vascular structure, musculature, and skull development.

Kennard (1938, 1940) was the first person to systematically study the effect of early brain damage. She found that infant monkeys with unilateral motor cortex lesions had milder impairments than adult monkeys with the same injury. Kennard hypothesized that infant monkeys had greater capacity for cortical reorganization following brain damage. This notion is based on the idea that the immature brain has large unused *equipotential* areas, which have the capacity to take over functioning from damaged tissue (Luria, 1963). The notion that "If you are going to have a brain injury, do it early," dubbed the "Kennard principle," (Teuber, 1962) became clinical folklore.

Hebb (1949) was the first to clearly contradict the Kennard principle, as he found that children with early frontal lobe injuries had more severe functional impairments than adults with similarly sized injuries. He proposed that early injuries prevent the development of appropriate intellectual capacity integral to normal development. The heuristic proposed by Dennis (1988) may best clarify this concept. According to this heuristic, if a skill or behavior associated with the affected brain region is in the early process of development (not yet expected to be mature), an injured child will not immediately look different from his or her peers. The child may appear to "recover" quite quickly. Problems are expected to emerge later, when the skill typically develops. There is considerable evidence from both animal research (e.g., Goldman-Rakic, Isseroff, Schwartz, & Bugbee, 1983) and human studies (e.g., Banich, Cohen-Levine, Kim, & Huttenlocher, 1990) to support this notion, which has been called "growing into deficit." Age at injury appears to be most important for those injured in the preschool or early childhood years, and less important in late childhood and early adolescence (Anderson & Pentland, 1998).

In addition to differences in cognitive development, infants and young children have certain structural and neurological features that may affect the outcome of a brain injury. Infants have weak neck muscles, which, when combined with their proportionally large heads, make them more susceptible to jarring forces. In addition, the relatively thin skull of a young child is more susceptible to skull fractures than that of an adult. On the other hand, young children are less likely to suffer contusions, lacerations, and subdural hematomas, likely due to the flexibility and open sutures in the young skull (Anderson et al., 2001). Children's brains are less myelinated, and thus softer and better able to absorb the force of an impact. However, unmyelinated fibers are more vulnerable to shearing effects, leading to a higher likelihood of diffuse axonal injury (Anderson et al., 2001). Finally, although young children are less likely to lose consciousness, children are approximately twice as likely as adults to suffer from posttraumatic seizures, particularly in the first weeks after severe TBI (Yablon, 1993). The immature brain, with its numerous neural connections, requires considerable energy expenditure. This makes the brain more susceptible to seizures as well as anoxia.

The most common neuropsychological sequelae following brain injury in children are the same as in adults: deficits in attention, concentration, memory, and executive function (Sohlberg & Mateer, 2001b). Children are still developing skills, and skill development is dependent upon adequate executive and attention skills (e.g., efficient approach to a task, attention in a learning environment); thus children are more susceptible to a broad range of impairments from brain damage, especially prefrontal damage (Anderson, Jacobs, & Harvey, 2005). IQ scores in children are often generally depressed both in the acute phase (Catroppa & Anderson, 1999) and in the long term (circumscribed prefrontal lesions—Anderson et al., 2005; moderate to severe TBI—Anderson & Pentland, 1998). In addition to depression of overall intellectual function, moderate deficits were found across a number of neuropsychological domains, including measures of construction skills, expressive language, learning, memory, attention, and executive function, when children with moderate to severe brain injuries were compared to orthopedic controls (Taylor et al., 2002).

In addition to neuropsychological deficits, TBI in children is associated with socioemotional problems, behavioral problems, and impaired academic performance. Recent research has attempted to distinguish sequelae that can be directly attributed to brain injury from outcomes that are moderated by other variables, such as family factors or adjustment issues. One robust finding is that moderate to severe TBI is related to poor outcomes across a variety of neuropsychological domains, with a dose–response relationship between severity of injury and neuropsychological functioning (Anderson et al., 2006; Yeates et al., 2002). Severity of injury is also related to behavioral and academic problems (Taylor et al., 2002). Family factors, such as socioeconomic status, are important moderators of group differences in long-term behavioral and academic outcome. Children from more disadvantaged families show greater long-term decline in academic performance, less rapid short-term progress in social skills, and greater long-term behavioral sequelae (Taylor et al., 2002). However, unlike injury severity, family factors do not appear to have a direct impact on recovery of cognitive function (Yeates et al., 2002).

Work by Anderson and Buffery (1982, as cited in Anderson et al., 2001) helped differentiate which emotional and behavioral outcomes in children were direct results of brain injury and which outcomes were more likely to reflect psychosocial adjustment to the changes following TBI. Aggressive, hyperactive, and impulsive behavior, as well as difficulty in expressing and perceiving emotions, were specific to children with right anterior pathology, and therefore believed to be direct results of a frontal injury. Depression and anxiety were common symptoms regardless of injury site, and were therefore believed to be reactions to the changes associated with TBI.

In addition to severity of injury, other important factors in predicting the outcome of brain injury are the focalized nature and laterality of the lesion. These factors are especially important in the developing brain, as evidence suggests that normal postnatal development involves a gradual change from diffuse, bilateral representation of function to an increasingly localized representation. Localization of function in the mature brain is thought to increase the efficiency and accuracy of information processing by decreasing the interference seen when more than one task uses the same brain area at the same time. In addition, restricting functions to certain areas frees up space for later-developing functions, such as reading and higher mathematics (Huttenlocher, 2002). Therefore, a focal lesion in infants or young children will lead to a less specific deficit than a similar lesion in an adult, but will be associated with more global dysfunction. When a healthy region of the young brain takes over the function of a damaged region, the healthy region has less capacity to serve its intended function. In addition, there are fewer synaptic sites available to be taken up by new, emerging skills, leading to a "crowding" of functions. This has been shown in individuals who had early lesions involving left-hemisphere speech areas. Whereas a significant minority of children injured young (before age 5) showed a shift of language function to the right hemisphere (Rasmussen & Milner, 1977), there were costs to this recovery: a deficit in "right-hemisphere functions," such as copying a figure and imitating complex arm movements; an overall drop in IQ; and limitations in the development of complex language structures (Kolb & Milner, 1981; Mateer & Dodrill, 1983; Woods & Teuber, 1973).

Animal research has found that even large unilateral frontal lesions in perinatal rats are associated with good functional recovery. However, recovery from unilateral lesions can be entirely eliminated by the addition of even a very small injury to the contralateral hemisphere (Kolb, Gibb, & Gorny, 2000). A human correlate of this was a case study of a 6½-year-old boy with a small lesion in the sensory–motor strip in the right hemisphere, in addition to a lesion in Broca's area in the left hemisphere. In this case, speech did not move from the left to the right hemisphere, despite the intact homologue to Broca's area on the right side (Vargha-Khadem, Watters, & O'Gorman, 1985).

Cancer and Its Treatment

Leukemia is the most common cancer in childhood and adolescence, accounting for one-third of cancers in children under the age of 15. Acute lymphoblastic leukemia (ALL) is the most common leukemia of childhood, with annual incidence varying from 2 to 8 per 100,000, depending on the specific age group. The 5-year survival rate for ALL is now 80%, due to advances in treatment in the last decades. With a growing population of ALL survivors, there has been much attention to the long-term effects of cancer treatment. Next to ALL, CNS malignancies constitute the second most frequently diagnosed form of pediatric cancer, with an annual incidence of 2.7 per 100,000. Survival rates of brain tumors vary considerably among tumor types (Ries et al., 1999).

Prophylactic CNS cancer treatments are designed to reach cancer cells that may survive behind the protection of the blood–brain barrier. They are typically given once remission is achieved, as the CNS is a common site of relapse (Anderson, Godber, Smibert, & Ekert, 1997). In the past, prophylactic treatment typically involved cranial irradiation therapy (CRT) in combination with intrathecal (IT) chemotherapy (chemotherapy delivered directly to the CNS), sometimes CRT in combination with steroids, or IT chemotherapy alone. In recent years, evidence has been mounting for the neuropathological and neuropsychological aftereffects of CRT, whereas evidence for the aftereffects of IT chemotherapy by itself has been less consistent (for reviews, see Butler & Mulhern, 2005; Moleski, 2000). Because IT chemotherapy appears to be as effective as CRT in the prevention of CNS relapse, with less evidence of harm, it has become the standard prophylactic treatment. CRT is typically reserved for treatment of CNS relapse or for very high-risk individuals, including children with CNS malignancies. IT chemotherapy, although generally considered less harmful than CRT, is associated with some degree of cognitive impairment in at least 30% of children who receive it (Copeland, Moore, Francis, Jaffe, & Culbert, 1996). Evidence has also emerged that certain corticosteroids typically administered with chemotherapy may cause an increase in cognitive difficulties. Specifically, dexamethasone, which has become more commonly used because of its effectiveness, has been found to be more neurotoxic than prednisone (Waber et al., 2000).

Butler and Mulhern (2005) summarized the impact of CNS cancer treatment by dividing sequelae into *core deficits*, which include deficits in executive functions, attention, speed of processing, and working memory, and *secondary deficits*, which are primarily deficits in knowledge-based (crystallized) abilities. Research into the pathology underlying core deficits has found that CRT is associated with white matter hypodensity, calcifications, and widening of the ventricles and subarachnoid space. Demyelination and vascular lesions have been implicated as the causes of these cerebral abnormalities. The location of intracerebral calcifications tends to be bilateral, with the basal ganglia (associated with attention and expressive language) a frequent site of injury (Anderson et al., 1997). A study of childhood survivors of brain tumor treated with CRT found that deficits in attention could explain a significant amount of the relationship between reduced volumes of normal-appearing white matter in the brain and reduced IQ (Reddick et al., 2003).

Early studies suggested that deficits take some time to emerge following treatment, which may parallel findings of delayed neuropathology following CRT with IT chemotherapy (Riccardi, Brouwers, Di Chiro, & Poplack, 1985). These declines in ability are particularly associated with specific risk factors, such as younger age at treatment, higher doses of CRT (Anderson, Godber, Smibert, Weiskop, & Ekert, 2000), and higher doses of chemotherapy (Buizer, De Sonneville, Van Den Heuvel-Eibrink, Njiokiktjien, & Veerman, 2005). However, it is possible that long-term declines may also be related to a failure to acquire age-appropriate skills.

Schatz, Kramer, Ablin, and Mattay (2000) developed a model to explain the emergence of deficits over time. Their work is based on the assumption that improvements in processing speed may be necessary for the development of working memory, which in turn is necessary for development of fluid intelligence. They hypothesized that CRT affects processing speed, which in turn affects working memory, which then lowers IQ. From an examination of 23 children with ALL treated with CRT plus IT chemotherapy or IT chemotherapy alone, Schatz et al. concluded that delayed IQ deficits following CRT are indeed affected by deficits in processing speed, but that deficits in working memory are above what would be expected from processing speed deficits alone. Ultimately, they concluded that both processing speed and working memory deficits lead to impairment in IQ.

Attention-Deficit/Hyperactivity Disorder

ADHD occurs in approximately 3–7% of the school-age population (American Psychiatric Association [APA], 2000). It is one of the most commonly diagnosed disorders of childhood, accounting for nearly 50% of child referrals to outpatient clinics (Adams & Sutker, 2001). The disorder typically manifests itself before age 7, is present in two or more settings (e.g., home and school), and is relatively persistent (APA, 2000). The current version of the *Diagnostic and Statistical Manual of Mental Disorders* (DSM-IV-TR) specifies three subtypes of ADHD: predominantly inattentive, predominantly hyperactive–impulsive (relatively rare, typically seen in preschool age), and combined inattentive and hyperactive–impulsive (APA, 2000). There are currently no cognitive, neuropathological, or neuropsychological indicators that are capable of clearly identifying individuals affected by ADHD. Therefore, diagnosis is typically based on parent and teacher report.

There is strong evidence for heritability in ADHD, but environmental causes (e.g., lead poisoning, dietary factors) are suspected of being causal in a small percentage of children with ADHD (Adams & Sutker, 2001), indicating that the same pattern of behavioral and cognitive deficits can arise from multiple pathways. Several decades of research provide much evidence for abnormalities in the dopamine-mediated prefrontal–striatal–cerebellar circuits in the combined type of ADHD (Barkley, 1997). Although their exact mechanism is unknown, stimulant medications that facilitate release and block reuptake of norepinephrine and dopamine have been found to be effective in treating ADHD (Pliszka, 2006). However, the benefits of stimulant medications are typically considered not to be maintained once medications are discontinued (though see Plizka, Lancaster, Liott, Semrud-Clikeman, 2006, as described later in this chapter). Neuropathological research reports that ADHD is associated with differences in the corpus callosum, the striatum (particularly the caudate nucleus), the anterior cingulate cortex, the cerebellum (particularly the vermis), and the frontal lobe (see Krain & Castellanos, 2006, for a review). Moreover, a meta-analysis found strong support for the notion that children with ADHD have reduced overall brain volumes (Castellanos & Acosta, 2004).

Many have suggested that the predominantly inattentive type of ADHD has distinctly different characteristics and underlying neuropathology/neurochemistry, and therefore should be considered a separate disorder (Barkley, 1997). Diamond (2005) has suggested that the predominantly inattentive type is an example of childhood-onset dysexecutive syndrome, with a core deficit in working memory. In contrast to the combined type of ADHD, the inattentive type is associated with deficits primarily in the prefrontal cortex, with frontoparietal circuits additionally affected. Examination of differences among subtypes is relatively new, and more research is clearly necessary (see Baeyens, Roeyers, & Walle, 2006, for a review).

REHABILITATION

A classification outlined by Robertson and Murre (1999) provides a helpful framework within which to approach rehabilitation. In children with mild injuries, neurons or networks of neurons that were disconnected may regain their original patterns of connections through the normal dynamic learning processes. Therefore, children with these types of injuries typically recover without intervention. In children with severe lesions, there may be little or no recovery, and therefore intervention should focus on compensation by intact brain areas. This type of supportive intervention includes such approaches as memory books, external cueing systems, visual aids, and organizers, as well as training in specific skills (such as vocational activities). Between the groups with mild and severe injuries, there is a middle group of individuals for whom recovery depends on rehabilitative, experience-dependent input. Also included in this group are children with developmental disorders who show similar levels of impairment in cognitive functioning. The children in this middle group are the ones addressed in this chapter. These individuals have impairments, but also have residual abilities that can be capitalized on by focused interventions.

A central thesis of this chapter is that attention in children can be improved with direct, focused intervention, and that underlying this improvement are changes in the neurocircuitry supporting attention. Attention is a key function, and therefore its improvement can have a broad impact on cognitive functioning. However, because brain injuries and developmental disorders are complex and highly individualized, attention rehabilitation should be but one aspect of a broader intervention that should include various additional services (as needed). These services may include psychoeducation, implementation of new teaching strategies, environmental modifications and support, speech and language therapy, direct academic remediation, and provision of emotional support for the affected individual and the family.

The Process Approach

How and Why?

Beginning in the late 1980s, there has been an increasing interest in providing direct training to rehabilitate basic attention processes (the *process approach*) after acquired brain injury. This type of training typically involves a series of repetitive drills or exercises, which become increasingly difficult as the client's skills improve. The theoretical basis of the process approach is that repeated activation and stimulation of basic attentional processes strengthens and/or reconnects neural pathways necessary for attention function, thereby improving cognitive capacity.

The process approach is exemplified by the Attention Process Training (APT) program (Sohlberg & Mateer, 2001a). The Pay Attention! program (Thomson, Kerns, Seidenstrang, Sohlberg, & Mateer, 2001) is a modification of APT for young children, in which the content have been modified so that the basic cognitive skills are at a child's level and the materials have been made more engaging for children.

A key principle of the process approach to attention training is that the treatment must be grounded in attention theory (Sohlberg & Mateer, 2001b; Thomson et al., 2001). The APT and Pay Attention! programs are based on Sohlberg and Mateer's (1987) clinical model of attention. This model was developed through observation and analysis of task performance, errors, and subjective complaints by persons with brain injury, in concert with cognitive theories of attention. In this model, attention is divided into five hierarchical components: *focused attention* (basic responding to stimuli, a function of basic arousal—not typically addressed in process training); *sustained attention* (vigilance, working memory); *selective attention* (ability to withstand distraction); *alternating attention* (mental flexibility); and *divided attention* (response to two or more tasks simultaneously). Experimental evidence to support training specific aspects of attention rather than attention in general comes from Sturm, Wilmes, and Orgass (1997), who showed that training specific aspects of attention led to specific improvements in those components.

In APT and Pay Attention!, one or two components of attention are chosen for training. Three or four tasks may be utilized at once within each component. For example, within the sustained visual attention component of Pay Attention!, a child is presented with a deck of cards; each card presents a different "person" with variously salient characteristics (e.g., gender, age, hair color, family name). Various tasks are completed with the cards. For example, the child may be asked to sort the cards into two stacks—one for each gender, or one for individuals with brown hair color and one for all other hair colors. Or, at a more complex level, the child may be required to sort based on two characteristics—for example, separating the cards into different stacks by gender, while placing all characters with blonde hair face down.

With any process-specific training, exercises should be organized hierarchically (Sohlberg & Mateer, 2001b). An important feature of the clinical model is that intact lower-level attentional skills (e.g., focused and sustained attention) are necessary for the function of higher-level attentional skills (e.g., alternating and divided attention). Therefore, intervention should begin with lower-level components, gradually increasing the difficulty level, and moving to higher-order attentional skills once mastery of the lower-order skills is demonstrated. Treatment must be based on the individual client's skill level (Sohlberg & Mateer, 2001b). The appropriate starting level is determined by a preintervention assessment. Again, experimental evidence in support of this principle in adults comes from Sturm et al. (1997), who demonstrated that training in sustained attention increased basic as well as more complex attentional processes. However, if higher levels of attention were trained before lower levels were established, attention did not improve, and even declined in some cases.

A case example highlighting the importance of this principle is found in Thomson and Kerns (2000). A 9-year-old girl of above-average intelligence received eight 1-hour APT sessions 2 years after a TBI. During the initial sessions, she put forth adequate effort, but appeared quite frustrated and was making little improvement. When the therapist went back to tasks that were simpler and lower in the hierarchy, she began to show the expected trend in improvement, and eventually worked well beyond the tasks with which she originally had made no gains. In the Pay Attention! program, children generally begin with sustained attention and work toward alternating and divided attention. Tasks within each attentional component become more difficult as a child becomes more proficient (e.g., distractors are added or the tasks are made more complex). As a general guideline, when a child reaches 90–100% accuracy on three consecutive sessions, the therapist progresses to the next task.

Another guiding principle of process training is that the training must provide sufficient repetition to reestablish neural pathways underlying attention skills (Sohlberg & Mateer, 2001b). There is evidence from motor rehabilitation therapy that highly repetitive hand and finger movements improved hand function significantly better than therapy consisting of a range of movements (Butefisch, Hummelsheim, Denzler, & Mauritz, 1995). Similar to this approach to physical rehabilitation, the process approach to attention training is based on the Hebbian principle (Hebb, 1949) that "neurons that fire together, wire together." Coactivation of neurons produces changes in the synapses, making it more likely that the neurons will fire together in the future. Repetition is required to link these pathways firmly.

Finally, a key component of the process approach is the incorporation of activities intended to facilitate generalization of skills from therapy to real-world activities (Sohlberg & Mateer, 2001b). Clients should be encouraged to practice attention skills in their everyday environment. For children, this typically will require collaboration with a "coach" in the school or home. Measurement of the extent of generalization to everyday activities provides an assessment of the success of the intervention. For example, measurements at school may include number of off-task behaviors during a certain time period, or time taken to complete a homework sheet.

Research Support

A growing body of literature supports the efficacy of the process approach to attention rehabilitation during the postacute stage following acquired brain injury in adults (for reviews, see Cappa et al., 2005; Cicerone et al.,

2005; Lincoln, Majid, & Weyman, 2005; Michel & Mateer, 2006; Park & Ingles, 2001; Sohlberg et al., 2003).

In children, there is a much smaller body of literature (see Penkman, 2004, for a review). The Pay Attention! program has been used successfully for young children with ADHD (Kerns, Eso, & Thomson, 1999). Fourteen children ages 7–11 participated in two 30-minute sessions per week for 8 weeks. Results showed that the children who participated in Pay Attention! did significantly better on untrained tasks of attention and academic efficiency than a control group who participated in a "sham" condition (non-attention-training, computer-based activities). However, teacher reports showed no change in either group, while parent reports indicated that both groups improved. Tamm, Hughes, Ames, Pickering, Silver, et al. (2010) found similar results in 19 children with ADHD (ages 8–14) using the Pay Attention! Program.

APT materials were also used successfully for children with ADHD (Semrud-Clikeman et al., 1999). Twenty-one school-recruited children ages 8–12 participated in APT and problem-solving training in small groups (2 hours per week for approximately 18 weeks). These children improved to the level of nonclinical (untreated) controls on untrained measures of visual and auditory attention. Twelve children with ADHD who did not receive treatment showed only minimal change. Parent and teacher reports were only collected before the intervention; therefore, the impact of the intervention on everyday functioning was not determined.

APT has also been used in children with acquired brain injury. Thomson and Kerns (2000) reported two case studies using APT materials. A 9-year-old (see above) and a 17-year-old with mild TBI underwent 8 weeks of 1-hour training sessions. Both individuals showed considerable improvement on untrained tests of attention, and in some cases on executive function and memory tasks. Thomson (1995), using APT materials, conducted a small-group, multiple-baseline study with six adolescents ages 14–17. Following 12 weeks of three 30-minute sessions per week, participants in treatment showed improvements in sustained attention, reading speed, and math performance.

Other direct approaches utilize computerized materials for process-specific attention training. Brett and Laatsch (1998) implemented a cognitive rehabilitation program in a public high school for 10 students (9 with TBI, 1 with viral encephalopathy). Treatment was provided by specially trained teachers and was held during 40-minute blocks, approximately biweekly over about a 20-week period (the total number of sessions varied from 18 to 42). Training included individualized or small-group computerized, hierarchical attention training and metacognitive strategy training. Significant posttreatment improvement was found for verbal memory skills, but intellectual functioning and performance on other tasks did not change significantly. Despite demonstrating the ability to bring rehabilitation into the school setting, this study was not able to demonstrate its utility. This study also highlighted the challenges of having teachers provide rehabilitation (i.e., training and support needs).

Computerized Progressive Attentional Training (CPAT) is a computerized program with gradual progression across difficulty levels and direct, immediate feedback on progress. CPAT is based on Posner and Petersen's (1990) theory of attention networks. Each unit within the individualized training program intensively exercises one of four networks: sustained attention, selective attention, orienting attention, or executive attention. In a recent study using CPAT (Shalev, Tsal, & Mevorach, 2007), 20 children with ADHD (ages 6–13), participated in 8 weeks of training, with two 1-hour sessions per week. A control group participated in various computer and paper-and-pencil tasks, also with multiple levels of difficulty and feedback. Pre- and posttests included academic measures of math, reading comprehension, and passage copying, as well as parent rating scales. Compared to the control group, the treatment group showed significantly greater improvement in reading comprehension, passage copying, and parent-rated inattention symptoms. The CPAT was also used in a group of 10 children (ages 6–15) with a Fetal Alcohol Spectrum Disorder (Kerns, MacSween, Vander Wekken, & Gruppuso, 2010). Following approximately 16 hours of training, including provision of metacognitive strategies, there was significant pre- to posttest improvement in several neuropsychological measures of attention and working memory, as well as generalization to measures of reading and math fluency.

Klingberg and colleagues have also developed a computerized process training approach for children with ADHD. Their approach focuses on training a specific aspect of executive functioning proposed to be of particular importance in ADHD: working memory (Barkley, 1997). High-intensity working memory training in adults was associated with improvement on untrained measures of working memory. In addition, functional magnetic resonance imaging (fMRI) showed training-induced increases in neural activity in prefrontal and parietal cortices (Olesen, Westerberg, & Klingberg, 2004). The approach taken by Klingberg and colleagues rests on the theory that working memory underlies other cognitive abilities, such as logical reasoning and problem solving, and therefore improvement in working memory should lead to improvement across a number of key functions.

Klingberg and colleagues conducted high-intensity working memory training with two groups of children with ADHD (off medication) over a 5-week period: a small study with 14 children (Klingberg, Forssberg, & Westerberg, 2002), and a larger, randomized, double-blind study with 53 children (Klingberg et al., 2005). The treatment group included increasingly difficult working memory training, while the control group's activities remained at a simple level throughout. In addition to including a larger sample size, a 3-month follow-up, and parent/teacher ratings, the 2005 study equalized the amount of training between groups, so that the treatment and control groups both completed the same number of trials daily. In both studies, the treatment group showed significantly better improvement than the control group on untrained working memory, executive, and problem-solving tasks. Importantly, all of these improvements remained at the 3-month follow-up (although some decreased in strength). In the 2002 study, the treatment group showed a significant decrease in head movements compared to the control group, which was associated with improvement on working memory tasks. However, this finding was not replicated in the 2005 study. In the 2005 study, parent ratings (but not teacher ratings) of inattention and hyperactivity showed significant improvements in the treatment group. These are important findings, suggesting that working memory training transfers to long-lasting improvement in executive functions, as well as everyday functioning.

In addition to showing the efficacy of working memory training in children with ADHD, this study provides experimental evidence for one of the foundations of process training: It is not simply the repetitive stimulation of basic processes (i.e., the control condition in this study) that activates change, but rather the individualized, increasingly challenging, hierarchical stimulation of processes. Klingberg and colleagues' research also provides an important link between process training and changes in neurophysiology in adults. A replication of the imaging data in children would provide a nice complement to these studies.

Another computerized cognitive rehabilitation program, Captain's Log (Sanford & Browne, 1988), contains several units that focus on training specific cognitive functions, including attention, visual–motor abilities, memory, and high-order conceptual skills. The attention modules, which increase in difficulty as a child progresses, were designed according to the Sohlberg and Mateer (1987) model. Kotwal, Burns, and Montgomery (1996) used the attention and concentration units of the program in a case study intervention with a 13-year-old boy with ADHD. Pre- and posttests included the Conners Parent and Teacher Rating Scales, measures of intellectual functioning, and electrophysiological measures (electromyography [EMG] and electroencephalographic [EEG] theta, beta, and theta–beta ratio). Thirty-five sessions of hierarchical training were conducted over 3 months. Postintervention assessment revealed significant improvement according to parent ratings. Teacher ratings were inconsistent across subscales, although verbal report was consistent with parent ratings. Parent ratings at a 7-month follow-up were nearly all maintained. There was no change in intellectual functioning with training. EEG outcomes were surprising in that although theta waves were reduced (as expected), beta waves were also reduced, leading to an overall increase in the theta–beta ratio. These changes remained, and even increased, at follow-up. Posttest reduction in another aspect of EEG was associated with reduction in facial EMG activity; this change was reversed on follow-up.

Integration into a Comprehensive Intervention

A common theme of these studies is that with training, improvement is found on trained and untrained measures of attention, suggesting that process-specific attention training does indeed improve underlying attentional processes. This effect appears to be specific to attention although in some cases it includes memory and executive functions. There is insufficient evidence to claim generalization to improvements in overall IQ or academic functions, or to changes in attention, hyperactivity, or impulsivity as observed by parents and teachers. Partly this is due to a lack of examination of these variables. It also suggests that intervention programs should attend more to generalization of skills to everyday environments by actively incorporating generalization activities into the program. The Cognitive Remediation Program (CRP) developed by Butler and colleagues is an example of an intervention program which does just that.

Butler and Copeland (2002) developed the CRP for children who had received CNS cancer treatment. It involves a three-part approach: (1) activities designed to strengthen attentional skills and processing speed (modified APT or Pay Attention!); (2) metacognitive strategies designed to improve preparedness, task approach, on-task behavior, and generalization; and (3) cognitive behavioral interventions intended to improve resistance to distraction through internal dialogue as well as provide specific mnemonic strategies. Generalization activities include asking the child to describe instances where strategies were used at school, having the child complete homework during training sessions, and providing homework to be completed between sessions. Parents and teachers are considered members of the treatment team; they are informed of the strategies used in sessions, so that they may help promote their use at home and school. Direct contact with the primary teacher also helps to address concerns and make recommendations for accommodations in the classroom.

The pilot project for the CRP consisted of 50 hours of direct treatment over 6 months. Children were seen once per week for 2-hour sessions. Participants included 21 cancer survivors with CNS involvement or with treatment likely to have affected the CNS (ages 6–22). The control group included 6 children with similar diagnoses/treatment, who were either on the waiting list for the CRP or could not participate because of distance from the training center. Pre- and posttest measures included the overall index from the Conners Continuous Performance Test (C-CPT), Digit Span from the Wechsler Intelligence Scale for Children—Third Edition, a sentence memory task, and a test of arithmetic skills (to measure generalization).

The groups were similar in gender composition, age, years posttreatment, and mean dosage of CRT. At pretest, the CRP group had a higher Digit Span scaled score, but otherwise the groups were not significantly different on the assessment measures. At posttest, approximately 6 months later, the CRP group significantly improved on each of the three attention measures, but not on the generalization measure. The control group, however, did not show any significant changes. The overall C-CPT index proved to be the most sensitive to change (estimated effect size d = 0.84), while the other attention measures showed moderate levels of change (Digit Span, d = 0.48; sentence memory, d = 0.55). Parent and teacher reports were not collected. A large, multisite randomized clinical control trial of the CRP (Butler, Copeland, Fairclough, Mulhern, Katz, et al., 2008) was completed in 161 school-aged children who had survived cancer. With 40 hours of intervention over 4 to 5 months, the CRP group attained modest improvement across a number of neuropsychological variables and parent-teacher ratings of attention. Some of these were specific to the CRP group (academic achievement, working memory, learning strategies, and teacher ratings of attention).

In addition to the work by Butler and Copeland, Penkman (2004) provided a single case study showing that the CRP can be used with children as young as 6 years of age. After receiving the CRP, the young boy in this case study (who had been treated with CRT plus IT chemotherapy) evidenced improvement on attention and processing speed, as well as parent report of attention. As he did not show changes on tasks of language and visual–motor function, the improvement was felt to be specific to attention. The Pay Attention! materials were reported to be sufficiently engaging for this child.

Another comprehensive program, similar to the CRP, is the Amsterdam Memory and Attention Training for children (AMAT-c; Hendriks & van den Broek, 1996). The AMAT-c program includes an attention training program based on a modified version of the Sohlberg and Mateer (1987) clinical model of attention. There are three levels of training: (1) sustained attention, (2) selective attention, and (3) mental tracking, which includes memory training. The program also includes metacognitive training with a focus on learning strategies. Unlike the CRP, which uses trained professionals as rehabilitation specialists, the AMAT-c is conducted with the help of a coach at home or school, but includes weekly meetings with a rehabilitation specialist. An initial series of three case studies of children with acquired brain injuries reported improvement in sustained and selective attention, as well as some improvement in memory (van't Hooft, Andersson, Sejersen, Bartfai, & von Wendt, 2003). Based on feedback from this project, van't Hooft et al. (2005) adapted the program by reducing its length to 30 minutes daily for 17 weeks, individualizing the difficulty level, and integrating a reward system. Forty children with acquired brain injury (the majority had TBI), ages 9–17, were randomly assigned to treatment or to a control condition (a freely chosen interactive activity). Immediate postintervention neuropsychological testing showed that the treatment group improved significantly more than the control group on measures of sustained and selective attention, complex memory, and everyday memory. Unfortunately, no measures of generalization (e.g., academic achievement, parent/teacher reports) were available. Many of the gains persisted at 6-month follow-up (van't Hooft et al., 2007). The AMAT-C was also employed with children with TBI (ages 8–16) in a school setting. Gains were made on measures of attention and memory, but not on measures of executive function (Sjö, Spellerberg, Weidner, & Kihlgren, 2010). In another study, Galbiati, Recla, Pastore, Liscio, and Bardoni (2009) provided rehabilitation to 45 children (ages 6–18) with severe brain injury for 6 months following discharge from a subacute treatment unit. The program combined metacognitive strategies and a computerized attention training program which utilized the process approach. Compared to baseline, the experimental participants made significantly more improvement on measures of sustained attention and parent-reported adaptive functioning 1 year posttreatment, compared to the nontreatment control group.

Novel Clinical Applications

CHILDREN WITH DYSLEXIA

Thomson et al. (2005) used structural equational modeling to look at the functional systems influencing reading and writing in 209 children and adolescents with dyslexia. Attention problems in these children fell along a continuum, with only 10.5% qualifying for a diagnosis of ADHD. Attentional skills, as measured by parent ratings, appeared to have an impact on specific language processes important for reading and writing (orthographic and rapid naming, but not phonological skills). Therefore, these authors proposed, attention training might have an impact on reading and writing ability.

To examine this hypothesis, Thomson et al. randomly assigned 20 children (fourth to sixth graders) with dyslexia to either attention training (Pay Attention!) or an active control condition consisting of reading fluency training. Training was conducted over ten 25-minute individual sessions, followed by 10 sessions of group composition training (which included attentional bridges and coaching). Interestingly, those children who received Pay Attention! were better able to learn from the composition training than those children who participated in a reading fluency group. After the first 10 sessions, both groups showed similar levels of progress on measures of attention and measures of reading ability. However, between the midpoint and the end of the final training period, there was a significant time × treatment interaction, such that 8 of 10 children in the Pay Attention! group showed significantly more progress on written expression than the reading fluency group (Chenault, Thomson, Abbott, & Berninger, 2006).

Further examination of the results of this study showed that pre- to posttest improvement in the group that received Pay Attention! was limited to orthography and rapid naming (skills associated with attention), and not phonological skills (skills not associated with attention). However, because the tests of reading/writing skills were not given at the midpoint of training, it is not possible to assess whether attention training had a direct impact on these skills (Thomson et al., 2005).

TYPICALLY DEVELOPING CHILDREN

The importance of attention in learning has led investigators to examine whether attention training is able to build attentional ability in typically developing children, and whether such improvement in ability is related to physiological change in the brain. Rueda, Rothbart, McCandliss, Saccomanno, and Posner (2005) implemented an executive attention training program for typically developing children ages 4 to 6—ages between which Posner's executive attention network (Posner & DiGirolamo, 1998) shows significant development. The goal of this program was to determine whether attention training might be a helpful component of preschool education. Training consisted of 9 or 10 exercises, divided into a number of different difficulty levels. After 5 days of training over a 2- to 3-week period, Rueda and colleagues showed that those children who were in the active treatment group showed more mature performance than those children in the control group (who either received no therapeutic contact or watched videos). Change was evident both on test scores and on an electrophyiosiological measure (evoked response potentials [ERPs]). The effect of treatment was similar to change that naturally occurs with development, so that trained 4-year-olds showed ERPs similar to those of untrained 6-year-olds, and trained 6-year-olds showed more adult-like ERPs. Some generalization of training effects was demonstrated by a small improvement in overall IQ, most of which could be accounted for by an improvement on the Matrices subscale of the Kaufman Brief Intelligence Test, a measure of nonverbal reasoning. The authors suggested that activation of the executive network and the cingulate accounted for this generalization effect.

In an ongoing study by Neville, Andersson, Bagdade, Bell, Currin, et al. (2008) with low-income preschool children enrolled in Head Start, children were randomly assigned to regular (large group) Head Start or to one of three types of small group pull out sessions for 40 minutes per day over the 8-week intervention (small group Head Start, attention training, or music training). Preliminary results show that while all groups made improvement in language, the small groups made larger gains across more cognitive variables. The authors suggested that increased adult attention and guidance may be the underlying element responsible for improving children's cognitive skills in the small groups.

Neurofeedback

Another approach to attention training is EEG biofeedback (or *neurofeedback*). Neurofeedback is an operant conditioning procedure in which an individual is trained to modify the amplitude, frequency, or coherence of his or her brain wave activity through the provision of immediate feedback on brain electrical activity. Through this process, the goal is to normalize activity through increased awareness of how the normalized pattern "feels." Thus a connection is made between certain brain states (e.g., attentive) and specific frequencies or combinations of frequencies. This may be particularly beneficial for children, who often have trouble understanding the abstract concept of what it means to "pay attention." Through biofeedback, children are given a concrete representation of the mental state of "attention." By reinforcing certain underlying brain patterns, neurofeedback (like process-specific attention training) is thought to change patterns of neural networks.

EEG research in individuals with ADHD reveals robust evidence for increased power in drowsy (particularly theta) waveforms, as well as reduced power in active, information-processing (beta) waveforms (for reviews, see Barry, Clarke, & Johnstone, 2003; Loo & Barkley, 2005). This finding is consistent with the view that ADHD is a disorder of neural regulation and underarousal. Biofeedback treatment in ADHD typically involves theta suppression/sensory–motor rhythm (SMR) enhancement and/or theta suppression/beta 1 enhancement. SMRs are at the low-frequency end of the beta waveform spectrum (12–15 Hz); beta 1 activity consists of 16- to 20-Hz waveforms. Some protocols also incorporate suppression of beta 2 waveforms (22–30 Hz; Monastra, 2005).

A review of the utility of EEG biofeedback in children with ADHD (Loo & Barkley, 2005) concluded that although the approach is promising (as indicated by many positive case reports and small studies), there has been a distinct lack of scientifically rigorous neurofeedback studies in ADHD. Small sample sizes, lack of randomized assignment, lack of active placebo-controlled groups, and other methodological weaknesses dominate the literature. There is also no clear evidence that the feedback, and not other, nonspecific support factors, accounts for improvement following neurofeedback. Studies in the last few years have been more encouraging. Preliminary results from a randomized, double-blind, placebo-controlled study found that biofeedback changed electrophysiology in the treatment group compared to the control group after 20 sessions (deBeus, Ball, deBeus, & Herrington, 2004). Gevensleben, Holl, Albrecht, Vogel, Schlamp, et al. (2009a) found that 36 sessions of EEG neurofeedback was associated with significantly more improvement in both parent and teacher ratings of ADHD symptomatology compared to an active control group (moderate effect sizes). Furthermore, predicted changes in brain activity were associated with improvements in ADHD symptomatology (Gevensleben, Holl, Albrecht, Schlamp, Kratz, et al., 2009b).

Another study demonstrated similar specific improvement in parent and teacher ratings of ADHD in a neurofeedback group (30 sessions) compared to a cognitive behavioral group therapy program of the same duration. However, neuropsychological measures of attention and impulsivity improved in both groups similarly (Drechsler, Straub, Doehnert, Heinrich, Steinhausen, et al., 2007). Of note, the latter two studies both included activities to facilitate generalization (homework).

An fMRI study investigated the neural substrates of change following biofeedback (Beauregard & Lévesque, 2006). A group of 15 children with ADHD participated in 40 biofeedback sessions, while 5 children with ADHD served as untreated controls. All sessions involved suppression of theta waves; half of the sessions also involved enhancement of beta 1 waves, and half involved enhancement of SMR waves. Results showed that the treatment group, but not the control group, improved on neuropsychological and parent report measures of inattention and hyperactivity. Moreover, the treatment group (but not the control group) showed changes in brain functioning on a task of shifting attention (counting Stroop) and a task of inhibition (go/no-go). Following treatment, fMRI data revealed new loci of activation while children were doing these tasks. The new loci were interpreted to be a reflection of normalizing of brain function, particularly in frontostriatal circuits mediated by dopamine.

TBI is also associated with EEG abnormalities. A review (Arciniegas, Anderson, & Rojas, 2005) found that such abnormalities are common, especially in the acute phase of injury and in children. There is also evidence for long-term abnormalities. Moreover, certain types of abnormalities, such as loss of beta and alpha power (Kane, Moss, Curry, & Butler, 1998), have been shown to be associated with poor outcome following TBI. EEG biofeedback has been used with some success as a treatment in adults with brain injury (for a review, see Thornton & Carmody, 2005), but no published research with children has been found to date—and, as with ADHD research, there is a general lack of methodologically strong research.

Role of Emotion/Motivation

Attention to motivational factors is especially important in children. Unlike adults, children do not typically present themselves for rehabilitation. In fact, they may not be able to conceptualize what they are working toward.

This is particularly true of children with developmental disorders, who do not have "preinjury" memories of themselves for comparison. In addition, motivational problems are hypothesized to be a core feature of at least one developmental disorder: ADHD, combined type (Diamond, 2005).

An effective rehabilitation program for children must be engaging and motivating. Emotional valence has an important impact on learning and synaptic change through the function of neuromodulators (neurotransmitters or neuropeptides manufactured in the brainstem or hypothalamus). Systems involved in processing emotions—the amygdala and the paralimbic areas of the anterior cingulate cortex and the orbitofrontal cortex—typically trigger the release of neuromodulators. Through this release, emotional processes are able to initiate global changes in neural processing by adjusting firing rates upward or downward, thereby facilitating or hindering long-term potentiation (Lewis, 2005). Reflections from an intervention study conducted in our laboratory suggests that a group format for intervention promotes motivation and interest in children (McLellan, 2003). Another method for maximizing interest in children is the use of a virtual-reality environment (Rizzo et al., 2006). Cho et al. (2002) found that teenagers who completed attention training in a virtual classroom were motivated, while those who used a regular computer monitor found the tasks tedious and uncomfortable. All trained children showed improvement on a continuous performance task, compared to untrained controls; however, the virtual-reality group showed the most improvement.

Family Factors

Following brain injury, there is a reciprocal relationship between family adjustment and child outcomes over time (Taylor et al., 2001). Not surprisingly, postinjury cognitive and behavior problems have an impact on family adjustment, while problems with family adjustment make it more difficult for families to deal with their child. Families of children with developmental disorders may show a similar pattern. This suggests that rehabilitation programs that improve child outcomes will have a positive impact on overall family functioning. However, it also suggests that improvements in basic cognitive skills may be stymied—or, if they occur, may prove meaningless—if the family is highly distressed or dysfunctional. Therefore, it is key that interventions include attention to family issues. Ideally, family functioning should be addressed early (immediately after injury or diagnosis), to prevent the downward spiral that can occur. Family interventions may include increasing coping mechanisms, implementing stress reduction techniques, providing assistance in dealing with loss, or providing education about the child's disorder (including appropriate parenting techniques). These types of interventions may work synergistically with child-focused interventions to maximize recovery.

Medication

Although their exact mechanism is unknown, psychostimulant medications that facilitate release and block reuptake of the neurotransmitters norepinephrine and dopamine are accepted as empirically supported treatments that ameliorate the core features of ADHD. Psychostimulants have been found to improve (although not necessarily normalize) behavior in 70–80% of children with ADHD (for reviews, see Conners, 2002; Pliszka, 2006).

Neuroimaging studies that have compared treatment-naïve children to chronically treated children with ADHD have found that treatment-naïve children have smaller whole brain gray and white matter volumes (Castellanos et al., 2002), as well as smaller right anterior cingulate cortices (Pliszka et al., 2006). This suggests that medication is associated with plastic changes in neurophysiology. Although the mechanism is as yet unknown, Pliszka and colleagues suggest that stimulant medication may "lower the threshold" for learning, allowing children to benefit more fully from other interventions.

There is considerably less research on the effect of medication in acquired brain injury. In a detailed review of the (primarily adult) literature, Whyte, Vaccaro, and Grieb-Neff (2002) concluded that medication does not have a very strong effect on specific attentional abilities. Rather, medication's largest effect seems to be in the area of processing speed. Therefore, medication may provide an incremental benefit when used in combination with attention training, which does not typically affect processing speed (Whyte et al., 2004). A dearth of research in children means that caution must be taken in applying these findings to children. Two experimental studies provide contrasting results, adding to the uncertainty. One crossover study of 14 children with mild to moderate TBI found that children in the treatment group improved significantly more than children in the placebo group on all six measures of attention, concentration, and processing speed (Mahalick et al., 1998). The placebo group did not differ significantly from the baseline condition, indicating a lack of placebo and test–retest effects. Another double-blind, placebo-controlled crossover design involved 10 children with TBI ranging from mild to severe (Williams, Ris, Ayyangar, Schefft, & Berch, 1998). In contrast to the previous study, this study showed no difference between placebo and treatment conditions on measures of behavior, attention, memory, and processing speed.

In addition to psychostimulants, which aim to treat the behavioral symptoms of brain injury/dysfunction, a new line of research is focusing on pharmacological approaches to reducing the damage in the immediate aftermath of TBI, promoting recovery through the prevention of neuronal loss, and promoting growth and plasticity (e.g., through neurotrophic factors). For a review, see Browning (2004). Medications that promote neural plasticity may be particularly helpful in combination with process-specific attention training or neurofeedback. While medication may increase new synaptic development, direct approaches to improving attentional functioning may help sculpt the development to provide maximum functionality.

Broad-Based Interventions: Physical Activity and Tactile Stimulation

Process-specific attention training and neurofeedback aim to improve overall functioning by targeting specific underlying processes in children with developmental or acquired brain dysfunction. In contrast, two broad-based interventions using vastly different methods and underlying philosophies—physical activity and tactile stimulation—have also shown promise in improving cognitive function in similar populations.

Experimental research in laboratory animals showed that voluntary exercise was associated with better spatial and working memory performance. Moreover, exercised animals showed increased neurogenesis and long-term potentiation in the dentate gyrus of the hippocampus (van Praag, Christie, Sejnowski, & Gage, 1999).

Underlying the increase in neuronal plasticity may be an association between exercise and an increase in the production of molecules (e.g., trophic substances, growth factors) that promote plasticity (Gomez-Pinilla, So, & Kesslak, 1998; Griesbach, Hovda, Molteni, Wu, & Gomez-Pinilla, 2004b). Exercise may also improve performance though an increase in the flow of nutrients to the brain by causing the formation of new blood vessels (Black, Isaacs, Anderson, Alcantara, & Greenough, 1990).

Like healthy animals, cortically lesioned animals also benefit from exercise, showing an improvement in spatial learning and memory, along with an increase in the production of plasticity-associated factors. However, when voluntary exercise occurred during the acute phase after lesion surgery, it led to a decrease in plasticity-associated factors, as well as to impairment in spatial learning and memory. Therefore, exercise must be used with caution in the acute stage of injury (Griesbach, Gomez-Pinilla, & Hovda, 2004a; Griesbach et al., 2004b).

In another interesting line of research, investigators have examined the effect of exercise on animals prenatally exposed to alcohol. Christie et al. (2005) noted that deficits displayed in these rats are "virtually the diametric opposite" (p. 1719) of benefits incurred with voluntary exercise wheel activity. With voluntary exercise, long-term potentiation increased in alcohol-exposed rats, up to just above the level of nonexercised controls (Christie et al., 2005). Hippocampal cellular proliferation and neurogenesis also increased in the dentate gyrus (Redila et al., 2006). These changes were associated with improvement in both working and reference memory, as measured by performance on the Morris water maze.

Complex motor learning (acrobatic training) has been shown to ameliorate the coordination and balance deficits associated with fetal alcohol exposure in rats (Klintsova et al., 1998). Such training was associated with experience-induced plasticity in the paramedian lobule of the cerebellum (Klintsova et al., 2002). In contrast, simple exercise (running) was associated with the addition of new blood vessels, but not with synaptic change in the cerebellum (Black et al., 1990).

In another broad approach to rehabilitation, tactile stimulation has been shown to be helpful in animal and human infant studies. It has been suggested that touch is particularly important in early infancy, as the tactile system develops earlier than the visual and auditory systems. Moreover, it is postulated that the skin has an early and close relationship to the CNS, as both develop from the same blastocytic ectodermal layer (Schanberg & Field, 1987). Stroking infant rats with a camel hair paintbrush three times daily from day 7 to day 21 of life led to enhanced performance on a skilled reaching task in adulthood, compared to that of control animals (Kolb & Gibb, 2001, as cited in Kolb et al., 2000). Similar studies have been conducted with cortically lesioned rats. Animals were given frontal or posterior parietal lesions at 4 days of age, followed by tactile stimulation (stroking) until weaning occurred. Those animals that received stimulation showed a large attenuation of the behavioral effects typically seen as a result of the lesion, performing nearly as well as control rats. Examination of their brains showed a lack of the atrophy typically seen in the brains of lesioned animals (Kolb, Gorny, & Gibb, 1994), suggesting that, as with physical activity, improvement is mediated by neuroplastic changes.

There is also evidence that touch can be a useful therapy for human neonates. An experiment by Wheeden et al. (1993) randomly assigned 30 preterm cocaine-exposed neonates to a massage treatment condition (three 15-minute massage treatments over 3 consecutive hours for 10 days) or a noncontact control group. Group assignment was stratified based on gestational age, birth weight, duration in intensive care, and weight at the start of the study. Infants in the treatment group averaged 28% greater weight gain per day (with caloric intake equal to that of controls). Massaged infants also showed fewer medical complications, fewer stress behaviors, and more mature motor behavior than controls did at the end of the study. Results were similar to those of an earlier study with preterm neonates (Field et al., 1986).

Many questions remain regarding tactile stimulation and physical activity as interventions in humans. However, given the multiple possible pathways of positive benefits, their low cost, and their ease of application, their addition to an intervention plan seems to be warranted. Timing of these interventions seems to be quite important. Physical activity in the acute stage of brain injury is to be avoided. Although tactile stimulation is not contraindicated at any particular age or stage of recovery, research particularly supports its use in neonates, particularly preterm infants.

SUMMARY

Problems with attention and executive functioning are common to a number of acquired and developmental disorders of childhood. The premise of this chapter is that targeted, direct interventions can improve attention, and that this improvement is mediated by changes in underlying brain functions. The interventions discussed in this chapter include process-specific attention training, neurofeedback, medication, physical activity, and tactile stimulation.

One frequently studied method, the process approach to attention training, is theorized to repeatedly activate the neural networks underlying specific attentional processes. With massed, increasingly challenging practice, the repeated coactivation of neurons is believed to strengthen (or reconnect) the neural pathways responsible for the process, leading to improved attentional function. Attention training is well accepted as a treatment in the postacute stage of TBI and stroke in adults, and research over the last decade has shown it to be a useful intervention method for children and adolescents as well. Randomized, placebo-controlled research has found that process-specific attention training improves attention functioning in children with TBI (van't Hooft et al., 2005), ADHD (Kerns et al., 1999; Klingberg et al., 2005; Shalev et al., 2007), Fetal Alcohol Spectrum Disorders (Kerns et al., 2010), as well as in typically developing preschoolers (Rueda et al., 2005). In a novel application, written expression improved more in children with dyslexia who were given prior attention training than in children given prior reading fluency training (Chenault et al., 2006). In some but not all studies, the effects of attention training generalized to aspects of executive functioning, memory, academic skills, and parent ratings of attention and hyperactivity.

Neurofeedback is also frequently researched, but is a far more controversial intervention approach than attention training. Neurofeedback for attention problems involves the provision of immediate feedback on brain wave activity. Participants are positively reinforced for activity that indicates "paying attention," with the goal of permanently altering the patterns of brain wave activity. Following decades of research and a large body of publications, the field of neurofeedback is only beginning to demonstrate methodologically rigorous research (e.g., random assignment, placebo controls).

Other approaches, such as physical activity, tactile stimulation, and medication, have been shown to have an impact on functioning (presumably through neuroplastic mechanisms) and may be useful adjuncts to an intervention program.

In the last decade, there have been several exciting studies showing that the intervention approaches discussed in this chapter are associated with brain-based functional and structural changes. However, almost all of this work has been done exclusively in adults. Animal studies provide more evidence for experience-dependent plasticity, as interventions have been associated with increased synaptic/dendritic growth, neurogenesis, and long-term potentiation in addition to behavioral change in young and adult animals.

FUTURE DIRECTIONS

Child-specific attention rehabilitation research has advanced dramatically in the last few years, but a number of questions remain. For example, with the exception of the 3-month follow-up by Klingberg et al. (2005), which showed the maintenance of nearly all intervention gains, there has been a lack of follow-up to track the long-term impact of interventions. This is especially important, given the dynamic changes occurring in brain development and cognition during childhood.

In addition, there is a great need for child-specific studies that utilize neurophysiological outcome measurements (e.g., changes in fMRI or EEG). Again, child-specific research is important, given the differences between the developing and the adult brain. This type of measurement provides valuable data to complement cognitive testing, and helps link behavioral and cognitive changes to changes in brain function and structure.

Another looming question is the importance of timing of interventions, both in relation to the onset of injury (or identification of dysfunction) and the age of the child. Certainly children have an advantage in increased neuroplasticity compared to adults, but are there "critical periods" for intervention, or times when children would be expected to make maximum gains? Rueda et al. (2005) have shown that it is possible to improve executive attention in typically developing children as young as 4 years of age, at an age when executive attention is normally under development. This suggests that it is possible to differentiate the benefits of treatment from the normal developmental processes. Attention training may also be of use for very young children who have attention problems or are at risk for attention problems. This leads to the question: Can early intervention help to prevent later problems? Research suggests that certain groups of children are likely to have problems with attention and executive functions as they develop. Young children who suffer brain damage may not initially show problems with attention, but as their peers begin to develop mature functioning, such deficits may become readily apparent. The same may be true of other groups of children who are identified early with developmental disorders (e.g., autism, problems associated with low birth weight, fetal alcohol spectrum disorders, etc.). Given what we know about the ubiquity of problems with attention and executive function in certain groups of children, perhaps early intervention could be utilized to prevent the onset of attention problems. This type of research would be expensive and time-consuming, as it would require following participants over the long term to determine whether they have a better developmental outcome than non-treated individuals. In addition, perhaps children would need additional courses of intervention as they develop and reach new stages.

Although the goals are similar, the intervention methods discussed in this chapter work through very different physiological mechanisms. Given the diverse causes of attention problems, some individuals may benefit more from one method than from another. As our understanding of the neurophysiological changes associated with rehabilitation grows, such knowledge will enable us to fine-tune our approach to rehabilitation. For example, a physiological screen may be able to help predict which individuals would most benefit from attention training, versus those who would be best served by a behavioral compensation approach or who may benefit greatly from an exercise plan. Functional imaging may also be used to monitor progress in individual patients and to adjust intervention plans accordingly. However, it is important to note that many (if not most) individuals would maximally benefit from a combination of approaches, given each approach's different mechanisms of action.

Attention intervention has been greatly enriched by the wealth of plasticity research in the last few decades. With a combination of advances in neurophysiological measurement and elaboration of theories of attention, now is an opportune moment for attention research to inform and enrich our understanding of plasticity.

REFERENCES

Adams, H., & Sutker, P. (Eds.). (2001). *Comprehensive handbook of psychopathology*. New York: Kluwer Academic/Plenum.

American Psychiatric Association. (2000). *Diagnostic and statistical manual of mental disorders* (4th ed., text rev.). Washington DC: Author.

Anderson, V. A., Catroppa, C., Dudgeon, P., Morse, S. A., Haritou, F., & Rosenfeld, J. V. (2006). Understanding predictors of functional recovery and outcome 30 months following early childhood head injury. *Neuropsychology, 20*(1), 42–57.

Anderson, V. A., Godber, T., Smibert, E., & Ekert, H. (1997). Neurobehavioral sequelae following irradiation and chemotherapy in children: An analysis of risk factors. *Pediatric Rehabilitation, 1*(2), 63–76.

Anderson, V. A., Godber, T., Smibert, E., Weiskop, S., & Ekert, H. (2000). Cognitive and academic outcome following cranial irradiation and chemotherapy in children: A longitudinal study. *British Journal of Cancer, 82*(2), 255–262.

Anderson, V. A., Jacobs, R., & Harvey, A. S. (2005). Prefrontal lesions and attentional skills in childhood. *Journal of the International Neuropsychological Society, 11*(7), 817–831.

Anderson, V. A., Northam, E., Hendy, J., & Wrennall, J. (2001). *Developmental neuropsychology: A clinical approach.* Philadelphia: Psychology Press.

Anderson, V. A., & Pentland, L. (1998). Residual attention deficits following childhood head injury: Implications for ongoing development. *Neuropsychological Rehabilitation, 8*(3), 283–300.

Arciniegas, D. B., Anderson, C. A., & Rojas, D. C. (2005). Electrophysiological techniques. In J. M. Silver, T. W. McAllister, & S. C. Yudofsky (Eds.), *Textbook of traumatic brain injury* (pp. 135–157). Washington, DC: American Psychiatric Publishing.

Baeyens, D., Roeyers, H., & Walle, J. V. (2006). Subtypes of attention-deficit/hyperactivity disorder (ADHD): Distinct or related disorders across measurement levels? *Child Psychiatry and Human Development, 36*(4), 403–417.

Banich, M. T., Cohen-Levine, S., Kim, H., & Huttenlocher, P. R. (1990). The effects of developmental factors on IQ in hemiplegic children. *Neuropsychologia, 28*, 35–47.

Barkley, R. A. (1997). *ADHD and the nature of self-control.* New York: Guilford Press.

Barry, R. J., Clarke, A. R., & Johnstone, S. J. (2003). A review of electrophysiology in attention-deficit/hyperactivity disorder: I. Qualitative and quantitative electroencephalography. *Clinical Neurophysiology, 114*(2), 171–183.

Beauregard, M., & Lévesque, J. (2006). Functional magnetic resonance imaging investigation of the effects of neurofeedback training on the neural bases of selective attention and response inhibition in children with attention-deficit/hyperactivity disorder. *Applied Psychophysiology and Biofeedback, 31*(1), 3–20.

Black, J. E., Isaacs, K. R., Anderson, B. J., Alcantara, A. A., & Greenough, W. T. (1990). Learning causes synaptogenesis, whereas motor activity causes angiogenesis, in cerebellar cortex of adult rats. *Proceedings of the National Academy of Sciences USA, 87*, 5568–5572.

Brett, A. W., & Laatsch, L. (1998). Cognitive rehabilitation therapy of brain-injured students in a public high school setting. *Pediatric Rehabilitation, 2*(1), 27–31.

Browning, R. A. (2004). Neurotransmitters and pharmacology. In M. J. Ashley (Ed.), *Traumatic brain injury: Rehabilitative treatment and case management* (2nd ed., pp. 57–118). Boca Raton, FL: CRC Press.

Buizer, A. I., De Sonneville, L. M. J., Van Den Heuvel-Eibrink, M. M., Njiokiktjien, C., & Veerman, A. J. P. (2005). Visuomotor control in survivors of childhood acute lymphoblastic leukemia treated with chemotherapy only. *Journal of the International Neuropsychological Society, 11*(5), 554–565.

Butefisch, C., Hummelsheim, H., Denzler, P., & Mauritz, K. H. (1995). Repetitive training of isolated movements improves the outcome of motor rehabilitation of the centrally paretic hand. *Journal of the Neurological Sciences, 130*(1), 59–68.

Butler, R. W., & Copeland, D. R. (2002). Attentional processes and their remediation in children treated for cancer: A literature review and the development of a therapeutic approach. *Journal of the International Neuropsychological Society, 8*(1), 115–124.

Butler, R. W., Copeland, D. R., Fairclough, D. L., Mulhern, R. K., Katz, E. R., Kazak, A. E., et al. (2008). A multicenter, randomized clinical trial of a cognitive remediation program for childhood survivors of a pediatric malignancy. *Journal of Consulting and Clinical Psychology, 76*(3), 367–378.

Butler, R. W., & Mulhern, R. K. (2005). Neurocognitive interventions for children and adolescents surviving cancer. *Journal of Pediatric Psychology, 30*(1), 65–78.

Cappa, S. F., Benke, T., Clarke, S., Rossi, B., Stemmer, B., & van Heugten, C. M. (2005). EFNS guidelines on cognitive rehabilitation: Report of an EFNS task force. *European Journal of Neurology, 12*(9), 665–680.

Castellanos, F. X., & Acosta, M. T. (2004). The neuroanatomy of attention deficit/hyperactivity disorder. *Revista de Neurologia, 38*(Suppl. 1), 131–136.

Castellanos, F. X., Lee, P. P., Sharp, W., Sharp, W., Jeffries, N. O., Greenstein, D. K., et al. (2002). Developmental trajectories of brain volume abnormalities in children and adolescents with attention deficit/hyperactivity disorder. *Journal of the American Medical Association, 288*, 1740–1748.

Catroppa, C., & Anderson, V. A. (1999). Attentional skills in the acute phase following pediatric traumatic brain injury. *Child Neuropsychology, 5*(4), 251–264.

Chenault, B. M., Thomson, J. B., Abbott, R. D., & Berninger, V. W. (2006). Effects of prior attention training on child dyslexics' response to composition training. *Developmental Neuropsychology, 29*(4), 243–260.

Cho, B.-H., Ku, J., Pyojang, D., Kim, S., Lee, Y. H., Kim, I. Y., et al. (2002). The effect of virtual reality cognitive training for attention enhancement. *CyberPsychology and Behavior, 5*(2), 129–137.

Christie, B. R., Swann, S. E., Fox, C. J., Froc, D., Lieblich, S. E., Redila, V., et al. (2005). Voluntary exercise rescues deficits in spatial memory and long-term potentiation in prenatal ethanol-exposed male rats. *European Journal of Neuroscience, 21*(6), 1719–1726.

Cicerone, K. D., Dahlberg, C., Malec, J. F., Langenbahn, D. M., Felicetti, T., Kneipp, S., et al. (2005). Evidence-based cognitive rehabilitation: Updated review of the literature from 1998 through 2002. *Archives of Physical Medicine and Rehabilitation, 86*(8), 1681–1692.

Conners, C. K. (2002). Forty years of methylphenidate treatment in attention-deficit/hyperactivity disorder. *Journal of Attention Disorders, 6*(Suppl. 1), S17–S30.

Copeland, D. R., Moore, B. D., Francis, D. J., Jaffe, N., & Culbert, S. J. (1996). Neuropsychological effects of chemotherapy on children with cancer: A longitudinal study. *Journal of Clinical Oncology, 14*, 2826–2835.

deBeus, R., Ball, J. D., deBeus, M. E., & Herrington, R. (2004). Attention training with ADHD children: Preliminary findings in a double-blind placebo-controlled study. *Journal of Neurotherapy, 8*(2), 145–147.

Dennis, M. (Ed.). (1988). *Language and the young damaged brain.* Washington, DC: American Psychological Association.

Diamond, A. (2005). Attention-deficit disorder (attention-deficit/hyperactivity disorder without hyperactivity): A neurobiologically and behaviorally distinct disorder from attention-deficit/hyperactivity disorder (with hyperactivity). *Development and Psychopathology, 17*(3), 807–825.

Drechsler, R., Straub, M., Doehnert, M., Heinrich, H., Steinhausen, H.-C., & Brandeis, D. (2007). Controlled evaluation of a neurofeedback training of slow cortical potentials in children with Attention Deficit/Hyperactivity Disorder (ADHD). *Behavioral and Brain Functions, 3.*

Field, T. M., Schanberg, S. M., Scafidi, F., Bauer, C. R., Vega-Lahr, N., Garcia, R., et al. (1986). Tactile/kinesthetic stimulation effects on preterm neonates. *Pediatrics, 77*(5), 654–658.

Galbiati, S., Recla, M., Pastore, V., Liscio, M., & Bardoni, A. (2009). Attention remediation following traumatic brain injury in childhood and adolescence. *Neuropsychology, 2*, 40–49.

Gevensleben, H., Holl, B., Albrecht, B. R., Vogel, C., Schlamp, D., Kratz, O., et al. (2009a). Is neurofeedback an efficacious treatment for ADHD? A randomised controlled clinical trial. *Journal of Child Psychology and Psychiatry, 50*(7), 780–789.

Gevensleben, H., Holl, B., Albrecht, B., Schlamp, D., Kratz, O., Studer, P., et al. (2009b). Distinct EEG effects related to neurofeedback training in children with ADHD: A randomized controlled trial. *International Journal of Psychophysiology, 74*(2), 149–157.

Goldman-Rakic, P. S., Isseroff, A., Schwartz, M. L., & Bugbee, N. M. (1983). The neurobiology of cognitive development. In P. H. Mussen (Series Ed.) & M. M. Haith & J. J. Campos (Vol. Eds.), *Handbook of child psychology: Vol. 2. Infancy and developmental psychobiology* (4th ed., pp. 311–344). New York: Wiley.

Gomez-Pinilla, F., So, V., & Kesslak, J. P. (1998). Spatial learning and physical activity contribute to the induction of fibroblast growth factor: Neural substrates for increased cognition associated with exercise. *Neuroscience, 85*(1), 53–61.

Griesbach, G. S., Gomez-Pinilla, F., & Hovda, D. A. (2004a). The upregulation of plasticity-related proteins following TBI is disrupted with acute voluntary exercise. *Brain Research, 1016*(2), 154–162.

Griesbach, G. S., Hovda, D. A., Molteni, R., Wu, A., & Gomez-Pinilla, F. (2004b). Voluntary exercise following traumatic brain injury: Brain-derived neurotrophic factor upregulation and recovery of function. *Neuroscience, 125*(1), 129–139.

Hebb, D. O. (1949). *The organization of behavior: A neuropsychological theory.* New York: Wiley.

Hendriks, C. M., & van den Broek, T. M. (1996). *AMAT-c manual and workbook.* Lisse, The Netherlands: Swets & Zeitlinger.

Huttenlocher, P. R. (2002). *Neural plasticity: The effects of environment on the development of the cerebral cortex.* Cambridge, MA: Harvard University Press.

Kane, N. M., Moss, T. H., Curry, S. H., & Butler, S. R. (1998). Quantitative electroencephalographic evaluation of non-fatal and fatal traumatic coma. *Electroencephalography and Clinical Neurophysiology, 106*, 244–250.

Kennard, M. (1938). Reorganization of motor function in the cerebral cortex of monkeys deprived of motor and premotor areas in infancy. *Journal of Neurophysiology, 1*, 477–496.

Kennard, M. (1940). Relation of age to motor impairment in man and in subhuman primates. *Archives of Neurology and Psychiatry, 44*, 377–397.

Kerns, K. A., Eso, K., & Thomson, J. B. (1999). Investigation of a direct intervention for improving attention in young children with ADHD. *Developmental Neuropsychology, 16*(2), 273–295.

Kerns, K. A., MacSween, J., Vander Wekken, S., & Gruppuso, V. (2010). Investigating the efficacy of an attention training programme in children with foetal alcohol spectrum disorder. *Developmental Neurorehabilitation, 13*(6), 413–422.

Kerns, K. A., & Mateer, C. A. (Eds.). (1996). *Walking and chewing gum: The impact of attentional capacity on everyday activities.* Delray Beach, FL: GR Press/St Lucie Press.

Klingberg, T., Fernell, E., Olesen, P. J., Johnson, M., Gustafsson, P., Dahlström, K., et al. (2005). Computerized training of working memory in children with ADHD: A randomized, controlled trial. *Journal of the American Academy of Child and Adolescent Psychiatry, 44*(2), 177–186.

Klingberg, T., Forssberg, H., & Westerberg, H. (2002). Training of working memory in children with ADHD. *Journal of Clinical and Experimental Neuropsychology, 24*(6), 781–791.

Klintsova, A. Y., Cowell, R. M., Swain, R. A., Napper, R. M., Goodlett, C. R., & Greenough, W. T. (1998). Therapeutic effects of complex motor training on motor performance deficits induced by neonatal binge-like alcohol exposure in rats: I. Behavioral results. *Brain Research, 800*(1), 48–61.

Klintsova, A. Y., Scamra, C., Hoffman, M., Napper, R. M., Goodlett, C. R., & Greenough, W. T. (2002). Therapeutic effects of complex motor training on motor performance deficits induced by neonatal binge-like alcohol exposure in rats: II. A quantitative stereological study of synaptic plasticity in female rat cerebellum. *Brain Research, 937*(1–2), 83–93.

Kolb, B., Gibb, R., & Gorny, G. (2000). Cortical plasticity and the development of behavior after early frontal cortical injury. *Developmental Neuropsychology, 18*(3), 423–444.

Kolb, B., Gorny, G., & Gibb, R. (1994). Tactile stimulation enhances recovery and dendritic growth in rats with neonatal frontal lesions. *Society for Neuroscience Abstracts, 20*, 1430.

Kolb, B., & Milner, B. (1981). Performance of complex arm and facial movements after focal brain lesions. *Neuropsychologia, 19*(4), 491–503.

Kotwal, D. B., Burns, W. J., & Montgomery, D. D. (1996). Computer-assisted cognitive training for ADHD. *Behavior Modification, 20*, 85–96.

Krain, A. L., & Castellanos, F. X. (2006). Brain development and ADHD. *Clinical Psychology Review, 26*(4), 433–444.

Kraus, J. F. (1995). Epidemiological features of brain injury in children: Occurrence, children at risk, causes and manner of injury, severity, and outcomes. In S. H. Broman & M. E. Michel (Eds.), *Traumatic head injury in children* (pp. 23–39). New York: Oxford University Press.

Kraus, J. F., & Chu, L. D. (2005). Epidemiology. In J. M. Silver, T. W. McAllister, & S. C. Yudofsky (Eds.), *Textbook of traumatic brain injury* (pp. 3–26). Washington, DC: American Psychiatric Publishing.

Langlois, J. A., Rutland-Brown, W., & Thomas, K. E. (2005). The incidence of traumatic brain injury among children in the United States: Differences by race. *Journal of Head Trauma Rehabilitation, 20*(3), 229–238

Lewis, M. D. (2005). Self-organizing individual differences in brain development. *Developmental Review, 25*(3), 252–277.

Lincoln, N. B., Majid, M. J., & Weyman, N. (2005). *Cognitive rehabilitation for attention deficits following stroke* (Vol. 2). Oxford: Update Software.

Loo, S. K., & Barkley, R. A. (2005). Clinical utility of EEG in attention deficit hyperactivity disorder. *Applied Neuropsychology, 12*(2), 64–76.

Luerssen, T. (1991). Head injury in children. *Neurosurgery Clinics of North America, 2*(2), 399–410.

Luria, A. R. (1963). *Restoration of function after brain injury.* New York: Macmillan.

Lynch, J. K. (2004). Cerebrovascular disorders in children. *Current Neurology and Neuroscience Reports, 4*(2), 129–138.

Lynch, J. K., & Nelson, K. B. (2001). Epidemiology of perinatal stroke. *Current Opinion in Pediatrics, 13*(6), 499–505.

Mahalick, D. M., Carmel, P. W., Greenberg, J. P., Molofsky, W., Brown, J. A., Heary, R. F., et al. (1998). Psychopharmacologic treatment of acquired attention disorders in children with brain injury. *Pediatric Neurosurgery, 29*(3), 121–126.

Mateer, C. A., & Dodrill, C. B. (1983). Neuropsychological and linguistic correlates of atypical language lateralization: Evidence from sodium amytal studies. *Human Neurobiology, 2*(3), 135–142.

Max, J. E., Fox, P. T., Lancaster, J. L., Kochunov, P., Mathews, K., Manes, F. F., et al. (2002). Putamen lesions and the development of attention-deficit/hyperactivity symptomatology. *Journal of the American Academy of Child and Adolescent Psychiatry, 41*(5), 563–571.

Max, J. E., Manes, F. F., Robertson, B. A. M., Mathews, K., Fox, P. T., & Lancaster, J. (2005). Prefrontal and executive attention network lesions and the development of attention-deficit/hyperactivity symptomatology. *Journal of the American Academy of Child and Adolescent Psychiatry, 44*(5), 443–450.

McLellan, E. (2003). *A group intervention approach to improving attention abilities in children.* Victoria, British Columbia, Canada: University of Victoria.

Michel, J. A., & Mateer, C. A. (2006). Attention rehabilitation following stroke and traumatic brain injury: A review. *Europa Medicophysica, 42*(1), 59–67.

Moleski, M. (2000). Neuropsychological, neuroanatomical, and neurophysiological consequences of CNS chemotherapy for acute lymphoblastic leukemia. *Archives of Clinical Neuropsychology, 15*(7), 603–630.

Monastra, V. J. (2005). Electroencephalographic biofeedback (neurotherapy) as a treatment for attention deficit hyperactivity disorder: Rationale and empirical foundation. *Child and Adolescent Psychiatric Clinics of North America, 14*(1), 55–82.

Neville, H., Andersson, A., Bagdade, O., Bell, T., Currin, J., Fanning, J., et al.

(2008). Effects of music training on brain and cognitive development in under-privileged 3- to 5-year-old children: Preliminary results. In C. Asbury & B. Rich (Eds.), *Learning, arts, and the brain* (pp. 105–116). New York: Dana Press.

Neville, H. J. (2006). *Experience shapes human development and function.* Paper presented at the Brain Development and Learning: Making Sense of the Science conference, Vancouver, British Columbia, Canada.

Olesen, P. J., Westerberg, H., & Klingberg, T. (2004). Increased prefrontal and parietal activity after training of working memory. *Nature Neuroscience, 7*(1), 75–79.

Park, N. W., & Ingles, J. L. (2001). Effectiveness of attention rehabilitation after an acquired brain injury: A meta-analysis. *Neuropsychology, 15*(2), 199–210.

Penkman, L. (2004). Remediation of attention deficits in children: A focus on childhood cancer, traumatic brain injury and attention deficit disorder. *Pediatric Rehabilitation, 7*(2), 111–123.

Pliszka, S. R. (2006). The neuropsychopharmacology of attention-deficit/hyperactivity disorder. *Journal of Biological Psychiatry, 57*(11), 1385–1390.

Pliszka, S. R., Lancaster, J., Liott, M., & Semrud-Clikeman, M. (2006). Volumetric MRI differences in treatment-naïve vs. chronically treated children with ADHD. *Neurology, 67,* 1023–1027.

Posner, M. I., & DiGirolamo, G. J. (1998). Executive attention: Conflict, target detection, and cognitive control. In R. Parasuraman (Ed.), *The attentive brain* (pp. 401–423). Cambridge, MA: MIT Press.

Posner, M. I., & Petersen, S. E. (1990). The attention system of the human brain. *Annual Review of Neuroscience, 13,* 25–42.

Rasmussen, T., & Milner, B. (1977). The role of early left-brain injury in determining lateralization of cerebral speech functions. *Annals of the New York Academy of Sciences, 299,* 355–369.

Reddick, W. E., White, H. A., Glass, J. O., Wheeler, G. C., Thompson, S. J., Gajjar, A., et al. (2003). Developmental model relating white matter volume to neurocognitive deficits in pediatric brain tumor survivors. *Cancer, 97*(10), 2512–2519.

Redila, V. A., Olson, A. K., Swann, S. E., Mohades, G., Webber, A. J., Weinberg, J., et al. (2006). Hippocampal cell proliferation is reduced following prenatal ethanol exposure but can be rescued with voluntary exercise. *Hippocampus, 16*(3), 305–311.

Riccardi, R., Brouwers, P., Di Chiro, G., & Poplack, D. G. (1985). Abnormal computed tomography brain scans in children with acute lymphoblastic leukemia: Serial long-term follow-up. *Journal of Clinical Oncology, 3,* 12–18.

Ries, L. A. G., Smith, M. A., Gurney, J. G., Linet, M., Tamra, T., Young, J. L., et al. (1999). *Cancer incidence and survival among children and adolescents: United States SEER program 1975–1995* (NIH Publication No. 99-4649). Bethesda, MD: National Cancer Institute, SEER Program.

Rizzo, A. A., Bowerly, T., Buckwalter, J. G., Klimchuk, D., Mitura, R., & Parsons, T. D. (2006). A virtual reality scenario for all seasons: The virtual classroom. *CNS Spectrums, 11*(1), 35–44.

Robertson, I. H., & Murre, J. M. J. (1999). Rehabilitation of brain damage: Brain plasticity and principles of guided recovery. *Psychological Bulletin, 125*(5), 544–575.

Rueda, M. R., Rothbart, M. K., McCandliss, B. D., Saccomanno, L., & Posner, M. (2005). Training, maturation, and genetic influences on the development of executive attention. *Proceedings of the National Academy of Sciences USA, 102*(41), 14931–14936.

Sanford, J. A., & Browne, R. J. (1988). *Captain's Log* [Computer program]. Richmond, VA: Braintrain.

Schanberg, S. M., & Field, T. M. (1987). Sensory deprivation stress and supplemental stimulation in the rat pup and preterm human neonate. *Child Development, 58*(6), 1431–1447.

Schatz, J., Kramer, J. H., Ablin, A., & Mattay, K. K. (2000). Processing speed, working memory, and IQ: A developmental model of cognitive deficits following cranial radiation therapy. *Neuropsychology, 14*(2), 189–200.

Semrud-Clikeman, M., Nielsen, K. H., Clinton, A., Sylvester, L., Parle, N., & Connor, R. T. (1999). An intervention approach for children with teacher- and parent-identified attentional difficulties. *Journal of Learning Disabilities, 32*(6), 581–590.

Shalev, L., Tsal, Y., & Mevorach, C. (2007). Computerized progressive attention training (CPAT) program: Effective direct intervention for children with ADHD. *Child Neuropsychology, 13*(4), 382–388.

Sjö, N. M., Spellerberg, S., Weidner, S., & Kihlgren, M. (2010). Training of attention and memory deficits in children with acquired brain injury. *Acta Paediatric, 99*, 230–236.

Sohlberg, M. M., Avery, J., Kennedy, M., Ylvisaker, M., Coelho, C., Turkstra, L., et al. (2003). Practice guidelines for direct attention training. *Journal of Medical Speech–Language Pathology, 11*(3), xix–xxxix.

Sohlberg, M. M., & Mateer, C. A. (1987). Effectiveness of an attention-training program. *Journal of Clinical and Experimental Neuropsychology, 9*(2), 117–130.

Sohlberg, M. M., & Mateer, C. A. (2001a). *Attention Process Training (APT).* Wake Forest, NC: Lash & Associates Publishing/Training.

Sohlberg, M. M., & Mateer, C. A. (2001b). *Cognitive rehabilitation: An integrative neuropsychological approach.* New York: Guilford Press.

Sturm, W., Wilmes, K., & Orgass, B. (1997). Do specific attention deficits need specific training? *Neuropsychological Rehabilitation, 7*, 81–103.

Tamm, L., Hughes, C., Ames, L., Pickering, J., Silver, C. H., Stavinoha, P., et al. (2010). Attention training for school-aged children with ADHD: Results of an open trial. *Journal of Attention Disorders, 14*(1), 86–94.

Taylor, H. G., Yeates, K. O., Wade, S. L., Drotar, D., Stancin, T., & Burant, C. (2001). Bidirectional child–family influences on outcomes of traumatic brain injury in children. *Journal of the International Neuropsychological Society, 7*(6), 755–767.

Taylor, H. G., Yeates, K. O., Wade, S. L., Drotar, D., Stancin, T., & Minich, N. (2002). A prospective study of short- and long-term outcomes after traumatic brain injury in children: Behavior and achievement. *Neuropsychology, 16*(1), 15–27.

Teuber, M. L. (1962). Behavior after cerebral lesions in children. *Developmental Medicine and Child Neurology, 4*, 3–20.

Thomson, J. B. (1995). Rehabilitation of high school-aged individuals with traumatic brain injury through utilization of an attention training program. *Journal of the International Neuropsychological Society, 1*(2), 149.

Thomson, J. B., Chenault, B., Abbott, R. D., Raskind, W. H., Richards, T., Aylward, E., et al. (2005). Converging evidence for attentional influences on the orthographic word form in child dyslexics. *Journal of Neurolinguistics, 18*, 93–126.

Thomson, J. B., & Kerns, K. A. (2000). Mild traumatic brain injury in children. In S. A. Raskin & C. A. Mateer (Eds.), *Neuropsychological management of mild traumatic brain injury* (pp. 233–251). Oxford: Oxford University Press.

Thomson, J. B., Kerns, K. A., Seidenstrang, L., Sohlberg, M. M., & Mateer, C. A. (2001). *Pay Attention!: A children's Attention Process Training program.* Wake Forest, NC: Lash & Associates Publishing/Training.

Thornton, K. E., & Carmody, D. P. (2005). Electroencephalogram biofeedback for reading disability and traumatic brain injury. *Child and Adolescent Psychiatric Clinics of North America, 14*(1), 137–162.

van't Hooft, I., Andersson, K., Bergman, B., Sejersen, T., Von Wendt, L., & Bartfai, A. (2005). Beneficial effect from a cognitive training programme on children with acquired brain injuries demonstrated in a controlled study. *Brain Injury, 19*(7), 511–518.

van't Hooft, I., Andersson, K., Bergman, B., Sejersen, T., Von Wendt, L., & Bartfai, A. (2007). Sustained favourable effects of cognitive training in children with acquired brain injuries. *NeuroRehabilitation, 22*, 109–116.

van't Hooft, I., Andersson, K., Sejersen, T., Bartfai, A., & von Wendt, L. (2003). Attention and memory training in children with acquired brain injuries. *Acta Paediatrica, 92*(8), 935–940.

van Praag, H., Christie, B. R., Sejnowski, T. J., & Gage, F. H. (1999). Running enhances neurogenesis, learning, and long-term potentiation in mice. *Proceedings of the National Academy of Sciences USA, 96*, 13427–13431.

Vargha-Khadem, F., Watters, G. V., & O'Gorman, A. M. (1985). Development of speech and language following bilateral frontal lesions. *Brain and Language, 25*(1), 167–183.

Waber, D. P., Carpentieri, S. C., Klar, N., Silverman, L. B., Schwenn, M., Hurwitz, C. A., et al. (2000). Cognitive sequelae in children treated for acute lymphoblastic leukemia with dexamethasone or prednisone. *Journal of Pediatric Hematology/Oncology, 22*(3), 206–213.

Wheeden, A., Scafidi, F. A., Field, T., Ironson, G., Valdeon, C., & Bandstra, E. (1993). Massage effects on cocaine-exposed preterm neonates. *Journal of Developmental and Behavioral Pediatrics, 14*, 318–322.

Whyte, J., Hart, T., Vaccaro, M., Grieb-Neff, P., Risser, A., Polansky, M., et al. (2004). Effects of methylphenidate on attention deficits after traumatic brain injury: A multidisciplinary, randomized, controlled trial. *American Journal of Physical and Medical Rehabilitation, 83*, 401–420.

Whyte, J., Vaccaro, M., & Grieb-Neff, P. (2002). Psychostimulant use in the rehabilitation of individuals with traumatic brain injury. *Journal of Head Trauma Rehabilitation, 17,* 284–299.

Williams, S. E., Ris, M. D., Ayyangar, R., Schefft, B. K., & Berch, D. (1998). Recovery in pediatric brain injury: Is psychostimulant medication beneficial? *Journal of Head Trauma Rehabilitation, 13*(3), 73–81.

Woods, B. T., & Teuber, H. L. (1973). Early onset of complementary specialization of cerebral hemispheres in man. *Transactions of the American Neurological Association, 98,* 113–117.

Yablon, S. A. (1993). Postraumatic seizures. *Archives of Physical Medicine and Rehabilitation, 74*(9), 983–1001.

Yeates, K. O., Taylor, H. G., Wade, S. L., Drotar, D., Stancin, T., & Minich, N. (2002). A prospective study of short- and long-term neuropsychological outcomes after traumatic brain injury in children. *Neuropsychology, 16*(4), 514–523.

CHAPTER 10

Language Therapy

SUSAN A. LEON
LYNN M. MAHER
LESLIE J. GONZALEZ ROTHI

References to treatment of neurologically induced deficits of language processing can be found in the literature as far back as Biblical times. Though these early efforts focused on remedies such as herbal potions or the placing of stones in the mouth, it was not until World War I that investigators began to focus on behavioral manipulations for the management of aphasia. Between 1965 and 1985, research focused on establishing that aphasia treatment is efficacious in order to answer the question posed by Darley (1972, p. 7): "Does language rehabilitation accomplish measurable gains in language function beyond what can be expected to occur as a result of spontaneous recovery?" Siegel (1987, p. 306) suggested that these early efficacy studies were pursued "not to learn about therapy, but rather to satisfy the skeptics who look at communication therapy with a jaundiced eye and a shrinking purse." Paired with a newly emerging emphasis on the translation of basic discoveries into clinical applications, research shifted its focus from establishing "treatment efficacy" to searching for "efficacious treatments."

This focus on treatment innovation and evolution through the process of clinical trials is ultimately yielding the information needed for successful evidence-based practice in aphasia rehabilitation. Several comprehensive databases analyzing the efficaciousness of treatments are now available, and the reader is referred to these sources (Evidence-Based Treatment Outcomes in Aphasia, Veteran Affairs Field Advisory Council; Speech and Language Therapy for Aphasia Following Stroke, Cochrane Database).

COMMON APPROACHES TO APHASIA TREATMENT

Because this volume is devoted to neuroplasticity, we focus in this section on therapies aimed at reconditioning language function, rather than on those aimed at teaching compensation for lost language function. We describe a sample of treatments; these are selected exemplars rather than exhaustive lists.

The first category of treatments we discuss addresses deficits in phonology and the lexicon. *Phonology* is the sound system of language, while the *lexicon* is the vocabulary. We describe treatments targeting remediation at the phonological level, as well as therapies aimed at improving naming and word retrieval. The second category consists of treatments at the level of syntax, which governs the way that words can be arranged in a sentence. The therapies described here are aimed at remediation of sentence-level production deficits. *Verbal generation* or communicative intention is the focus of the third category, which encompasses treatments targeting initiation and elaboration of verbal responses. Treatments for retraining *comprehension* constitute the fourth category.

In the following section, we briefly review a selection of studies that have provided functional magnetic resonance imaging (fMRI) evidence suggesting a correlative relationship between neural map changes and functional change in the context of aphasia treatment. We then address the principles of experience-dependent learning as they apply to language rehabilitation, and discuss the use or nonuse of these principles in the described language therapies. The final major section of the chapter focuses on a newly emerging approach to aphasia rehabilitation that is designed to maximize the advantages offered by what is known about experience-dependent neuroplasticity. We conclude the chapter with a discussion of the "new frontier" in language treatment—that of adjunctive treatments. These adjuncts are designed to layer onto behavioral treatments, in hopes of optimizing the yield of the behavioral attempts at rehabilitation.

Phonology and the Lexicon

Retrieving the phonological representation of a word targeted for production begins with the meaning one is trying to communicate to a receiver. The first treatment we describe here attempts to refine the ability to specify the meaning of an object or idea clearly and accurately. Next is a semantic treatment that targets the linkage between a meaning and a word form more specifically. Finally, we describe a phonologically based treatment that targets the word form itself.

Semantic Feature Analysis

Semantic feature analysis is a treatment based on the concept of activating a greater portion of an item's semantic network to boost activation of the item itself, thereby increasing the chance that a person with aphasia will be able to retrieve it. The person with aphasia is guided by questioning from a clinician to produce the most salient and distinguishing features for the target concept. For example, if a person has been unsuccessful in retrieving the word *dog*, he or she might be asked to describe elements of the targeted item (such as *tail* or *fur*), or might be asked what sound this animal makes or where this animal usually lives. Producing words that are semantically related to the target word is thought to activate the entire semantic network surrounding the target, thus spreading activation throughout the network and boosting the activation of the target item itself above threshold level. This type of treatment has been used for individuals with aphasia with moderate success; most showed word retrieval improvement for treated items and limited generalization to untreated items (Boyle & Coelho, 1995; Coelho, McHugh, & Boyle, 2000; Lowell, Beeson, & Holland, 1995).

Semantic Cueing Treatment

Semantic cueing treatment, usually used for persons with anomic aphasia, specifically targets the lexical–semantic level of processing. A clinician provides cues or prompts to guide a person with aphasia toward producing the target. Tasks that may be used include semantic relatedness judgments, provision of antonyms or synonyms for a given word, categorization of objects or pictures, or matching of pictures to words (Wambaugh et al., 2001). Semantic cueing therapy is not a unitary treatment, however, and some semantic tasks may produce more benefit than others. Nickels and Best (1996) suggest that word-to-picture matching may be more effective than semantic relatedness judgments in producing transfer of production to untreated items. In addition, some studies have shown that semantic cueing was inferior to phonological cueing (Saito & Takeda, 2001), or that semantic cueing treatments did not result in as much generalization to untreated items as did phonological cueing (Greenwald, Raymer, Richardson, & Gonzalez Rothi, 1995). However, other studies have obtained equivocal results when comparing semantic cueing to phonological cueing (Howard, Patterson, Franklin, Orchard-Lisle, & Morton, 1985), and some researchers suggest that a combination of semantic and phonological cueing may in fact be most beneficial (Drew & Thompson, 1999).

Phonological Cueing Treatment

Phonological cueing treatment is also used for individuals with naming deficits and targets the lexical–phonological level of processing. Tasks used in this type of treatment include rhyme generation, rhyme judgments, repetition of oral models of the target, and production of targets following cueing of the initial sound of the word (Wambaugh et al., 2001). One study evaluated the use of phonological cueing treatment to determine whether it could produce lasting improvements in word retrieval (Hickin, Best, Herbert, Howard, & Osborne, 2002), and found that both phonological and orthographic cues were effective in facilitating naming.

Summary

All of these treatments target skills required to arrive at single-word-level representation. These treatments also all involve the use of cueing by the therapist to aid the individual with aphasia in production. As stated previously, these have been selected merely as exemplars for remediating phonological and lexical systems; there are other treatments worth noting as well. One such treatment focuses on the use of actions to prompt intentional systems to influence language production activity. An intentional movement involving a lateralized hand gesture, paired with language production activity, caused a shift in neural activation on fMRI from the left to the right hemisphere during naming tasks (Crosson et al., 2005). Another promising treatment at the phonological level, reported by Kendall, Conway, Rosenbek, and Gonzalez Rothi (2003), utilizes the Lindamood Phoneme Sequencing (LIPs) Program (Lindamood & Lindamood, 1998) developed for use with individuals with developmental dyslexia. The LIPS Program explicitly trains individuals to discriminate between different phonemes by using visual and auditory cues, as well as pictorial representations of the mouth movements used to produce each of the different phonemes.

Syntax

Syntax Stimulation

Syntax stimulation treatments have been devised and administered to individuals with aphasia who show deficits in grammatical sentence production. The foremost of these is the Helm Elicited Program for Syntax Stimulation, which is a hierarchically structured approach that uses a story completion format as well as picture description (Helm-Estabrooks & Ramsberger, 1986). The treatment aim is to elicit verbal productions of targeted syntactical structures organized in a hierarchy of linguistic difficulty. The clinician reads to the individual with aphasia a short story (usually two sentences) that ends with a question, followed by a response sentence that uses a targeted structure. The clinician then rereads the story without the targeted response, and the person supplies the final sentence. Here is an example of such a story: "Rob's grandchild is bored. Rob gets a book, and he reads his grandchild a story. What does he do? He reads his grandchild a story." The first two sentences are then repeated, and the individual with aphasia is asked to produce the target sentence aloud.

This treatment has been shown to result in significant posttreatment improvement on a standardized syntax screening test (Helm-Estabrooks & Ramsberger, 1986), in generalization by some participants to untreated sentences of the same structure, and in generalization to untreated sentence structures (Fink et al., 1995). Syntax stimulation treatment has also been shown to be effective in chronic aphasia (Murray & Ray, 2001).

Structure-Level Training

Structure-level training for syntax focuses on training persons with aphasia to use a particular syntactic structure within a sentence. One of the best known is linguistic-specific treatment, later referred to as treatment of underlying forms (Thompson, 1998). This treatment focuses a person's attention on the individual elements in the sentence (such as noun phrases) by teaching him or her first how to identify the structures, and then how to move the structures to create more complex types of sentences. A treatment designed to target the structure and use of *wh-* questions (questions beginning with *What, Where, Who*, etc.) by using story completion items resulted in improved use of these structures in both trained and untrained versions (Wambaugh & Thompson, 1989). This treatment was then expanded so that participants were also trained to recognize the lexical and syntactic properties of declarative sentences and to understand what movements were necessary to create the interrogative form (*wh-* question). For example, a person might be given a sentence such as "The girl went to the store" and trained to create a *wh-* question such as "Who went to the store?" Other structural elements may also be targeted with this treatment. This treatment has resulted in improved use of *wh-* structures and use of more complex sentence structures (Thompson, Shapiro, Tait, Jacobs, & Schneider, 1996). In later versions of this treatment approach, Thompson and colleagues applied the same strategies to train complex syntactic structures. They demonstrated that treatment of complex sentences requiring particular syntactic operations generalizes to other complex sentences using the same operations, as well as to less complex structures contained within the more complex sentence (Thompson, Shapiro, Kiran, & Sobecks, 2003).

Mapping Therapy

Mapping therapy is a treatment for a syntactic or word order deficit in aphasia resulting from difficulty in thematic role assignment (i.e., accurate placement of the arguments around the verb) (Caramazza, Capasso,

Capitani, & Miceli, 2005; Chatterjee & Maher, 2000; Saffran, Schwartz, & Marin, 1980; Schwartz, Saffran, & Marin, 1980). It is based on the premise that some deficits in sentence production and comprehension are due to difficulties in "mapping" the underlying thematic roles to sentence structure, resulting in problems with comprehending or communicating knowledge of who is doing what to whom. Performance is often worsened with reversible sentences (i.e., ones in which it is plausible to reverse the actor and the recipient of the action).

Mapping problems may be explained by a deficit at the early stage of sentence production, during which the thematic relationship of sentence elements is established (Berndt, 1998; Chatterjee & Maher, 2000; Garrett, 1980, 1984). Mapping therapies have been designed to address assignment of thematic roles in sentences and to explicitly strengthen the association between thematic roles and word order (Byng, 1988; Byng & Black, 1995; Chatterjee, Maher, & Heilman, 1995; Maher, Chatterjee, Gonzalez, Rothi, & Heilman, 1995; Schwartz, Saffran Fink, Myers, & Martin, 1994). Individuals with aphasia are trained to identify verbs, agents, and themes with color-coded and spatially coded templates, in an effort to strengthen the association between the thematic roles and word order. Mapping therapy has been demonstrated to be effective in improving sentence comprehension and production in some individuals with agrammatism (Byng et al., 1994; Schwartz et al., 1994; Wierenga et al., 2006).

Summary

These treatments target the more complex language level of sentence production. Not all of the treatments require the participants to produce verbal responses, and they involve less direct "cueing" by the therapist than in the phonological and lexical treatments do. However, all have the same essential goal—to retrain the use and comprehension of syntactically complex sentences.

Verbal Generation

Melodic Intonation Therapy

Melodic intonation therapy (MIT; Alberts, Sparks, & Helm, 1973) was designed to recruit the nondominant hemisphere through an explicit focus on the melodic line and rhythm of spoken utterances. This therapy is often used for those individuals with aphasia who are severely nonfluent but who have moderately preserved auditory comprehension. MIT is a hierarchically structured treatment involving three levels, arranged from simplest to most difficult in terms of syntactic complexity. In the first two levels, single multisyllabic words and then short phrases are produced by the person, using musical intonation. The clinician acts as a metronome, tapping out the syllables on the person's left hand while he or she is intoning the words or phrases. At the third level, the participant moves to longer, more complex phrases—first using melodic intonation, then using exaggerated prosodic contours, and finally producing complex phrases with normal prosodic contours. All utterances are selected before a treatment session begins, and the pitch, stress, and rhythm patterns are noted. The clinician models the utterance, making sure to intone very slowly and to maintain voicing throughout. MIT has resulted in marked improvements in naming as well as increases in phrase length for individuals with aphasia (Sparks, Helm & Albert, 1974; Sparks & Holland, 1976).

Response Elaboration Training

Response elaboration training is used to expand the quantity of the verbal output of those with aphasia. It uses a structured questioning technique to elicit and expand verbal productions. The treatment was intended to emphasize communication functionality over language form, focusing on the interactive aspect of communication to a greater extent than highly structured training programs do (Kearns, 1985). Picture stimuli are used to elicit verbal responses from the person, who then is encouraged to respond spontaneously. The response solicitation does not specify words or language structures to target. After response, the clinician encourages the individual with aphasia to elaborate, using a series of *wh*- questions. This treatment has been reported to generalize across clinicians, and treated items using these methods have been shown to generalize to novel settings (Kearns & Potechin Scher, 1989).

Promoting Aphasics' Communicative Effectiveness

Promoting Aphasics' Communicative Effectiveness (PACE; Davis & Wilcox, 1985) was designed as a naturalistic way to improve the communication performances of an individual with aphasia. It involves reciprocal exchanges of ideas between a therapist and an individual. PACE is based on four principles, the first of which stresses that the ideas communicated between a clinician and an individual with aphasia must involve an exchange of new information. The second principle stresses that the participation in communication must be equal; that is, the therapist is not to exert undue influence in shaping it. The third principle is that the individual with aphasia may use any communication mode desired, and the final principle is that the feedback given to the person must be functional. This therapy has been used for different types of aphasias and varying levels of deficit. At least one study has shown PACE to be effective in producing "observable improvement" on confrontation naming and picture description by a severely aphasic individual (Li, Kitselman, Dusatko, & Spinelli, 1988).

Additional Comments

The therapies just described are designed to encourage verbal elaboration or to improve the fluency of verbal output of individuals with aphasia. There are other noteworthy therapies aimed at improving language output by improving other factors that influence output, such as perseveration or difficulty in initiating speech. Voluntary control of involuntary utterances (Helm & Barresi, 1980) uses spontaneous and involuntary utterances as the basis for treatment of individuals with severe aphasia. An individual with aphasia is assisted in bringing the involuntary utterances (stereotypies) under voluntary control, leading to more volitional use of language. A similar treatment for verbal perseveration, called treatment of aphasic perseveration, has been developed (Helm-Estabrooks, Emory, & Albert, 1987).

Auditory Comprehension

Sentence-Level Auditory Comprehension

Sentence-level auditory comprehension (SLAC) is a three-level treatment for auditory comprehension. The treatment starts at the single-word level, requiring the person to discriminate between auditorily presented word pairs (same vs. different). The next level involves matching a prerecorded target word to a written word, and the last level involves matching a prerecorded word embedded in a sentence to a written word. SLAC has been shown to improve auditory comprehension in some people with chronic aphasia (Naesar, Haas, Mazurski, & Laughlin, 1986).

Token Test

Auditory comprehension treatments using the format of the Token Test (DeRenzi & Vignola, 1962) have also been devised. The Token Test requires a person to follow verbally presented directions of increasing length and complexity to form patterns using tokens of different sizes and colors. The training based upon this format exposes the participant to similarly increasing lengths and syntactic complexities of verbal directions, and with its use, improvement in performance on the Token Test has been shown (Holland & Sonderman, 1974; West, 1973).

Summary

These are two commonly used treatments for auditory comprehension difficulties in individuals with aphasia. Both treatments start at levels of less complex language comprehension (i.e., single words or single-step commands) and progress to more complex language comprehension tasks. This simple-to-complex hierarchy has been a traditional strategic approach to language treatment in aphasia; however, the value of this tradition is now questioned. Thompson's (2007) data suggest that treatments targeting simpler language forms (in the case of Thompson's data, syntax and grammar) result in no generalization to untreated forms, whereas starting with more complex forms results in generalization of treatment effects to less complex stimuli or behaviors.

Therapies for Aphasia: Conclusions

What can we learn from our experience with these therapies for aphasia? Most importantly we learn that aphasia is treatable. This conclusion has been supported by a meta-analysis of aphasia treatment which showed "that aphasia treatment is efficacious, resulting in superior performance by persons receiving language therapy" (Robey, 1994).

We also learn that aphasia rehabilitation has an important limitation—namely, that there is often little generalization to untreated language behaviors or contexts. *Generalization* in aphasia treatment is the process whereby the effects of a given treatment extend to untreated behaviors, stimuli, or contexts. The mechanisms of generalization in language treatment are still poorly understood (Nadeau, Gonzalez Rothi, & Rosenbek, 2008). In addition, measurement and focus of generalization vary among researchers, depending on the objective of the given treatment.

Finally, we learn that treatment gains often drop off after therapy has ended. *Maintenance* is the process wherein improved performance on a treated behavior is retained after the treatment ends.

A more in-depth discussion of treatment generalization and maintenance can be found in Leon et al. (2008). Creating therapies where treatment gains are maintained and generalize to untreated stimuli, behavior, and contexts remains the key challenge of language rehabilitation research. It is possible that many treatments result in poor generalization and maintenance because they fail to result in lasting neural reorganization. It has been suggested that the brain must change to alter behavior in enduring ways (Kolb, Cioe, & Williams, Chapter 2, this volume). Can the yield of rehabilitation be increased by using principles of plasticity such as those suggested by Kolb et al. in Chapter 2, or by Kleim and Jones (2008)? In the remainder of this chapter, we highlight only the principles of plasticity most salient to language rehabilitation, while recognizing that this list is not exhaustive.

NEUROPLASTICITY AND APHASIA

Neuroscience has made major advances in understanding how brain structure can be encouraged or enabled to remodel—a process generally instantiated by learning. This remodeling is not a single event, but rather a complex chain of molecular, cellular, structural, and physiological events that depend upon one another (Kleim & Jones, 2008). Neural remodeling is usually referred to as *neuroplasticity*, and is thought to involve neurons' altering their structure and function in response to a variety of conditions, including drugs or such experiences as behavioral therapies (see Kolb & Whishaw, 1998, for a review). Research has shown that learning results in a remodeling of neural circuitry (i.e., change in the number or functioning of synapses) to encode the new experience or behavior (Friel, Heddings, & Nudo, 2000; Nudo & Milliken, 1996). However, much of the research completed to date has used animal models, and although the findings may be intuitively applicable to humans, this has yet to be confirmed. Thanks to a recent emphasis on translational neuroscientific investigation focused on rehabilitation issues, we may see these basic discoveries studied in humans in the decade ahead. In the meantime, researchers are tentatively applying some of these emerging principles to rehabilitation of aphasia and other cognitive disorders that are chronic consequences of stroke. We focus in this chapter on the treatment of aphasia, because of the large corpus of treatment studies that target this cognitive domain; however, the findings may apply to other cognitive domains in some instances.

Most of what we currently suspect about neuroplasticity and aphasia treatment comes from studies utilizing functional imaging. Since we cannot directly examine cellular or molecular neural changes in humans following stroke (as is commonly done in animal models), we infer neuroplasticity from the changes in activity seen via imaging techniques such as functional MRI or transcranial magnetic imaging. Most studies on neuroplasticity and aphasia examine how brain activity during language use differs between individuals with aphasia and normal controls on different tasks (e.g., naming vs. comprehension). A smaller number of studies examine whether a particular treatment is able to induce both functional and representational change; however, this is a relatively new application of this tool, and only a few studies with small subject samples have been completed.

Not surprisingly, neuroimaging studies of individuals who display recovery of some amount of language function after stroke-induced aphasia have shown that activation is found in perilesional areas and/or contralesional regions (for reviews, see Crosson et al., 2007b; Price & Crinion, 2006; Thompson, 2000). When increased contralesional activity is noted with recovery, it is often in areas that are homologues of normally involved left-hemisphere language structures (e.g., Abo et al., 2004; Calvert et al., 2000; Léger et al., 2002; Naeser et al., 2004; Thulborn, Carpenter, & Just, 1999; Warburton, Price, Swinburn, & Wise, 1999). Whereas Wierenga et al. (2006) showed primarily left ipsilesional activation associated with recovery of function in the context of a mapping treatment in two individuals with agrammatical aphasia, Thompson (2000) showed more right- than left-hemisphere activity following a linguistic-specific version of sentence-level treatment for aphasia. Consistent with Thompson's (2000) findings, Musso et al. (1999) showed increased activity in the right superior temporal gyrus (homologue activity) following a brief comprehension-based treatment for aphasia.

There has been controversy in the literature regarding whether the increased right-hemisphere activations seen in some studies is maladaptive. Some have suggested that greater recruitment of the unaffected right hemisphere is associated with poor recovery (Heiss, Kessler, Thiel, Ghaemi, & Karbe, 1999). This finding may be due to the fact that those with larger lesions or lesions affecting more critical language areas are forced to recruit right-hemisphere homologues more, but the homologues are not sufficient for complete recovery of language function (Rijntjes, 2006). Others suggest that neural substrates in both hemispheres can play a positive role in functional recovery; however, the time course of involvement may differ (Crosson et al., 2007a). Crosson et al. (2005) designed a treatment that involved using a left-handed gesture to recruit right-hemisphere intentional mechanisms during picture-naming tasks. They found that although there was activation in both hemispheres before and after therapy, the amount of activity in the right hemisphere decreased from pretreatment to posttreatment.

Rijntjes (2006) suggests that there are three phases of hemispheric reorganization following stroke. The first phase, which occurs directly after stroke, results in depression of the entire network. In the second phase, there is up-regulation and overactivation of some areas, particularly in the unaffected hemisphere. In the final phase, activation decreases and may balance between the hemispheres. The precise time course of these phases is not yet clear, but some preliminary data from a longitudinal fMRI study (Saur et al., 2006) support the hypothesis. Evidence from a study investigating recovery following MIT may also be supportive. Positron emission tomography was used to examine seven individuals with chronic nonfluent aphasia who had shown dramatic improvement after receiving MIT (Belin et al., 1996). After treatment, the participants showed greater left- than right-hemisphere activation when intoning words with melodic intonations, whereas they showed greater right-sided activation when they intoned words with no melody. Although MIT is thought to work by recruiting right-hemisphere melody and rhythm abilities, activation following the treatment appeared to be a more "normal" pattern, with reactivation of essential left-sided language areas (Belin et al., 1996).

EXPERIENCE-DEPENDENT LEARNING AND APHASIA

Basic principles have been outlined that govern plasticity in both healthy and damaged brains (for a review, see Kleim & Jones, 2008). A subset of these principles can be used to inform aphasia rehabilitation research (Raymer et al., 2008). These principles include timing, learned nonuse (also called "use it or lose it"), repetition, intensity, specificity, transfer or generalization, saliency, and interference.

Timing of treatment refers to how soon after stroke or injury language rehabilitation is started. There is some evidence from animal studies that starting rehabilitation too quickly may have negative consequences for functional return (Kleim, Jones, & Schallert, 2003). However, it remains to be established at exactly what time after injury the period of possible harm ends. Because there is a tremendous amount of change already happening in the damaged brain, the timing factor may be critical in rehabilitation. Unfortunately, it is also one of the least well-understood principles in humans, due in part to innate timing differences between shorter-lived laboratory animals and humans. If the phases of reorganization (Rijntjes, 2006) are considered, then it is possible that treatment may affect the language system differently in different phases. For instance, treatment during the second phase, when greater activation is seen in the unaffected hemisphere, may result in more recruitment of right-hemisphere language homologues.

Learned nonuse refers to the common finding that failure to use a specific brain function may lead to degradation of that function (Taub, Uswatte, & Elbert, 2002). Lack of use is very important from a rehabilitation standpoint. If a neural system is left unused for long periods, degradation of function can occur. Evidence from these studies has shown that deprivation can result in a loss or reallocation of representation, as well as a decrease in numbers of synapses at the cortex (e.g., Merzenich et al., 1983).

Repetition and *intensity* of the language treatment also have implications for the strength of the response to the intervention. Induction of plasticity requires sufficient repetition, particularly when a therapist is trying to induce change in a behavior as complex as language. Often in rehabilitation a behavior is trained until the person reaches some criterion level, at which point we assume that the person has acquired the behavior. However, animal studies have shown that rats trained on a skilled task require training beyond acquisition to show increases in synaptic strength (Monfils & Teskey, 2004), synapse number, or map reorganization, all of which are indicators of neuroplasticity (Kleim et al., 2004).

Repetition itself is not sufficient; intensity is also crucial to neuroplasticity. In a rehabilitation setting, *intensity* most naturally refers to how often a given treatment is administered. In most clinical settings, language rehabilitation treatment is administered only two or three times a week at best; however, more intensive treatment may result in greater gains for a person. Intensity may be a double-edged sword, though, as overuse has been shown to worsen some motor functions in rats (Kozlowski, James,

& Schallert, 1996). Nevertheless, it is important to remember that studies suggesting that overuse may be dangerous have not been looking at cognitive functions and have shown that there must be an extreme amount of overuse (Kleim & Jones, 2008).

Repeating a previously acquired skill may also not be sufficient to promote plasticity. Learning or acquisition of a new skill may be crucial. Plautz, Milliken, and Nudo (2000) and Kleim, Cooper, and VandenBerg (2002) found that rats repeating previously acquired motor movements did not show significant markers of plasticity, such as synapse addition or cortical map extension. This finding illustrates the principle of *specificity*. Evidence suggests that plasticity is induced by learning a new skilled motor task, rather than by merely repeating an unskilled or previously acquired task. However, it is unclear at this point how these findings may apply to a cognitive function such as language, rather than a motor function.

As noted earlier, *transfer* or *generalization* refers to improvement on a task that has not been trained in treatment. Often in language therapy generalization occurs between related tasks, such as being able to name items in an untrained category that is linked semantically to items that were specifically trained. Using the principles of experience-dependent learning to inform language rehabilitation may also maximize generalization gains for individuals with aphasia.

Saliency is another principle that can be applied to aphasia rehabilitation. *Saliency* in language recovery refers to a treatment's relevance to a person. Although a person may be able to be trained to name items from a list, for example, the task may have little relevance. More personal, and therefore more functional, language rehabilitation may prove to be not only more useful, but also more apt to promote plasticity.

Table 10.1 illustrates that some of these principles have been applied in the course of the common language therapies previously described, but that many others have not been utilized. Might we reap far more from language rehabilitation by considering these principles in designing a treatment program? An example of one current language treatment that does attempt to take advantage of these principles more inclusively (see the bottom row of Table 10.1) is constraint-induced language therapy (CILT).

CILT (also referred to as constraint-induced aphasia therapy or CIAT by Pulvermüller et al., 2001) is modeled after an intervention for chronic hemiplegia, constraint-induced movement therapy (CIMT; Kunkel et al., 1999; Miltner, Bauder, Sommer, Dettmers, & Taub, 1999; Taub, 2000). CIMT was designed to address the principle of learned nonuse, which suggests that the potential rehabilitation of an affected limb is negatively affected by the compensatory use of the unaffected limb (Dromerick, Edwards, & Hahn, 2000; Kopp et al., 1999; Taub, 2000). Learned nonuse is treated by restriction of use (i.e., constraint) of the unimpaired limb, yielding forced use of the impaired limb for intensive amounts of time. A

TABLE 10.1. Common Language Therapies' Use of the Principles Governing Neuroplasticity

Treatments	Timing	Learned nonuse	Transfer (generalization)	Repetition	Intensity	Saliency	Specificity
Phonology and the lexicon							
Semantic feature analysis			+				+
Semantic cueing				+			+
Phonological cueing				+			+
Syntax							
Syntax stimulation			+	+			+
Mapping therapy				+			+
Structure-level training			+	+			+
Verbal fluency and elaboration							
MIT			+	+			
PACE						+	
Response elaboration training						+	
Auditory comprehension							
SLAC				+			+
Token Test				+			+
CILT		+		+	+	+	+

number of studies have shown gains on measures of use of the impaired limb following CIMT, and some have shown increases in motor function as well. These gains have persisted well beyond the termination of therapy (Dettmers et al., 2005; Miltner et al., 1999; Taub, Uswatte, & Pidikiti, 1999). Furthermore, studies have shown not only that persons with chronic hemiparesis benefited clinically from CIMT, but that there was evidence for reorganization of motor cortex after this treatment (Liepert et al., 2000; Taub et al., 1999).

In addition to the principle of learned nonuse, CIMT incorporates other neuroplasticity principles, including repetition, intensity, salience, and specificity. The typical CIMT protocol involves restraint of the unaffected limb in a sling for all waking hours, as well as 6 hours of daily practice in using the affected limb, with a focus on completing functional activities important for daily living (Kunkel et al., 1999; Taub et al., 1999). Although further investigations have yielded conflicting results with respect to the amount of restraint and repetition needed (Page, Sisto, Levine, Johnston, & Hughes, 2001; Page, Sisto, Levine, & McGrath, 2004; Sterr et al., 2002), these principles form the basis of experience-dependent learning in motor rehabilitation following brain damage.

Many of the core principles of use-dependent learning are now being applied in aphasia rehabilitation research (Maher, Kendall, Swearengen, Rodriguez, Leon, et al., 2006; Meinzer, Elbert, Wienbruch, Djunda, Barthel, & Rockstroh, 2005; Pulvermüller, Neininger, Elbert, Elbert, Mohr, et al., 2001). In these studies, constraint was operationalized in the context of language by limiting the participants' response modality to speech through the use of visual barriers. Participants take turns in dyads or triads requesting and responding to requests in a dual card matching paradigm. Because of the placement of visual barriers, the participants were forced to use only the speech modality to request a card and forced to use speech in responding that they did or did not have the card being requested. All other means of communication (e.g., gesturing, pointing, writing, etc.) were prevented (i.e., "constrained") from use.

The results of preliminary studies of CIAT/CILT have been encouraging. Pulvermüller et al. (2001) studied 17 patients with chronic aphasia who had received prior language therapy and were believed to have exhausted their recovery potential. Ten subjects participated in small-group CIAT intensively for 3–4 hours per day over a 2-week period. When compared to another group who received "conventional" speech–language therapy over a distributed period of time for the same total number of hours in therapy, the group receiving CIAT demonstrated significantly greater gains in the amount and quality of communication, as measured by a communicative activity log and a standard aphasia battery. These results were confirmed in a further study using the standard CILT and a modification of the intervention that included writing assignments for homework and training of communication partners outside the therapy (Meinzer et al., 2004).

Maher et al. (2006) examined the influence of intensity on CILT outcome by comparing a group of four CILT participants to a group of five participants who received PACE therapy (Davis & Wilcox, 1985) at the same intensity. Both groups received intervention for 3 hours a day, 4 days a week, for 2 weeks. Although both groups demonstrated significant change from pre- to posttherapy on standard aphasia measures, individual case data suggested that three of the four participants in the CILT group showed significant change and that this gain was further increased at the 1-month follow-up, whereas only one member of the PACE group evinced the same amount of posttreatment change and there was no evidence of continued gains during the follow-up interval for any of the PACE participants. In addition, while linguistic analyses of narrative samples at the same testing intervals revealed an increase in the number of words, utterances, and sentences produced after treatment for the majority of the participants in both groups, results of subjective assessments of the narratives by experienced speech–language pathologists unaware of group membership or sample order suggested that the overall pattern of improvement in narrative discourse was stronger for the CILT group.

Two additional participants received the same amount of CILT but a less intense schedule—3 hours a week for 8 weeks (Maher, Schmadeke, Swearengen, & Gonzalez Rothi, 2005). One of those participants achieved gains comparable to those observed in the intensive version of CILT. These results suggest that at least for some individuals, CILT may be administered successfully in a distributed schedule, and these gains may be retained up to 1 month after treatment. Taken together, the results of these pilot studies suggest that while intensity of intervention may be potent, other aspects of the CILT approach appear to confer benefits beyond those achieved by intensity alone. The principle of saliency has been utilized in CILT by devising rehabilitative language activities that occurred in functionally relevant communication contexts (Maher et al., 2006). The responses required either a request for an item or a response to a request much like that of a typical activity. The "game" atmosphere of the activity created a relevance to completing the task correctly as participants competed to see who could collect the most pairs of cards. Progressively more difficult responses were "shaped" by manipulating the characteristics of the stimulus items, response requirements and reinforcement contingencies adhering to the specificity principle. Initially participants were required to produce only the target word or a brief request. As the participants progressed in therapy, the response demands increased to include full sentences with additional adjectives modifying the target noun. Certain social conventions were also added such as names of co-players, gratitude, and so on. Additional difficulty was introduced by adding low frequency target words to the task, such that the participants were continuously challenged to produce more difficult sentences (Maher et al., 2006).

The study by Maher and colleagues (2006) also incorporated the principles of repetition and specificity. Repetition was incorporated by using a limited number of tasks and through repeated practice of requests and responses on a dual card task. Specificity was addressed in that response requirements were individually determined based on ability, such that one participant might have received positive feedback for achieving one-word responses, whereas a more advanced participant would have been reinforced only if they achieved the entire sentence.

More recently, the principle of specificity has been investigated using constraint induced therapies targeting specific language deficits. Szflarski and colleagues (2008) modified the standard treatment to include individualized skill hierarchies for semantic, syntactic, or phonological abilities of individuals with chronic aphasia. Although the study was too small to determine whether this form of specified constraint induced therapy was more effective than the standard therapy, two of three participants with chronic aphasia showed improvements in verbal skills and comprehension on a standardized language battery. Goral and Kempler (2009) also conducted a single-case study using a modified form of CILT emphasizing the production of verbs. This individual, who had been aphasic for 10 years, was able to produce a significantly greater number of verbs in a narrative generation task following the treatment.

Timing refers to how soon after an injury rehabilitation is begun. The principle of timing was also recently addressed using CILT. Kirmess and Maher (2010) report utilization of CILT with individuals who were in the more acute phases of recovery from stroke (1–2 months). No negative influences of beginning this intensive treatment in the acute phase were observed or reported and all participants showed improvements on language assessments after therapy and at followup.

CONCLUSIONS

There is mounting evidence that interventions for aphasia can produce observable and in some cases lasting changes in language performance, and there is preliminary evidence that those behavioral changes are accompanied by changes in the neural organization of a broadly defined language network. CILT is a good example of such an intervention; however, it is important to remember that there is nothing magical about CILT. This treatment is best characterized as immersion in the acts of speaking and of receiving spoken language. An additional potent principle of plasticity may be the intensity of the treatment schedule (how often and how long), which in common practice today is not necessarily planned, but instead is likely to be determined by availability, convenience, or funding. Although more research is needed to determine exactly how long and how often treatment is needed, there is evidence that intensity can affect treatment outcome. Other aspects are proving to be potent in the treatment of language deficits as well, but intensity has received the most research attention thus far.

Finally, the "new frontier" of language rehabilitation may lie in the study and use of adjunctive therapies. These are therapies that are intended to layer onto behavioral therapies and are designed to optimize neuroplastic potential. These may include drugs such as donapezil, diamphetamine, bromocriptine, piracetam, nerve growth factor, and others still in development, all of which have shown varying levels of effectiveness in promoting recovery from aphasia in placebo-controlled trials (Berthier, 2005). Adjunctive measures may also include therapies such as transcranial magnetic stimulation, which has been found to create favorable changes in individuals with aphasia (Naeser et al., 2005a, 2005b). A great deal of research remains to be done regarding neuroplasticity and language rehabilitation, but the preliminary findings do suggest that the combination of these principles with language treatments will result in greater gains in recovery for individuals suffering from aphasia.

REFERENCES

Abo, M., Senoo, A., Watanabe, S., Miyano, S., Doseki, K., Sasaki, N., et al. (2004). Language-related brain function during word repetition in post-stroke aphasics. *NeuroReport, 15*, 1891–1894.

Alberts, M. L., Sparks, R. W., & Helm, N. A. (1973). Melodic intonation therapy for aphasia. *Archives of Neurology, 29*, 130–131.

Belin, P., Van Eckhout, P., Zilbovicus, M., Remy, Ph., Francois, C., Guillame, S., et al. (1996). Recovery from nonfluent aphasia after melodic intonation therapy: A PET study. *Neurology, 47*, 1504–1511.

Berndt, R. S. (1998). Sentence processing in aphasia. In M. T. Sarno (Ed.), *Acquired aphasia* (3rd ed., pp. 229–268). San Diego, CA: Academic Press.

Berthier, M. L. (2005). Poststroke aphasia: Epidemiology, pathophysiology and treatment. *Drugs and Aging, 22*, 163–182.

Boyle, M., & Coelho, C. (1995). Application of semantic feature analysis as a treatment for aphasic dysnomia. *American Journal of Speech–Language Pathology, 4*(4), 94–98.

Breier, J., Maher, L. M., Castillo, E., Novak, B., & Papanicolaou, A. (2006). Functional imaging before and after constraint induced language therapy for aphasia using magnetoencephalography. *Neurocase, 12*, 322–331.

Byng, S. (1988). Sentence processing deficits: Theory and therapy. *Cognitive Neuropsychology, 5*, 629–676.

Byng, S. (1992). Testing the tried: Replicating sentence-processing therapy for agrammatic Broca's aphasia. *Clinics in Communication Disorders, 2*(1), 34–42.

Byng, S., & Black, M. (1995). What makes a therapy?: Some parameters of therapeutic intervention in aphasia. *European Journal of Disorders of Communication, 30*(3), 303–316.

Calvert, G. A., Brammer, M. J., Morris, R. G., Williams, S. C. R., King, N., & Matthews, P. M. (2000). Using fMRI to study recovery from acquired dysphasia. *Brain and Language, 17*, 391–399.

Caramazza, A., Capasso, R., Capitani, E., & Miceli, G. (2005). Patterns of comprehension performance in agrammatic Broca's aphasia: A test of the trace deletion hypothesis. *Brain and Language, 94*(1), 43–53.

Chatterjee, A., & Maher, L. (2000). Grammar and agrammatism. In S. E. Nadeau, L. J. Gonzalez Rothi, & B. Crosson (Eds.), *Aphasia and language: Theory to practice* (pp. 133–156). New York: Guilford Press.

Chatterjee, A., Maher, L. M., & Heilman, K. M. (1995). Spatial characteristics of thematic role representation. *Neuropsychologia, 33*, 643–648.

Coelho, C. A., McHugh, R. E., & Boyle, M. (2000). Semantic feature analysis as a treatment for aphasic dysnomia: A replication. *Aphasiology, 14*, 133–142.

Crosson, B., Fabrizio, K. S., Singletary, F., Cato, M. A., Wierenga, C. E., Parkinson, R. B., et al. (2007a). Treatment of naming in nonfluent aphasia through manipulation of intention and attention: A phase 1 comparison of two novel treatments. *Journal of the International Neuropsychological Society, 13*(4), 582–594.

Crosson, B., McGregor, K., Gopinath, K. S., Conway, T. W., Benjamin, M., Chang, Y., et al. (2007b). Functional MRI of language in aphasia: A review of the literature and methodological challenges. *Neuropsychology Review, 17*, 157–177.

Crosson, B., Moore, A. B., Gopinath, K., White, K. D., Wierenga, C. E., Gaiefsky, M. E., et al. (2005). Role of the right and left hemispheres in recovery of function during treatment of intention in aphasia. *Journal of Cognitive Neuroscience, 17*(3), 392–406.

Darley, F. L. (1972). The efficacy of language rehabilitation in aphasia. *Journal of Speech and Hearing Disorders, 37*, 3–21.

Davis, G. A., & Wilcox, M. J. (1985). *Adult aphasia rehabilitation: Applied pragmatics.* San Diego, CA: College-Hill Press.

DeRenzi, E., & Vignola, L. (1962). The Token Test: A sensitive test to detect receptive disturbances in aphasia. *Brain, 65*, 665–678.

Dettmers, C., Teske, U., Hamzei, F., Uswatte, G., Taub, E., & Weiller, C. (2005). Distributed form of constraint-induced movement therapy improves functional outcome and quality of life. *Archives of Physical Medicine and Rehabilitation, 86*, 204–209.

Drew, R. L., & Thompson, C. K. (1999). Model-based semantic treatment for naming deficits in aphasia. *Journal of Speech and Hearing Research, 42*, 972–989.

Dromerick, A., Edwards, D., & Hahn, M. (2000). Does the application of constraint-induced movement therapy during acute rehabilitation reduce arm impairment after ischemic stroke? *Stroke, 31*, 2984–2988.

Fink, R. B., Schwartz, M. F., Rochon, E., Myers, J. L., Socolof, G. S., & Bluestone, R. (1995). Syntax stimulation revisited: An analysis of generalization of treatment effects. *American Journal of Speech–Language Pathology, 4*(4), 99–104.

Friel, K. M., Heddings, A. A., & Nudo, R. J. (2000). Effects of postlesion experience on behavioral recovery and neurophysiologic reorganization after cortical injury in primates. *Neurorehabilitation and Neural Repair, 14*, 197–198.

Garrett, M. F. (1980). Levels of processing in sentence production. In B. Butterworth (Ed.), *Language production* (pp. 177–221). New York: Academic Press.

Garrett, M. F. (1984). The organization of processing structure for language production: Application to aphasic speech. In D. Caplan, A. R. Lecours, & A. Smith (Eds.), *Biological perspectives on language* (pp. 172–193). Cambridge, MA: MIT Press.

Goral, M., & Kempler, D. (2009). Training verb production in communicative context: Evidence from a person with chronic non-fluent aphasia. *Aphasiology, 23*(12), 1383–1397.

Greenwald, M. L., Raymer, A. M., Richardson, M. E., & Gonzalez Rothi, L. J. (1995). Contrasting treatments for severe impairments of picture naming. *Neuropsychological Rehabilitation, 5*, 17–49.

Heiss, W. D., Kessler, J., Thiel, A., Ghaemi, M., & Karbe, H. (1999). Differential capacity of left and right hemispheric areas for compensation of post-stroke aphasia. *Annals of Neurology, 45*, 430–438.

Helm, N. A., & Barresi, B. (1980). Voluntary control of involuntary utterances: A treatment approach for severe aphasia. In R. H. Brookshire (Ed.), *Clinical Aphasiology Conference proceedings* (Vol. 10, pp. 308–315). Minneapolis, MN: BRK.

Helm-Estabrooks, N., Emory, P., & Albert, M. L. (1987). Treatment of Aphasic Perseveration (TAP) program. *Archives of Neurology, 44*, 1253–1255.

Helm-Estabrooks, N., & Ramsberger, G. (1986). Treatment of agrammatism in long-term Broca's aphasia. *British Journal of Communication Disorders, 21*, 39–45.

Hickin, J., Best, W., Herbert, R., Howard, D., & Osborne, F. (2002). Phonological therapy for word finding difficulties: A re-evaluation. *Aphasiology, 16*(10), 981–999.

Holland, A. L., & Sonderman, J. C. (1974). Effects of a program based on the Token-Test for teaching comprehension skills to aphasics. *Journal of Speech and Hearing Research, 17*, 589–598.

Howard, D., Patterson, K., Franklin, S., Orchard-Lisle, V., & Morton, J. (1985). The facilitation of picture naming in aphasia. *Cognitive Neuropsychology, 2*, 49–80.

Kearns, K. P. (1985). Response elaboration training for patient initiated utterances. In R. H. Brookshire (Ed.), *Clinical Aphasiology Conference proceedings* (Vol. 15, pp. 196–204). Minneapolis, MN: BRK.

Kearns, K. P., & Potechin Scher, G. (1989). The generalization of response elaboration training. In T. E. Prescott (Ed.), *Clinical aphasiology* (Vol. 18, pp. 223–245). Boston: College-Hill Press.

Kendall, D., Conway, T., Rosenbek, J., & Gonzalez Rothi, L. J. (2003). Phonologic rehabilitation of acquired phonologic alexia. *Aphasiology, 17*(11), 1073–1095.

Kirmess, M., & Maher, L. M. (2010). Constraint induced language therapy in early aphasia rehabilitation. *Aphasiology, 24*(6–8), 725–736.

Kleim, J. A., Cooper, N. R., & VandenBerg, P. M. (2002). Exercise induces angiogenesis but does not alter movement representations within rat motor cortex. *Brain Research, 934*, 1–6.

Kleim, J. A., Hogg, T. M., VandenBerg, P. M., Cooper, N. R., Bruneau, R., & Remple, M. (2004). Cortical synaptogenesis and motor map reorganization occur during late, but not early, phase of motor skill learning. *Journal of Neuroscience, 24*, 628–633.

Kleim, J. A., & Jones, T. A. (2008). Principles of experience dependent neural plasticity: Implications for rehabilitation after brain damage. *Journal of Speech, Language, and Hearing Research, 51*(1), S225–S239.

Kleim, J. A., Jones, T. A., & Schallert, T. (2003). Motor enrichment and the induction of plasticity before or after brain injury. *Neurochemical Research, 24*, 1757–1769.

Kolb, B., & Whishaw, I. Q. (1998). Brain plasticity and behavior. *Annual Review of Psychology, 49*, 43–61.

Kopp, B., Kunkel, A., Muhlnickel, W., Villringer, K., Taub, E., & Flor, H. (1999)

Plasticity in the motor system related to therapy-induced improvement of movement after stroke. *NeuroReport, 10*, 807–810.

Kozlowski, D. A., James, D. C., & Schallert, T. (1996). Use-dependent exaggeration of neuronal injury after unilateral sensorimotor cortex lesions. *Journal of Neuroscience, 16*, 4776–4786.

Kunkel, A., Kopp, B., Muller, G., Villringer, K., Villringer, A., Taub, E., et al. (1999). Constraint-induced movement therapy for motor recovery in chronic stroke patients. *Archives of Physical Medicine and Rehabilitation, 80*, 624–628.

Léger, A., Démonet, J. F., Ruff, S., Aithamon, B., Touyeras, B., Puel, M., et al. (2002). Neural substrates of spoken language rehabilitation in an aphasic patient: An fMRI study. *NeuroImage, 17*, 174–183.

Leon, S. A., Nadeau, S. E., de Riesthal, M., Crosson, B., Rosenbek, J. C., & Gonzalez Rothi, L. J. (2008). Aphasia. In D. T. Stuss, G. Winocur, I. Robertson (Eds.), *Cognitive neurorehabilitation: Evidence and applications* (2nd ed., pp. 435–448). Cambridge, UK: Cambridge University Press.

Li, E. C., Kitselman, K., Dusatko, D., & Spinelli, C. (1988). The efficacy of PACE in the remediation of naming deficits. *Journal of Communication Disorders, 21*, 111–123.

Liepert, J., Bauder, H., Wolfgagn, H. R., Miltner, W., Taub, E., & Weiller, C. (2000). Treatment-induced cortical reorganization after stroke in humans. *Stroke, 31*(6), 1210–1216.

Lindamood, P. C., & Lindamood, P. D. (1998). *The Lindamood Phoneme Sequencing Program for reading, spelling, and speech.* Austin, TX: PRO-ED.

Lowell, S., Beeson, P. M., & Holland, A. L. (1995). The efficacy of semantic cueing procedures on naming performance of adults with aphasia. *American Journal of Speech–Language Pathology, 4(4), 109–114.*

Maher, L. M., Chatterjee, A., Gonzalez Rothi, L. J., & Heilman, K. M. (1995). Agrammatic sentence production: The use of a temporal-spatial strategy. *Brain and Language, 49*, 105–124.

Maher, L. M., Kendall, D., Swearengin, J. A., Rodriguez, A., Leon, S. A., Pingel, K., et al. (2006). A pilot study of use-dependent learning in the context of constraint induced language therapy. *Journal of the International Neuropsychological Society, 12*, 843–852.

Maher, L. M., Schmadeke, S., Swearengin, J., & Gonzalez Rothi, L. J. (2005). Intensity variation for constraint induced language therapy for aphasia. *The ASHA Leader: 2005 Convention Program, 166.*

Meinzer, M., Elbert, T., Wienbruch, C., Djundja, D., Barthel, G., & Rockstroh, B. (2004). Intensive language training enhances brain plasticity in chronic aphasia. *BCM Biology, 2*(20). Retrieved from *www.biomedcentral.com/1741-7007/2/20*

Merzenich, M. M., Kaas, J. H., Wall, J., Nelson, R. J., Sur, M., & Felleman, D. (1983). Topographic reorganization of somatosensory cortical areas 3b and 1 in adult monkeys following restricted deafferentiation. *Neuroscience, 8*, 33–55.

Miltner, W., Bauder, H., Sommer, M., Dettmers, C., & Taub, E. (1999). Effects of constraint-induced movement therapy on patients with chronic motor deficits after stroke: A replication. *Stroke, 30*(3), 586–592.

Monfils, M. H., & Teskey, G. C. (2004). Skilled-learning-induced potentiation in rat sensorimotor cortex: A transient form of behavioral long-term potentiation. *Neuroscience, 125*, 329–336.

Murray, L. L., & Ray, A. H. (2001). A comparison between relaxation training and syntax stimulation for chronic nonfluent aphasia. *Journal of Communication Disorders, 34*, 87–113.

Musso, M., Weiller, C., Kiebel, S., Müller, S. P., Bülau, P., & Rijntjes, M. (1999). Training-induced brain plasticity in aphasia. *Brain, 122*, 1781–1790.

Nadeau, S., Gonzalez Rothi, L. J., & Rosenbek, J. (2008). Language rehabilitation from a neural perspective. In R. Chapey (Ed.), *Language intervention strategies in adult aphasia* (pp. 689–734). Baltimore: Williams & Wilkins.

Naeser, M. A., Haas, G., Mazurski, P., & Laughlin, S. (1986). Sentence level auditory comprehension treatment program for aphasic adults. *Archives of Physical Medicine and Rehabilitation, 67*, 393–399.

Naeser, M. A., Martin, P. I., Baker, E. H., Hodge, S. M., Sczerzenie, S. E., Nicholas, M., et al. (2004). Overt propositional speech in chronic nonfluent aphasia studied with the dynamic susceptibility contrast fMRI method. *NeuroImage, 22*, 29–41.

Naeser, M. A., Martin, P. I., Nicholas, M., Baker, E. H., Seekins, H., Helm-Estabrooks, N., et al. (2005a). Improved naming after TMS treatments in a chronic, global aphasia patient: Case report. *Neurocase, 11*(3), 182–193.

Naeser, M. A., Martin, P. I., Nicholas, M., Baker, E. H., Seekins, H., Kobayashi, M., et al. (2005b). Improved picture naming in chronic aphasia after TMS to part of right Broca's area: An open protocol study. *Brain and Language, 93*(1), 95–105.

Nickels, L., & Best, W. (1996). Therapy for naming disorders: Part II. Specifics, surprises, and suggestions. *Aphasiology, 10*, 109–136.

Nudo, R. J., & Milliken, G. W. (1996). Reorganization of movement representations in primary motor cortex following focal ischemic infarcts in adult squirrel monkeys. *Journal of Neurophysiology, 75*, 2144–2149.

Page, S. J., Sisto, S. A., Levine, P., Johnston, M. V., & Hughes, M. (2001). Modified constraint induced therapy: A randomized feasibility and efficacy study. *Journal of Rehabilitation Research and Development, 38*, 583–590.

Page, S. J., Sisto, S. A., Levine, P., & McGrath, R. E. (2004). Efficacy of modified constraint-induced movement therapy in chronic stroke: A single-blind randomized controlled trial. *Archives of Physical Medicine and Rehabilitation, 85*, 14–18.

Plautz, E. J., Milliken, G. W., & Nudo, R. J. (2000). Effects of repetitive motor training on movement representations in adult squirrel monkeys: Role of use versus learning. *Neurobiology of Learning and Memory, 74*, 27–55.

Price, C. J., & Crinion, J. (2005). The latest on functional imaging studies of aphasic stroke. *Current Opinion in Neurology, 18*, 429–434.

Pulvermüller, F., Neininger, B., Elbert, T. R., Mohr, B., Rockstroh, B., Koebbel, P., et al. (2001). Constraint-induced therapy of chronic aphasia after stroke. *Stroke, 32*, 1621–1626.

Raymer, A. M., Kendall, D., Maher, L., Martin, N., Murray, L., Rose, M., et al. (2008). Translational research in aphasia: From neuroscience to neurorehabilitation. *Journal of Speech, Language, and Hearing Research, 51*, 259–275.

Rijntjes, M. (2006). Mechanisms of recovery in stroke patients with hemiparesis or aphasia: New insights, old questions and the meaning of therapies. *Current Opinion in Neurology, 19*, 76–83.

Robey, R. R. (1994). The efficacy of treatment for aphasic persons: A meta-analysis. *Brain and Language, 47*, 582–608.

Saffran, E. M., Schwartz, M. F., & Marin, O. S. (1980). The word order problem in agrammatism: II. Production. *Brain and Language, 10*(2), 263–280.

Saito, A., & Takeda, K. (2001). Semantic cueing effects on word retrieval in aphasic patients with lexical retrieval deficit. *Brain and Language, 77*, 1–9.

Saur, D., Lange, R., Baumgaertner, A., Schraknepper, V., Willmes, K., Rijntjes, M., et al. (2006). Dynamics of language reorganization after stroke. *Brain, 129*, 1371–1384.

Schwartz, M. F., Saffran, E. M., Fink, R. B., Myers, J. L., & Martin, N. (1994). Mapping therapy: A treatment programme for agrammatism. *Aphasiology, 8*, 19–54.

Schwartz, M. F., Saffran, E. M., & Marin, O. S. (1980). The word order problem in agrammatism. I. Comprehension. *Brain and Language, 10*(2), 249–262.

Siegel, G. M. (1987). The limits of science in communication disorders. *Journal of Speech and Hearing Disorders, 52*, 306–312.

Sparks, R., Helm, N., & Albert, M. (1974). Aphasia rehabilitation resulting from melodic intonation therapy. *Cortex, 10*(4), 303–316.

Sparks, R. W., & Holland, A. L. (1976). Treatment: Melodic intonation therapy for aphasia. *Journal of Speech and Hearing Disorders, 41*, 287–297.

Sterr, A., Elbert, T., Berthold, I., Kolbel, S., Rockstroh, B., & Taub, E. (2002). Longer versus shorter daily constraint induced movement therapy of chronic hemiparesis: An exploratory study. *Archives of Physical Medicine and Rehabilitation, 83*, 1374–1377.

Szflarski, J. P., Ball, A. L., Grether, S., Al-Fwaress, F., Griffith, N. M., Neils-Strunjas, J., et al. (2008). Constraint-induced aphasia therapy stimulates language recovery in patients with chronic aphasia after ischemic stroke. *Medical Science Monitor, 14*(5), 243–250.

Taub, E. (2000). Constraint-induced movement therapy and massed practice. *Stroke, 31*, 986–988.

Taub, E., Uswatte, G., & Elbert, T. (2002). New treatments in neurorehabilitation founded on basic research. *Nature Reviews: Neuroscience, 3*, 228–236.

Taub, E., Uswatte, G., & Pidikiti, R. (1999). Constraint-induced movement therapy: A new family of techniques with broad application to physical rehabilitation. A clinical review. *Journal of Rehabilitation Research and Development, 36*(3), 237–251.

Thompson, C. K. (1998). Treating sentence production in agrammatic aphasia. In N. Helm-Estabrooks & A. Holland (Eds.), *Approaches to treatment of aphasia* (pp. 113–151). San Diego, CA: Singular.

Thompson, C. K. (2000). Neuroplasticity: Evidence from aphasia. *Journal of Communication Disorders, 33*, 357–366.

Thompson, C. K. (2007). Complexity in language learning and treatment. *American Journal of Speech–Language Pathology, 16*, 3–5.

Thompson, C. K., Shapiro, L. P., Kiran, S., & Sobecks, J. (2003). The role of syntactic complexity in treatment of sentence deficits in agrammatic aphasia: The complexity account of treatment efficacy (CATE). *Journal of Speech, Language, and Hearing Research, 46*, 591–607.

Thompson, C. K., Shapiro, L. P., Tait, M. E., Jacobs, B. J., & Schneider, S. L. (1996). Training wh- question production in agrammatic aphasia: Analysis of argument and adjunct movement. *Brain and Language, 52*, 175–228.

Thulborn, K. R., Carpenter, P. A., & Just, M. A. (1999). Plasticity of language-related function during recovery from stroke. *Stroke, 30*, 749–754.

Wambaugh, J. L., Linebaugh, C. W., Doyle, P. J., Martinez, A. L., Kalinyak-Fliszar, M., & Spencer, K. A. (2001). Effects of two cueing treatments on lexical retrieval in aphasic speakers with different levels of deficit. *Aphasiology, 15*, 933–950.

Wambaugh, J. L., & Thompson, C. K. (1989). Training and generalization of agrammatic aphasic adults' wh- interrogative productions. *Journal of Speech and Hearing Disorders, 54*, 509–525.

Warburton, E., Price, C. J., Swinburn, K., & Wise, R. J. (1999). Mechanisms of recovery from aphasia: Evidence from positron emission tomography studies. *Journal of Neurology, Neurosurgery and Psychiatry, 66*, 155–161.

West, J. A. (1973). Auditory comprehension in aphasic adults: Improvement through training. *Archives of Physical Medicine and Rehabilitation, 54*, 78–86.

Wierenga, C. E., Maher, L. M., Moore, A. B., White, K. D., McGregor, K., Soltysik, D. A., et al. (2006). Neural substrates of syntactic mapping treatment: An fMRI study of two cases. *Journal of the International Neuropsychological Society, 12*(1), 132–146.

CHAPTER 11

Plasticity of High-Order Cognition

A Review of Experience-Induced Remediation Studies for Executive Deficits

REDMOND G. O'CONNELL
IAN H. ROBERTSON

As other chapters in this volume indicate, there is now a wealth of evidence demonstrating that normal associative learning and experience can evoke substantial changes in the efficiency of neural networks, and that consequently the human brain is amenable to change across the lifespan (see Lillie & Mateer, Chapter 12, Shaywitz & Shaywitz, Chapter 8). Perhaps one of the most exciting findings to emerge from the field of cognitive neuroscience is that the same mechanisms underlying experience-evoked neural plasticity also promote both spontaneous and guided recovery following brain injury. To date, much of the literature on cortical plasticity has focused on the potential for reorganization within primary sensory and motor circuits in the cortex. This chapter considers whether or not these same principles can also be applied to our higher cognitive abilities.

The term *executive functions* (EFs) encompasses the collection of high-order cognitive abilities that allow us to behave in a flexible and goal-directed manner by inhibiting our inappropriate behaviors and thoughts, planning our future behavior, directing our attention, and monitoring our actions (Pennington & Ozonoff, 1996). Functions such as working memory, response inhibition, sustained attention, and conflict resolution provide the fundamental building blocks for learning and for adaptive, purposeful interaction with our physical and social environment. Disturbance of these abilities can lead to functional impairments in a broad range of everyday settings and is thought to play a prominent role in a number of common clinical conditions, including acquired brain injury, schizophrenia, Tourette's syndrome, autism, and attention-deficit/hyperactivity disorder (ADHD), among others (Bradshaw, 2001).

Although it was initially thought that the principles of guided recovery applied only to low-level sensory, perceptual, and motor functions, some researchers have investigated the possibility that EFs may also be amenable to experience-dependent restitution through direct targeted practice, which we refer to as *cognitive remediation training* (CRT). Effectiveness of EFs is achieved by distributed networks originating in the frontal lobes and projecting to other cortical and subcortical structures (Alexander, DeLong, & Strick, 1986; Bradshaw, 2001; Chow & Cummings, 1999). These networks can be at least partially dissociated according to the EFs that they mediate, suggesting that it may be possible to selectively target specific brain regions by "exercising" particular cognitive functions. That is, repeated use of a particular cognitive process during training should strengthen connections in the underlying neural circuitry, and consequently should produce an increase in cognitive capacity. The rationale for CRT is simple, but the aim is ambitious. The key prediction is that benefits should generalize to any unpracticed task that recruits the same underlying cognitive functions, and so the ultimate goal is to produce improvements that are transferable beyond a controlled laboratory setting to alleviate functional impairments in everyday life activities.

The vast majority of EF training programs have been targeted toward patients with acquired brain injury (Cicerone et al., 2000; Park & Ingles, 2001), but more recently the same approach has been adopted with other clinical groups, including patients with schizophrenia (Twamley, Jeste, & Bellack, 2003), ADHD (Klingberg, 2010; O'Connell, Bellgrove, & Robertson, 2007) and age-related cognitive decline (Aamodt, 2007). A similar principle has also inspired the recent emergence of commercial "brain-training" packages that have been marketed for the general population as a means of keeping our brains "sharper." Although CRT programs have been in existence for several decades, systematic evaluation of these methods and their efficacy is a more recent development, and to date only a limited number of empirical investigations have been conducted with sufficient methodological rigor to allow a proper assessment of their findings. Comprehensive reviews of CRT evaluation studies have already been conducted separately for acquired brain injury (Park & Ingles, 2001; Ponsford & Willmott, 2004; Rohling, Faust, Beverly, & Demakis, 2009), schizophrenia (Bellack, Gold, & Buchanan, 1999; McGurk, Twamley, Slitzer,

McHugo, & Mueser, 2007; Silverstein & Wilkniss, 2004; Twamley et al., 2003), and ADHD (O'Connell et al., 2007), but very few randomized controlled trials have been conducted with any single clinical group. For this reason, the present chapter reviews the CRT literature as a whole, in order to gain a clearer picture of the available evidence base. In particular, we evaluate the evidence that EF training can lead to functional improvements in everyday life activities. We also discuss brain imaging studies that have elucidated the changes at the neuronal level accompanying changes in cognitive performance. Finally we will explore some pertinent critical issues that may have limited the possible impact of CRT, and conclude by exploring new avenues for maximizing the efficacy of this approach.

COGNITIVE PRACTICE AND THE HEALTHY BRAIN

A substantial literature has explored the effects of short-term cognitive practice on the brains of neurologically healthy individuals. A review of the work on practice effects (Kelly & Garavan, 2005) concludes that the changes in neural activity following cognitive practice are diverse and are not limited to simple increases in activity within a particular region. In fact, with sufficient experience, the normal brain is also capable of enhancing its efficiency by expanding the spatial extent of activations within a region, decreasing activations within a neural network, improving connectivity between brain regions, and even reorganizing the cortical areas that are employed (see Lillie & Mateer, Chapter 12, this volume, for a detailed discussion of the processes).

Hence the mechanisms by which plastic changes occur within frontal circuitry appear to be different from those observed in sensory or motor regions (Kelly, Foxe, & Garavan, 2006). Training on sensory or motor tasks is most likely to result in expanded cortical representations of the specific skills or processes required to perform the training tasks (e.g., Munte, Altenmuller, & Jancke, 2002). In contrast, high-order cognitive tasks recruit a distributed network of regions whose activation is not determined by the specific sensory or motor requirements of the task. Consequently, increased efficiency of this network may be best achieved by increasing connectivity between regions and enhancing neural efficiency within regions. The distinction between highly task-specific representations of sensory and motor skills and neural networks serving generalized top-down cognitive control processes appears to provide a neurophysiological basis for the prediction that the beneficial effects of CRT should lead to broad functional improvements that can be transferred to a range of situations.

It is well established that most neurologically healthy people can substantially improve their performance on a cognitive task with sufficient practice (see Kelly & Garavan, 2005), but a transfer of these improvements to untrained tasks must be demonstrated in order to prove that improved performance reflects an enhancement of underlying cognitive capacity, rather than the simple acquisition of a set of skills specific to the practiced task. Moreover, improvements should be evident on any task that recruits the targeted cognitive function, even if that task bears little resemblance to the trained task. We are aware of only two studies that have investigated generalization of practice effects in neurologically healthy individuals.

After 5 weeks of intensive practice on three visual–spatial working memory tasks, participants in a study by Olesen, Westerberg, and Klingberg (2004) not only showed improvements on untrained measures of working memory, but also achieved significantly higher scores on measures of inhibition (Stroop) and general fluid intelligence (Raven's Advanced Progressive Matrices). These changes were also accompanied by clear increases in activity in the middle frontal gyrus and inferior parietal cortices—areas that have been strongly implicated in working memory (Klingberg, Forssberg, & Westerberg, 2002a; Rypma & D'Esposito, 2000). Working memory is an important supportive process during problem solving and reasoning (Engle, Kane, & Tuholski, 1999), and so the findings of Olesen and colleagues support the hypothesis that improving a discrete cognitive function can also have benefits for more complex cognitive abilities.

Rueda, Rothbart, McCandliss, Saccomanno, and Posner (2005) examined the influence of a computerized training program for executive attention that was specifically adapted for children. Each training task exercised a particular EF, such as anticipation, conflict resolution, inhibitory control, or stimulus discrimination, and involved cartoon characters and concepts that were familiar to children. In order to control for the number of sessions involving child–adult interaction, a second group of children watched popular videos during which at varying intervals a video was paused and the image of a fish appeared on screen; the control children had to press a button to restart the video. Children who had participated in the training showed improvement in their ability to resolve conflict and exert executive control, compared to the group of children who had engaged in the control condition. The authors also found evidence of generalization of training benefits to measures of intelligence and reasoning ability. An electrophysiological analysis of these training effects also yielded interesting results.

Event-related potentials (ERPs) that index conflict resolution (prefrontal N2) were analyzed after the children were divided into separate groups according to their age (4 years and 6 years) and after a comparison group of adults was included. The results showed that 4-year-old children who received the training had an ERP pattern similar to that of untrained 6-year-olds, while the 6-year-olds who received training had a more adult-like pattern of activity. Whereas certain neuropsychological abilities are in place from early infancy, others are not performed efficiently until adulthood, when the protracted development of frontostriatal circuitry is finally complete. Developmental studies indicate that there is a dramatic leap in the ability to maintain attention and exert executive control between the ages of 3 and 8 (Luciana & Nelson, 1998; Paus, 2005; Rueda et al., 2004). This age range may therefore represent a sensitive period during which cognitive training would be most beneficial (interestingly, this is also the age at which symptoms of ADHD begin to become apparent; Drechsler, Brandeis, Foldenyi, Imhof, & Steinhausen, 2005). Although requiring replication, the findings of Rueda et al. (2005) point to the possibility that process-specific training at an early age may help to accelerate the development of EF networks.

Some of the imaging data from the literature on practice effects appears informative for the development of therapeutic training protocols. For example, research with healthy adults tells us that changes in brain activation with cognitive training follow a complex time course. An analysis of changes in cortical activity during training on a working memory task by Hempel et al. (2004) found that training-related activation changes in key frontoparietal working memory regions were best described by an inverse-U-shaped quadratic function, with initial activation increases at the time of improved performance giving way to decreases after consolidation of performance gains. Kelly and Garavan (2005) have noted the common process of *scaffolding*, in which activity in frontal control areas (prefrontal, anterior cingulate, and posterior parietal cortices) gradually decreases after a task has been well rehearsed. Hence greater familiarization with a task reduces the need for top-down monitoring of performance, as processing is delegated to the task-specific regions. This kind of scaffolding is not always accompanied by further improvements in performance (e.g., Shadmehr & Holcomb, 1997), which underlines the critical importance of brain imaging as a tool for evaluating training effects. These findings are also important in the context of therapeutic interventions that seek to target frontally driven EF processes. Evidence that frontal regions gradually deactivate with the attainment of automatic or asymptotic performance suggests that adapting task difficulty to current performance levels may be critical to maintaining demands on high-level executive processes.

In sum, there has been very little investigation of the effects of extended cognitive training on the normal brain, but the initial results are promising. The two studies that have attempted CRT with neurologically healthy participants reported gains in cognitive performance that transferred to untrained tasks and were accompanied by functional changes in underlying neural circuitry. These findings may be particularly important with respect to neurodevelopmental and neurodegenerative disorders, as they suggest that the benefits of CRT may not necessarily be limited to the recovery of dramatic losses of function, but may also be effective in the remediation of subtle cognitive impairments. We still have a great deal to learn about the potential plasticity of our higher cognitive abilities, and so further investigations with neurologically healthy participants will be of critical importance. The majority of CRT studies have been conducted with clinical populations, and this work is reviewed in the following sections.

COGNITIVE REHABILITATION OF ACQUIRED BRAIN INJURY

Impaired EFs are among the most common consequences of acquired brain injury. Even after complete recovery of sensory and motor deficits, persistent problems of concentration and impaired self-monitoring of behavior can present a significant barrier to independent living and returning to work (Turner & Levine, 2004). There is also evidence that these deficits interfere with rehabilitative efforts in noncognitive domains. For example, the capacity to self-sustain goal-directed attention has been shown to predict motor recovery following right-hemisphere stroke over a 2-year period (Robertson, Ridgeway, Greenfield, & Parr, 1997). Hence there is a strong imperative for the development of interventions that specifically target EF deficits.

Proper evaluation of the efficacy of CRT for acquired brain injury has been severely hampered by the methodological heterogeneity of the research conducted in this area. Some common methodological weaknesses have included a failure to accurately gauge levels of premorbid functioning and of spontaneous recovery; the absence of adequate control conditions; and a tendency to combine CRT with other therapeutic interventions, which precludes the assessment of CRT-specific effects. A comprehensive meta-analysis conducted by Park and Ingles (2001) yielded a total of 30 studies that specifically tested CRT. The training protocols typically involved extended practice on a set of mental tasks and drills in which participants responded to visual and/or auditory stimuli, designed to exercise different EFs separately. One of the most commonly studied protocols was Attention Process Training (APT; Sohlberg & Mateer, 1987), in which tasks are organized around a hierarchical model of attention, so that demands are placed on increasingly complex cognitive processes. (See Engle & Kerns, Chapter 9, this volume, for a fuller discussion of APT.) The training tasks range from simply pressing a buzzer when the number 3 is heard to complex semantic categorization, and each task is performed until mastery has been accomplished.

The vast majority of the studies reviewed by Park and Ingles (2001) reported positive effects of training on the training tasks themselves and on similar untrained tasks. The authors observed, however, that only a minority of these studies had included a control condition to exclude possible practice or placebo effects. Of the 12 studies that did include control measures, only 6 reported statistically significant improvements, and even then improvements were only seen on outcome measures that bore a strong resemblance to the training tasks. This suggests that, rather than reflecting an enhancement of cognitive function, these performance gains arose from skill acquisition; that is, participants become more adept at responding quickly and accurately to stimuli presented on a computer, or otherwise adopted more effective performance strategies. In addition, very little evidence was provided to support the contention that CRT could lead to improved real-world functioning for patients. Consequently, several authors have questioned the validity of this approach, suggesting that rehabilitative efforts should be concentrated instead on the use of environmental modifications, residual abilities, and self-management strategies designed to bypass the defective cognitive processor (Bellack et al., 1999; Park & Ingles, 2001; Ponsford & Willmott, 2004; Silverstein & Wilkniss, 2004).

The results of the Park and Ingles (2001) review are somewhat disappointing, but there are a number of reasons why the literature may have failed to demonstrate generalized CRT effects for acquired brain injury thus far. Perhaps chief among these is the variation in the severity of the lesions that patients have suffered. Basing their argument on computational models of cortical plasticity, Robertson and Murre (1999) have contended that the extent and nature of neural recovery following targeted intervention will depend largely on the severity of the injury. In the case of a large lesion, there may not be sufficient residual connectivity with which to reestablish a fully functioning network. In such cases, improvements may only be achieved via the compensatory recruitment of alternative brain regions or the use of alternative cognitive and behavioral strategies. Most of the studies reviewed by Park and Ingles (2001) included patients with severe brain injuries, who would not therefore necessarily be expected to benefit from CRT. In a similar vein, there is some evidence to suggest that patients with brain injury require training tailored to their specific needs. For example, an analysis of individual differences in responsiveness to APT (Sohlberg, McLaughlin, Pavese, Heidrich, & Posner, 2000) indicated that a patient's initial vigilance level influenced the extent of improvement with therapy on several tests of EFs. Only patients who had poor vigilance levels showed improvements in basic attentional skills, and only patients with higher vigilance levels showed improvement on more demanding attentional or working memory tasks. A tendency to include patients with brain injuries of varying severity and differing neuropsychological profiles in the same treatment group may explain in part why the results of CRT have been inconsistent. Further work is required to establish predictors of training efficacy, and future studies should delineate specific patient profiles in order to determine who is likely to benefit.

Another potential criticism of CRT studies, noted by Ponsford and Willmot (2004), is that the simplicity of many computerized cognitive training tasks means that they can be performed relatively automatically.

As mentioned in the preceding section, sufficient practice of a given task can lead to a reduction in the demands placed on the very executive systems that we are seeking to rehabilitate (Hempel et al., 2004). Seventeen percent of the studies reviewed by Park and Ingles (2001) did not adapt task difficulty to performance, which may have further diluted any potential benefits. A better understanding of the neural processes underlying practice-related improvements will be critical to the further development of effective training strategies, and advances in brain imaging technologies have opened new avenues for exploring the true potential of CRT.

Physical measures of brain structure and function are essential in allowing us to determine whether or not behavioral improvements arise from increased functioning within the targeted neuroanatomical structures. A good demonstration of what can be gained with this level of analysis was provided by Sturm et al. (2004), who conducted a positron emission tomography/functional magnetic resonance imaging activation study of the effects of alertness training on patients with right-hemisphere vascular brain damage. The computerized training procedure required participants to drive a simulated vehicle as quickly as possible while looking out for occasional obstacles on the road, and the difficulty level was adapted to performance. Previous work has established a right-lateralized frontoparietal alertness network (Paus et al., 1997; Sturm & Willmes, 2001). Before training, none of the patients activated the right superior, middle, or dorsolateral frontal cortex—areas implicated in the maintenance of an alert state. After training, however, patients who exhibited significant behavioral improvements in alertness showed reactivation of these right frontal regions. Patients who were included in a memory training control group did not show the same pattern of right-hemisphere activations after training. These findings have been replicated by Thimm, Fink, Kust, Karbe, and Sturm (2006), who found that increased activation was still evident at a 4-week follow-up, although the behavioral improvements were no longer apparent. This represents some of the first evidence that CRT can lead to persistent functional reorganization in the cortex.

Interestingly, when normal, healthy participants in Sturm et al.'s study completed the same training tasks, they exhibited *decreased* activation within the alertness network. As discussed in the preceding section, activation decreases are commonly seen when healthy participants practice cognitive tasks and are thought to reflect increased neural efficiency within the functional circuit (Kelly et al., 2006). The fact that patients and controls show opposite neural-level responses to training underlines the need for care in the interpretation of imaging results. It may be that initial performance levels will determine the nature of activation changes (Klingberg, 2010). Participants who already have high performance levels on the task may be more likely to exhibit activation decreases, whereas participants with low performance levels may be more likely to exhibit activation increases.

Hence the data relating to experience-induced rehabilitation of EF deficits following acquired brain injury are too equivocal to permit any firm conclusions. Further randomized controlled trials that take account of individual differences in lesion severity, initial performance levels, and changes in functional neuroanatomy will be required before the value of the CRT approach can be properly assessed.

Another, more complex approach to the rehabilitation of acquired brain injury is to target the affected region in an indirect manner by activating interconnected regions that are still intact. For example, Robertson, Mattingley, Rorden, and Driver (1998) reported that the spatial imbalance of stroke patients with unilateral neglect resulting from right ischemic lesions could be alleviated through the presentation of simple auditory alerts. This technique was informed by functional imaging and lesion data suggesting that the nonspatial alertness system is predominantly right-lateralized and receives ascending projections from subcortical arousal systems that are normally intact in cases of neglect (Paus et al., 1997; Rueckert & Graham, 1996). The resultant increase in awareness of left-sided stimuli in the Robertson et al. (1998) study suggests that the presentation of phasic alerts led to indirect stimulation of the affected spatial attention regions in the right hemisphere, producing a return of attention toward the left.

A similar rationale was used in the development of another training strategy for neglect, known as limb activation training, in which patients with left unilateral neglect are encouraged to make small movements of the left arm (Robertson, McMillan, MacLeod, Edgeworth, & Brock, 2002). Again, this approach was informed by theoretical models emerging from the field of cognitive neuroscience, which pointed to the existence of multiple representations of space in the brain that interact to produce a coherent spatial reference system (Rizzolatti & Camarda, 1987). As a result of the interconnections between these representations when the somatosensory spatial map is activated by limb movement, the damaged peripersonal spatial map will also be simultaneously activated. In two single cases reported by Wilson, Manly, Coyle, and Robertson (2000), patients who participated in an extended limb activation training program exhibited improved performance on neuropsychological measures of spatial attention and in the independent performance of everyday activities both during and after the training period. These improvements support the hypothesis that through repeated indirect activation of the damaged circuit, neural connections are reestablished, and the lost function gradually returns.

These studies provide an excellent illustration of how a detailed understanding of the neural processes underlying functional impairments resulting from brain injury can pave the way for the emergence of novel strategies for behaviorally inducing plastic reorganization of lesioned brain systems—strategies that provide an alternative to direct process-specific approaches. Several other methods for rehabilitation of spatial neglect that draw on similar network-based approaches have been developed; these have been reviewed by Singh-Curry and Husain (2008).

SLOWING DOWN AGE-RELATED COGNITIVE DECLINE

Age-related cognitive decline refers to the nonpathological losses in cognitive functioning that are an almost universal part of the aging process. Although not as dramatic as the other conditions discussed in this chapter, gradual reductions in EFs can have a substantial impact on one's quality of life in terms of independent living, social interaction, and engagement in cognitively demanding activities (Artero, Touchon, & Ritchie, 2001). The progressive decline in neural efficiency in the aging brain may arise in part from negative plasticity resulting from decreased use of cognitive abilities (e.g., Calero-Garcia, Navarro-Gonzalez, & Munoz-Manzano, 2007; Mahncke, Bronstone, & Merzenich, 2006). That is, a tendency to engage less as we grow old in active learning or activities that are cognitively demanding may lead to a progressive weakening of brain representations of those cognitive processes. Several studies have reported that maintaining an active lifestyle in old age through social interaction, physical exercise, and/or engagement in mentally stimulating activities has a protective effect on cognitive decline (Calero-Garcia et al., 2007; Hultsch, Small, Hertzog, & Dixon, 1999; Scarmeas & Stern, 2003). Hence age-related cognitive decline may be at least partially reversible and appears to be an ideal candidate for remediation by CRT (Gates & Valenzuela, 2010).

Three studies serve as examples of evaluations of CRT programs for elderly individuals. Mahncke et al. (2006) conducted a rigorously controlled trial of a memory training program. The training consisted of intensive practice on a range of cognitively stimulating and attention-demanding tasks that required stimulus recognition, discrimination, sequencing, and memory use. Specific efforts were made to target top-down executive control regions by increasing task difficulty according to performance. A total of 182 participants were assigned to one of three conditions: a computer-based training condition (60 minutes per day, 5 days per week, for 8–10 weeks), an active computer-based control condition (watching an educational DVD), and a nonactive control condition. Importantly, the training program was self-administered on a computer in each participant's own home, and all participants were able to use the program independently after initial instruction. The compliance level was 85%. Participants who received this training showed improvements on the training measures, which generalized to a standardized neuropsychological measure of global memory performance that bore little resemblance to the training procedure. In contrast, there was no change in memory performance in either of the control groups. A 3-month follow-up also indicated longer-term maintenance of this memory enhancement. Unfortunately, however, the transfer of these benefits to real-life measures was not investigated.

Another randomized controlled trial by Willis et al. (2006) paid particular attention to functional outcomes following cognitive training. A total of 2,832 older adults were divided into one of four training groups (memory training, reasoning training, speed-of-processing training, and nonactive control). The memory and reasoning trainings involved teaching of cognitive strategies and were not therefore primarily restorative in nature, but the speed-of-processing training involved repeated practice on tasks that required visual search and divided attention. Eighty-nine percent of participants were able to complete the treatment, and each training procedure produced significant improvement in the trained cognitive ability, which was retained across 5 years of follow-up testing. All three training groups reported improvements in their ability to handle day-to-day tasks, and the speed-of-processing group showed improvement on a performance-based measure of daily functioning.

In another study, Talassi et al. (2007) examined the effects of cognitive training on two separate groups of elderly patients diagnosed with mild dementia and mild cognitive impairment, respectively. The treatment group received computerized cognitive training (30–45 minutes, 4 days per week, for 3 weeks), while the control group was assigned to a physical rehabilitation program. Both groups also received occupational therapy and behavioral training. Only the training group exhibited statistically significant improvements on EF measures, and there were also improvements on self-ratings of functional impairment and mood.

Cognitive training as a possible intervention for age-related cognitive decline awaits further validation, but the three studies reviewed in this section provide some evidence to suggest that directly exercising specific cognitive processes may have protective value by reversing what may be a major contributing factor—decreased cognitive stimulation.

NEURODEVELOPMENTAL DISORDERS

Studies of patients with psychosis or clinically remitted schizophrenia indicate that executive dysfunction represents a primary core deficit in schizophrenia and is not simply the consequence of positive or negative symptoms (Bilder et al., 2000; Peuskens, Demily, & Thibaut, 2005). Many domains of cognitive functioning are disrupted in schizophrenia, including aspects of attention, problem solving, inhibition, verbal and visual–spatial working memory, and learning, leading to substantial functional impairment (Heinrichs & Zakzanis, 1998). In particular, deficient working memory may be a key vulnerability indicator and appears to be related to reduced metabolic activity in the dorsolateral prefrontal cortex (Bertolino et al.,

2006). Impairments in working memory have been found to correlate with formal thought disorder in schizophrenia (Spitzer, 1993). Moreover, EF deficits appear to be a strong predictor of long-term outcome. For example, Velligan et al. (1997) found that global measures of cognitive function predicted over 40% of the variance on an assessment of impaired functioning in daily living (see also Green, 1996, for further evidence). Although antipsychotic drugs have been shown to alleviate cognitive impairments, they do not eliminate them (Peuskens et al., 2005); as a result, many investigators have pursued nonpharmacological treatment methods.

Twamley et al. (2003) conducted a comprehensive quantitative review of CRT programs for patients with schizophrenia. Once again, there was wide variation in the methodologies used in terms of the training protocols, control conditions, patient profiles, and intensity/duration of training. The authors focused on the 17 studies that had conducted randomized controlled trials and implemented sound methodologies. The majority of these treatment programs involved computer-based training on multiple EF tasks. Of the 17 studies, 14 reported significant training-specific improvements on at least one outcome measure, and there was good evidence to suggest generalization of training effects in multiple areas. Mean effect sizes (Cohen's *d*) were small to medium for improvements in neuropsychological performance (0.32), symptom severity (0.26), and everyday life functioning (0.51). Selected CRT studies of schizophrenia have reported large effect sizes (e.g., Bell, Bryson, & Wexler, 2003; Wykes et al., 2003), suggesting that significant cognitive improvement can be achieved in schizophrenia when certain training protocols are implemented.

An fMRI study by Wexler, Anderson, Fullbright, and Gore (2000) has investigated the neuroanatomical correlates of CRT in schizophrenia. Eight patients were scanned before and after 10–15 weeks of verbal working memory exercises. It had previously been shown that poor performance on these tasks by patients with schizophrenia was accompanied by lower-than-normal activation of the left inferior frontal cortex (Stevens, Goldman-Rakic, Gore, Fullbright, & Wexler, 1998). Importantly, the degree of functional improvement on the memory tasks after training was significantly correlated with the percentage of increase in left inferior frontal activation.

The other neurodevelopmental disorder that has been the subject of numerous cognitive training studies is ADHD. ADHD is reliably associated with prominent deficits in such EFs as response inhibition, working memory, sustained attention, and temporal processing, tied to dysregulation of frontostriatal circuitry (Bush, Valera, & Seidman, 2005; Seidman, 2006). Although the primary symptoms of ADHD are behavioral, several of the most prominent explanatory models have proposed that neuropsychological impairments play a causal role in the development of this disorder (Barkley, 1997; Castellanos & Tannock, 2002; Sergeant, 2000;

Sonuga-Barke, 2000). Psychostimulant treatments not only have proven efficacious in dealing with the behavioral features of ADHD, but also lead to significant improvements in cognitive performance (Overtoom, Verbaten, Kemner, Kenemans, van Engeland, et al., 2003; Schweitzer, Lee, Hanford, Zink, Ely, et al., 2004; Shafritz, Marchione, Gore, Shaywitz, & Shaywitz, 2004; Tannock, Ickowicz, & Schachar, 1995). As in the case of schizophrenia, however, pharmacotherapy does not alter underlying neuropsychological abnormalities in a lasting manner (e.g., Schweitzer et al., 2004); this may explain in part why, despite long-term treatment, the symptoms of ADHD persist into adulthood in a significant proportion of cases (Faraone et al., 1998). As a result, there is still a need for new interventions that can directly target these deficits and bring about lasting improvements.

Elsewhere (O'Connell et al., 2007), we have reviewed the small number of studies that have attempted cognitive training in ADHD (Kerns, Eso, & Thomson, 1999; Klingberg et al., 2005; Klingberg, Forssberg, & Westerberg, 2002b; Semrud-Clikeman et al., 1999; Shaffer et al., 2000). Three of the studies targeted aspects of attention, and two targeted working memory. All five studies reported improvements on the training tasks and on similar untrained neuropsychological tasks. Four of the five studies reported a generalization of benefits to more complex cognitive domains, including measures of academic performance, reasoning, and language processing. Finally, three of the studies reported improvements in everyday behavioral symptoms.

One of the most thorough clinical trials of a cognitive training program designed for children was conducted by Klingberg et al. (2005), who investigated a computerized working memory program in a group of children with ADHD. Based on a training regimen previously used to induce cortical plasticity in sensory and motor cortices, the program was designed so that task difficulty was closely matched to each individual's performance on a trial-by-trial basis. Four subtests were presented during each training session: a visual–spatial working memory task, a backward digit span task, a letter span task, and a choice reaction time task. Fifty-three unmedicated children with ADHD, ages 7–12 (mean age = 9.8), were recruited from four clinical sites and randomly assigned to a treatment or comparison group. Participants in the control condition performed the same working memory training for the same duration as the intervention group, but without adjustment of difficulty; hence the possibility that improvements might arise simply from an increase in concentration levels or motivation could be ruled out. The training materials were saved on compact disc, allowing the children to complete the intervention independently either at home or at school.

After training, participants in the treatment group significantly outperformed the comparison group on each of the executive outcome measures (Span Board, Stroop, Digit Span, Raven's Progressive Matrices), and these differences remained at follow-up 3 months later. Importantly, the effect size for improvement on the untrained working memory task (0.93 on Span Board) represented a strong clinical effect and compares very favorably to those previously reported for stimulant medication. A comparison with previous studies of working memory and response inhibition indicated that the children's posttraining spatial working memory and Stroop performance was 0.3 standard deviations or less below normative levels. Most importantly, there was also a strong and specific clinical effect on parent ratings of ADHD symptoms when both *Diagnostic and Statistical Manual of Mental Disorders*, fourth edition (DSM-IV) criteria and the Conners Parent Rating Scale were used. Effect sizes of 1.21 for parent-rated attention and 0.47 for parent-rated hyperactivity–impulsivity are particularly impressive, given that all participants were unmedicated. Again, these differences were still evident at follow-up.

The results of studies conducted with neurodevelopmental disorders have provided some of the strongest evidence to date that CRT can lead to generalized improvements in both the short and the longer term.

SUMMARY

Because impairments in high-order cognitive abilities are serious concerns for various clinical and nonclinical groups, developing an effective nonpharmacological intervention that can be carried out easily at home or at school with a minimum of participation from clinicians an exciting prospect that is surely worthy of extensive investigation. But the recent increase in the marketing of brain-training products that purport to improve cognitive capacity has continued with little consideration of the available evidence base (Owen, Hampshire, Grahn, Stenton, Dajani, et al., 2010). The core aim of the CRT approach is highly ambitious, and a number of authors have understandably questioned whether extended training on a discrete set of cognitive tasks can really have an impact on the far more complex behaviors and skills that are required in our everyday lives. In this chapter, we have sought to evaluate the available evidence that experience-induced plasticity can be exploited to alleviate EF deficits.

The vast majority of CRT studies have reported significant improvements in trained and similar untrained cognitive tasks, and several studies have also reported a generalization of benefits to untrained cognitive tasks that are quite remote from the training measures. At present, however, there is not enough hard evidence to support the use of CRT in a clinical setting, since very few studies have either investigated or demonstrated a significant positive impact on everyday functional impairments. Nevertheless, selected studies (e.g., Bell et al., 2003; Klingberg et al., 2005) that have employed sound methodologies have indicated that clinically significant improvements in cognition and behavior are achievable. We have also cited the findings of brain imaging studies with clinical (Sturm et al., 2004; Thimm et al., 2006; Wexler et al., 2000) and nonclinical (Hempel et al., 2004; Olesen et al., 2004; Rueda et al., 2005) populations, indicating that training-related improvements in cognitive performance are accompanied by functional adaptations in underlying neural networks. We argue, therefore, that the CRT approach still represents a promising avenue for cognitive rehabilitation.

The results of studies with acquired brain injury have been the least convincing; they suggest that in cases of severe brain damage, direct retraining of cognitive abilities may not be the most appropriate treatment option. Instead, contextualized behavioral adaptation, overlearning of key skills, and the use of other compensatory strategies that reduce the load on the defective cognitive processes may be a more effective approach to rehabilitation. However, stronger evidence of generalized improvement following cognitive training in neurologically healthy participants and in clinical groups where substantial residual function remains (patients with age-related cognitive decline, schizophrenia, and ADHD) suggests that more studies should examine CRT in patients with less severe neurological abnormalities.

We conclude this chapter by outlining some of the critical issues that should be considered in future CRT studies.

FUTURE CONSIDERATIONS

CRT and Cognitive Neuroscience

A key challenge for CRT studies is selecting the ideal target for rehabilitation and identifying the most effective method by which this can be achieved. In cases of acquired brain injury, where relatively discrete lesions may be identified and linked to specific neuropsychological deficits, this may be relatively straightforward. Disorders such as schizophrenia or ADHD, however, involve a far more complex neuropathology and a multidimensional symptom profile. Consequently, cognitive impairments that are secondary to more fundamental, upstream neuropsychological processes may not be amenable to direct training (Bellack et al., 1999). For these reasons, several authors have advocated that CRT studies should be based more closely on the ideas emerging from cognitive neuroscience (Ponsford & Willmott, 2004; Robertson, 2002; Silverstein & Wilkniss, 2004). Strong explanatory models that are based on extensive pharmacological, brain imaging, and genetic evidence have been developed for several clinical conditions, but have yet to make any significant impact on the field of cognitive rehabilitation.

To give one example, recent neuropsychological models of ADHD postulate that separate pathophysiological mechanisms of disinhibition and poor motivation interact to produce the broad array of EF and behavioral deficits in this disorder (Castellanos, Sonuga-Barke, Milham, & Tannock, 2006). Hence this model identifies a candidate process for CRT and suggests that motivational influences should be considered in the design of training protocols, perhaps through the use of regular reinforcers. Another important, and related, issue is that many CRT studies have employed training tasks whose precise functional neuroanatomical correlates have not been established. Research in cognitive neuroscience has led to the development of increasingly process-specific paradigms with demonstrable brain–behavior relationships. Basing CRT protocols on the ideas emerging from cognitive neuroscience should provide a more coherent research framework and guide the selection of target processes for different clinical groups.

Individual Differences

One factor that is common to many clinical groups, and that may militate against significant training effects, is neuropsychological heterogeneity. Although group differences in EFs are consistently found when participants with schizophrenia or ADHD are compared to their neurologically healthy peers, these differences can mask the fact that only a subset of individuals will have a deficit in a given cognitive function. For example, Nigg, Willcutt, Doyle, and Sonuga-Barke (2005) found that out of 287 children with ADHD, only 50% performed in the abnormal range on any given EF measure when the 90th percentile was used as a cutoff. Similarly, there is evidence of significant interindividual variation in the neuropsychological profiles of patients with schizophrenia (Kremen, Seidman, Faraone, Toomey, & Tsuang, 2004). Bellack et al. (1999) point out that although there is clear evidence of cognitive dysfunction in schizophrenia, there is still controversy regarding which specific deficits account for a significant amount of the variance in functional impairments. Therefore, how do we choose the most appropriate EFs to target?

One possible solution is that candidates for CRT should be selected on the basis of individual symptom profiles and not solely on the basis of diagnostic category. Matching a treatment to individual needs may be as important as the actual components of the treatment itself, but individual differences are not addressed in the vast majority of studies reviewed in this chapter. Carefully matching cognitive treatments to individual impairments may be one way of maximizing treatment effects in future studies. Elucidating the relationship between neuropsychological deficits and real-world impairment remains a critical research question for clinical neuroscientists.

There are likely to be several other important predictors of treatment success. For example, Wykes et al. (2003) have indicated that medication type may be one such predictor for patients with schizophrenia. It is likely that a more sophisticated approach to CRT will be required, in which greater emphasis is placed on the treatment context. Factors such as mood, self-esteem, and motivation may also be expected to play an important role in determining treatment outcome.

Strategy Teaching

Another potentially fruitful line of enquiry for CRT studies may be the addition of strategy teaching to optimise cognitive performance. As noted by Bellack et al. (1999), experts (e.g., chess masters) are often distinguished from novices by the cognitive strategies that they employ on a given task, rather than by differences in their basic cognitive capacities or skills. There is evidence to suggest that the implementation of particular cognitive strategies does lead to functional adaptations in the brain. The prefrontal cortex is thought to play a central role in our ability to apply cognitive strategies, and Mioto et al. (2006) observed greater bilateral activation of the prefrontal cortex during a semantic memory task among participants who had received instruction in semantic organizational strategies. Hence Mioto et al. were able to manipulate the level of frontal activation during task performance. Although it is not primarily restorative in nature, strategy training may have synergistic effects when combined with extended cognitive practice by optimizing task performance and increasing the likelihood that benefits will be transferred to a range of settings.

Our research group has explored the value of strategy teaching in the context of sustained attention training. In our everyday lives, we are all more or less subject to momentary failures of attention that arise from a tendency to lapse into mindless, automatic action. Self-initiated increases in sustained attention are achieved by a frontoparietal cortical network that monitors and modulates activity in subcortical arousal systems to match current task demands (Sturm & Willmes, 2001), and we have previously shown that it is possible to train patients with sustained attention deficits to regulate sustained attention through self-instructional techniques (Robertson, Tegner, Tham, Lo, & Nimmo-Smith, 1995).

During such training, the goal is to encourage increased top-down maintenance of an alert, goal-directed state. Since repeated practice alone is unlikely to alter the way a sustained attention task is performed, some form of strategy training would appear to be necessary. In a more recent study (O'Connell et al., 2008), designed to test the role of arousal in mediating changes in behavior, participants learned to produce self-generated increases in alertness first in response to a periodic auditory cue and later in response to an internally generated cue. In order to strengthen the training effect, participants were provided with visual feedback conveying the magnitude of each self-alert event via online changes in electrodermal activity (EDA), an index of autonomic arousal. In the first trial of this brief training protocol, participants who implemented this strategy showed increased arousal levels (as indexed by EDA) during the performance of an untrained sustained attention task and made significantly fewer errors. In the second trial, we found the same pattern of improvement in a group of adults diagnosed with ADHD. We highlight this work in order to demonstrate not only the potential for the expansion of the CRT approach, but the important value of using the ideas emerging from the field of cognitive neuroscience to guide the development of new training protocols.

Multimodal Treatment

Since most neuropsychological conditions are multidimensional in nature, it is unlikely that a purely cognitive treatment will be sufficient to address the full spectrum of symptoms and impairments. It is far more likely that CRT will be at its most effective when administered in conjunction with other treatment modalities. For example, pharmacological treatments may provide the focus required to facilitate participation in a CRT program, and there is evidence that medication acting upon neurotransmitter systems can influence recovery from brain injury (Barrett & Gonzalez Rothi, 2002). This leads us to the hypothesis that pharmacological and neurocognitive interventions may have synergistic effects on neural plasticity. Although single-component analyses of CRT remain a priority in the short term, an interesting challenge for future work will be to investigate the potential adjunctive or synergistic effects that medical, psychosocial, and neurocognitive treatments have in combination. In addition, CRT strategies should be pitted against existing treatments, to allow a proper assessment of their unique value.

REFERENCES

Aamodt, S. (2007). Exercising to keep aging at bay. *Nature Neuroscience, 10*(3), 263.

Alexander, G. E., DeLong, M. R., & Strick, P. L. (1986). Parallel organisation of functionally segregated circuits linking basal ganglia and cortex. *Annual Review of Neuroscience, 9*, 357–381.

Artero, S., Touchon, J., & Ritchie, K. (2001). Disability and mild cognitive impairment: A longitudinal population-based study. *International Journal of Geriatric Psychiatry, 16*(11), 1092–1097.

Barkley, R. A. (1997). Behavioral inhibition, sustained attention, and executive functions: Constructing a unifying theory of ADHD. *Psychological Bulletin, 121*(1), 65–94.

Barrett, A. M., & Gonzalez Rothi, L. J. (2002). Theoretical bases for neuropsychological interventions. In P. Eslinger (Ed.), *Neuropsychological interventions: Clinical research and practice.* New York: Guilford Press.

Bell, M., Bryson, G., & Wexler, B. E. (2003). Cognitive remediation of working memory deficits: Durability of training effects in severely impaired and less severely impaired schizophrenia. *Acta Psychiatrica Scandinavica, 108*, 101–109.

Bellack, A. S., Gold, J. M., & Buchanan, R. W. (1999). Cognitive rehabilitation for schizophrenia: Problems, prospects, and strategies. *Schizophrenia Bulletin, 25*(2), 257–274.

Bertolino, A., Caforio, G., Petruzzella, V., Latorre, V., Rubino, V., Dimalta, S., et al. (2006). Prefrontal dysfunction in schizophrenia controlling for COMT Val-158Met genotype and working memory performance. *Psychiatry Research, 147*(2–3), 221–226.

Bilder, R. M., Goldman, R. S., Robinson, D., Reiter, G., Bell, L., Bates, J. A., et al. (2000). Neuropsychology of first-episode schizophrenia: Initial characterization and clinical correlates. *American Journal of Psychiatry, 157*(4), 549–559.

Bradshaw, J. L. (2001). *Developmental disorders of the frontostriatal system.* Philadelphia: Psychology Press/Taylor & Francis.

Bush, G., Valera, E. M., & Seidman, L. J. (2005). Functional neuroimaging of attention-deficit/hyperactivity disorder: A review and suggested future directions. *Biological Psychiatry, 57*(11), 1273–1284.

Calero-Garcia, M. D., Navarro-Gonzalez, E., & Munoz-Manzano, L. (2007). Influence of level of activity on cognitive performance and cognitive plasticity in elderly persons. *Archives of Gerontology and Geriatrics, 45*(3), 307–318.

Castellanos, F. X., Sonuga-Barke, E. J. S., Milham, M. P., & Tannock, R. (2006). Characterizing cognition in ADHD: Beyond executive dysfunction. *Trends in Cognitive Sciences, 10*(3), 117–123.

Castellanos, F. X., & Tannock, R. (2002). Neuroscience of attention-deficit/hyperactivity disorder: The search for endophenotypes. *Nature Neuroscience Reviews, 3*, 617–628.

Chow, T. W., & Cummings, J. L. (1999). Frontal–subcortical circuits. In B. L. Miller & J. L. Cummings (Eds.), *The human frontal lobes: Functions and disorders.* New York: Guilford Press.

Cicerone, K. D., Dahlberg, C., Kalmar, K., Langenbahn, D. M., Malec, J. F., Bergquist, T. F., et al. (2000). Evidence-based cognitive rehabilitation: Recommendations for clinical practice. *Archives of Physical Medicine and Rehabilitation, 81*, 1596–1615.

Drechsler, R., Brandeis, D., Foldenyi, M., Imhof, K., & Steinhausen, H. C. (2005). The course of neuropsychological functions in children with attention deficit hyperactivity disorder from late childhood to early adolescence. *Journal of Child Psychology and Psychiatry, 46*, 824–836.

Engle, R. W., Kane, M. J., & Tuholski, S. W. (1999). Individual differences in working memory capacity and what they tell us about controlled attention, general fluid intelligence, and functions of the prefrontal cortex. In A. Myake & P. Shah (Eds.), *Models of working memory: Mechanisms of active maintenance and executive control.* Cambridge, UK: Cambridge University Press.

Faraone, S. V., Biederman, J., Spencer, T., Wilens, T. E., Seidman, L. J., Mick, E., et al. (1998). ADHD in adults: An overview. *Biological Psychiatry, 48*(1), 9–20.

Gates, N., & Valenzuela, M. (2010). Cognitive exercise and its role in cognitive function in older adults. *Current Psychiatry Report*, 12.

Green, M. F. (1996). What are the functional consequences of neurocognitive deficits in schizophrenia? *American Journal of Psychiatry, 154*, 321–330.

Heinrichs, R. W., & Zakzanis, K. K. (1998). Neurocognitive deficit in schizophrenia: A quantitative review of the evidence. *Neuropsychology, 12*, 426–445.

Hempel, A., Gisel, F. J., Garcia Caraballo, N. M., Meyer, H., Wustenberg, T., Essig, M., et al. (2004). Plasticity of cortical activation related to working memory during training. *American Journal of Psychiatry, 161*(4), 745–747.

Hultsch, D., Small, B., Hertzog, C., & Dixon, R. (1999). Use it or lose it: Engaged lifestyle as a buffer of cognitive decline in aging? *Psychology and Aging, 14*, 245–263.

Kelly, C., Foxe, J. J., & Garavan, H. (2006). Patterns of normal human brain plasticity after practice and their implications for neurorehabilitation. *Archives of Physical Medicine and Rehabilitation, 87*(12, Suppl. 2), S20–S29.

Kelly, C., & Garavan, H. (2005). Human functional neuroimaging of brain changes associated with practice. *Cerebral Cortex, 15*(8), 1089–1102.

Kerns, K. A., Eso, K., & Thomson, J. (1999). Investigation of a direct intervention for improving attention in young children with ADHD. *Developmental Neuropsychology, 16*(2), 273–295.

Klingberg, T. (2010). Training and plasticity of working memory. *Trends in Cognitive Science, 14*, 317–324.

Klingberg, T., Fernell, E., Olesen, P. J., Johnson, M., Gustafsson, P., Dahlstrom, K., et al. (2005). Computerized training of working memory in children with ADHD: A randomized, controlled trial. *Journal of the American Academy of Child and Adolescent Psychiatry, 44*(2), 177.

Klingberg, T., Forssberg, H., & Westerberg, H. (2002a). Increased brain activity in frontal and parietal cortex underlies the development of visuo-spatial working memory capacity during childhood. *Journal of Cognitive Neuroscience, 14*, 1–10.

Klingberg, T., Forssberg, H., & Westerberg, H. (2002b). Training of working memory in children with ADHD. *Journal of Clinical and Experimental Neuropsychology, 24*(6), 781–791.

Kremen, W. S., Seidman, L. J., Faraone, S. V., Toomey, R., & Tsuang, M. T. (2004). Heterogeneity of schizophrenia: A study of individual neuropsychological profiles. *Schizophrenia Research, 71*(2–3), 307–321.

Luciana, M., & Nelson, C. A. (1998). The functional emergence of prefrontally-guided working memory systems in four- to eight-year-old children. *Neuropsychologia, 36*(3), 273–293.

Mahncke, H. W., Bronstone, A., & Merzenich, M. M. (2006). Brain plasticity and functional losses in the aged: Scientific bases for a novel intervention. In A. R. Moller (Ed.), *Progress in brain research: Vol. 157.* Amsterdam: Elsevier.

McGurk, S. R., Twamley, E. W., Slitzer, D. I., McHugo, G. J., & Mueser, K. T. (2007). A meta-analysis of cognitive remediation in schizophrenia. *American Journal of Psychiatry, 164*, 1791–1802.

Mioto, E. C., Savage, C. R., Evans, J. J., Wilson, B. A., Martins, M. G. M., Iaki, S., et al. (2006). Bilateral activation of the prefrontal cortex after strategic semantic cognitive training. *Human Brain Mapping, 27*, 288–295.

Munte, T. F., Altenmuller, E., & Jancke, L. (2002). The musician's brain as a model of neuroplasticity. *Nature Reviews Neuroscience, 3*, 473–478.

Nigg, J. T., Willcutt, E. G., Doyle, A. E., & Sonuga-Barke, E. J. S. (2005). Causal heterogeneity in attention-deficit/hyperactivity disorder: Do we need neuropsychologically impaired subtypes? *Biological Psychiatry, 57*(11), 1224–1230.

O'Connell, R. G., Bellgrove, M. A., Dockree, P. M., Lau, A., Fitzgerald, M., & Robertson, I. H. (2008). Self-alert training: Volitional modulation of autonomic arousal improves sustained attention. *Neuropsychologia, 46*(5), 1379–1390.

O'Connell, R. G., Bellgrove, M. A., & Robertson, I. H. (2007). Avenues for the neuro-remediation of ADHD: Lessons from clinical neurosciences. In M. A. Bellgrove, M. Fitzgerald, & M. Gill (Eds.), *Handbook of attention deficit hyperactivity disorder*. Chichester, UK: Wiley.

Olesen, P. J., Westerberg, H., & Klingberg, T. (2004). Increased prefrontal and parietal activity after training of working memory. *Nature Neuroscience, 7*(1), 75–79.

Overtoom, C. C. E., Verbaten, M. N., Kemner, C., Kenemans, J. L., van Engeland, H., et al. (2003). Effects of methylphenidate, desipramine, and L-dopa on attention and inhibition in children with ADHD. *Behavioural Brain Research, 145*, 7–15.

Owen, A., Hampshire, A., Grahn, J., Stenton, R., Dajani, S., et al. (2010). Putting brain training to the test. *Nature, 465*, 775–778.

Park, N. W., & Ingles, J. L. (2001). Effectiveness of attention rehabilitation after an acquired brain injury: A meta-analysis. *Neuropsychology, 15*(2), 199–210.

Paus, T. (2005). Mapping brain maturation and cognitive development during adolescence. *Trends in Cognitive Sciences, 9*(2), 60–68.

Paus, T., Zatorre, R. J., Hofle, N., Caramanos, Z., Gotman, J., Petrides, M., et al. (1997). Time-related changes in neural systems underlying attention and arousal during the performance of an auditory vigilance task. *Journal of Cognitive Neuroscience, 9*(3), 392–408.

Pennington, B. F., & Ozonoff, S. (1996). Executive functions and developmental psychopathology. *Journal of Child Psychology and Psychiatry, 37*(1), 55–87.

Peuskens, J., Demily, C., & Thibaut, F. (2005). Treatment of cognitive dysfunction in schizophrenia. *Clinical Therapeutics, 27*, 525–537.

Ponsford, J., & Willmott, C. (2004). Rehabilitation of non-spatial attention. In J. Ponsford (Ed.), *Cognitive and behavioral rehabilitation: From neurobiology to clinical practice*. New York: Guilford Press.

Rizzolatti, G., & Camarda, R. (Eds.). (1987). *Neural circuits for spatial attention and unilateral neglect*. Amsterdam: North-Holland.

Robertson, I. H. (2002). Cognitive neuroscience and brain rehabilitation: A promise kept [Editorial]. *Journal of Neurology, Neurosurgery and Psychiatry, 73*, 357.

Robertson, I. H., Mattingley, J. B., Rorden, C., & Driver, J. (1998). Phasic alerting of neglect patients overcomes their spatial deficit in visual awareness. *Nature, 395*, 169–172.

Robertson, I. H., McMillan, T. M., MacLeod, E., Edgeworth, J., & Brock, D. (2002). Rehabilitation by limb activation training (LAT) reduces impairment in unilateral neglect patients: A single-blind randomised control trial. *Neuropsychological Rehabilitation, 12*, 439–454.

Robertson, I. H., & Murre, J. J. (1999). Rehabilitation of brain damage: Brain plasticity and principles of guided recovery. *Psychological Bulletin, 125*(5), 544–575.

Robertson, I. H., Ridgeway, V., Greenfield, E., & Parr, A. (1997). Motor recovery after stroke depends on intact sustained attention: A 2-year follow-up study. *Neuropsychology, 11*(2), 290–295.

Robertson, I. H., Tegner, R., Tham, K., Lo, A., & Nimmo-Smith, I. (1995). Sustained attention training for unilateral neglect: Theoretical and rehabilitation implications. *Journal of Clinical and Experimental Neuropsychology, 17*, 416–430.

Rohling, M., Faust, M., Beverly, B., & Demakis, G. (2009). Effectiveness of cognitive rehabilitation following acquired brain injury: A meta-analytic re-examination of Cicerone et al.'s (2000, 2005) systematic reviews. *Neuropsychology, 23*, 20–39.

Rueckert, L., & Graham, J. (1996). Sustained attention deficits in patients with right frontal lesions. *Neuropsychologia, 34*, 953–963.

Rueda, M. R., Fan, J., McCandliss, B. D., Halparin, J., Gruber, D. B., Lercari, L. P., et al. (2004). Development of attentional networks in childhood. *Neuropsychologia, 42*, 1029–1040.

Rueda, M. R., Rothbart, M. K., McCandliss, B. D., Saccomanno, L., & Posner, M. I. (2005). Training, maturation, and genetic influences on the development of executive attention. *Proceedings of the National Academy of Sciences USA, 102*(41), 14931–14936.

Rypma, B., & D'Esposito, M. (2000). Isolating the neural mechanisms of age-related changes in human working memory. *Nature Neuroscience, 3*, 509–515.

Scarmeas, N., & Stern, Y. (2003). Cognitive reserve and lifestyle. *Journal of Clinical and Experimental Neuropsychology, 25*, 625–633.

Schweitzer, J. B., Lee, D. O., Hanford, R. B., Zink, C. F., Ely, T. D., Tagamets, M. A., et al. (2004). Effect of methylphenidate on executive functioning in adults with attention-deficit/hyperactivity disorder: Normalization of behavior but not related brain activity. *Biological Psychiatry, 56*(8), 597–606.

Seidman, L. J. (2006). Neuropsychological functioning in people with ADHD across the lifespan. *Clinical Psychology Review, 4*, 466–485.

Semrud-Clikeman, M., Nielsen, K. H., Clinton, A., Sylvester, L., Parle, N., & Connor, R. (1999). An intervention approach for children with teacher- and parent-identified attentional difficulties. *Journal of Learning Disabilities, 32*(6), 581–590.

Sergeant, J. (2000). The cognitive-energetic model: An empirical approach to attention-deficit hyperactivity disorder. *Neuroscience and Biobehavioral Reviews, 24*, 7–12.

Shadmehr, R., & Holcomb, H. H. (1997). Neural correlates of motor memory consolidation. *Science, 277*, 821–825.

Shaffer, R. J., Jacokes, L. E., Cassily, J. F., Greenspan, S. I., Tuchman, R. F., & Stemmer, P. J. (2000). Effect of interactive metronome training on children with ADHD. *American Journal of Occupational Therapy, 55*, 155–162.

Shafritz, K. M., Marchione, K. E., Gore, J., Shaywitz, S. E., & Shaywitz, B. A. (2004). The effects of methylphenidate on neural systems of attention in attention-deficit/hyperactivity disorder. *American Journal of Psychiatry, 161*, 1990–1997.

Silverstein, S. M., & Wilkniss, S. M. (2004). At issue: The future of cognitive rehabilitation of schizophrenia. *Schizophrenia Bulletin, 30*(4), 679–692.

Singh-Curry, V., & Husain, M. (2008). Rehabilitation of neglect. In D. T. Stuss, G. Winocur, & I. H. Robertson (Eds.), *Cognitive neurorehabilitation: Evidence and application* (2nd ed.). Cambridge, UK: Cambridge University Press.

Sohlberg, M. M., & Mateer, C. A. (1987). Effectiveness of an attention training program. *Journal of Clinical and Experimental Neuropsychology, 19*, 117–130.

Sohlberg, M. M., McLaughlin, K. A., Pavese, A., Heidrich, A., & Posner, M. I. (2000). Evaluation of attention process training and brain injury education in persons with acquired brain injury. *Journal of Clinical and Experimental Neuropsychology, 22*(5), 656–676.

Sonuga-Barke, E. J. S. (2000). Psychological heterogeneity in ADHD: A dual pathway model of behaviour and cognition. *Behavioural Brain Research, 130*, 29–36.

Spitzer, M. (1993). The psychopathology, neuropsychology, and neurobiology of associative and working memory in schizophrenia. *European Archives of Psychiatry and Clinical Neuroscience, 243*, 57–70.

Stevens, A. A., Goldman-Rakic, P. S., Gore, J. C., Fullbright, R. K., & Wexler, B. E. (1998). Cortical dysfunction in schizophrenia during auditory word and tone working memory demonstrated by functional magnetic resonance imaging. *Archives of General Psychiatry, 55*, 1097–1103.

Sturm, W., Longoni, F., Weis, S., Specht, K., Herzog, H., Vohn, R., et al. (2004). Functional reorganisation in patients with right hemisphere stroke after training of alertness: A longitudinal PET and fMRI study in eight cases. *Neuropsychologia, 42*(4), 434–450.

Sturm, W., & Willmes, K. (2001). On the functional neuroanatomy of intrinsic and phasic alertness. *NeuroImage, 14*, S76–S84.

Talassi, E., Guerreschi, M., Feriani, M., Fedi, V., Bianchetti, A., & Trabucchi, M. (2007). Effectiveness of a cognitive rehabilitation program in mild dementia (MD) and mild cognitive impairment (MCI): A case control study. *Archives of Gerontology and Geriatrics, 44*(Suppl.), 391–399.

Tannock, R., Ickowicz, A., & Schachar, R. (1995). Differential effects of methylphenidate on working memory in ADHD children with and without comorbid anxiety. *Journal of the American Academy of Child and Adolescent Psychiatry, 34*, 886–896.

Thimm, M., Fink, G. R., Kust, J., Karbe, H., & Sturm, W. (2006). Impact of alertness training on spatial neglect: A behavioural and fMRI study. *Neuropsychologia, 44*(7), 1230–1246.

Turner, G. R., & Levine, B. (2004). Disorders of executive functioning and self-awareness. In J. Ponsford (Ed.), *Cognitive and behavioral rehabilitation*. New York: Guilford Press.

Twamley, E. W., Jeste, D. V., & Bellack, A. S. (2003). A review of cognitive training in schizophrenia. *Schizophrenia Bulletin, 29*(2), 359–382.

Velligan, D. I., Mahurin, R. K., Diamond, P. L., Hazleton, B. C., Eckert, S. L., & Miller, A. L. (1997). The functional significance of symptomatology and cognitive function in schizophrenia. *Schizophrenia Research, 25*(1), 21–31.

Wexler, B. E., Anderson, M., Fullbright, R. K., & Gore, J. C. (2000). Preliminary evidence of improved verbal working memory performance and normalization of task-related frontal lobe activation in schizophrenia following cognitive exercises. *American Journal of Psychiatry, 157*, 1094–1097.

Willis, S. L., Tennstedt, S. L., Marsiske, M., Ball, K., Elias, J., Mann Koepke, K., et al. (2006). Long-term effects of cognitive training on everyday functional outcomes in older adults. *Journal of the American Medical Association, 296*(23), 2805–2814.

Wilson, F. C., Manly, T., Coyle, D., & Robertson, I. H. (2000). The effect of contralesional limb activation training for self-care programmes in unilateral spatial neglect. *Restorative Neurology and Neuroscience, 16*(1), 1–4.

Wykes, T., Reeder, C., Williams, C., Corner, J., Rice, C., & Everitt, B. (2003). Are the effects of cognitive remediation therapy (CRT) durable?: Results from an exploratory trial in schizophrenia. *Schizophrenia Research, 61*, 163–174.

CHAPTER 12

Neuroplasticity and the Treatment of Executive Deficits

Conceptual Considerations

REMA A. LILLIE
CATHERINE A. MATEER

Executive dysfunction is a common occurrence across a variety of neurological conditions, ranging from strokes, tumors, and traumatic brain injuries to dementing diseases and psychiatric disorders. The neural networks subserving executive abilities are diffusely located throughout frontal, prefrontal, and subcortical areas and are susceptible to damage following a variety of events, including encephalitis and hypoxia. The high connectivity of these regions with more posterior areas means that disruption of connections (e.g., white matter damage) can also lead to disturbances in executive abilities. Some have noted that executive dysfunction is the most common presenting problem in neuropsychological practice (e.g., Stuss & Levine, 2002).

Executive functioning can at times seem to be a catch-all term used to refer to any higher-order brain ability. Planning, concept formation, mental flexibility, insight, higher-level attentional skills, sequencing, working memory, behavioral regulation, and social cognition, among others, have all been subsumed under the heading of executive functions. Cicerone,

Levin, Malec, Stuss, and Whyte (2006) have advocated the use of four more clearly defined and circumscribed domains: (1) executive cognitive functions, (2) behavioral self-regulatory functions, (3) activation-regulating functions, and (4) metacognitive processes.[1] Most importantly for the present discussion, these divisions follow both anatomy and evolutionary development. We would argue that if current research on neuroplasticity is to inform rehabilitation efforts, it is imperative for models of cognitive functioning to be grounded in neuroanatomy. Whether such a high standard can be met in the area of executive functioning remains yet to be seen, but there is promising work suggesting that specific functional abilities can be linked to neuroanatomical substrates (e.g., Antonucci et al., 2006; Boghi et al., 2006; Dockery, Hueckel-Weng, Birbaumer, & Plewnia, 2009; Gunstad, Cohen, Paul, Luyster, & Gordon, 2006; Shafritz, Kartheiser, & Belger, 2005).

In recent years, major advances have been made in our understanding of the neural mechanisms involved in executive functioning and recovery from injury. However, rehabilitation efforts for treating executive deficits have yet to capitalize on this knowledge. In this chapter, we review relevant findings from current research on neuroplasticity and discuss possible implications for the rehabilitation of executive deficits. We hope that this information will introduce rehabilitation specialists to themes in the neuroscience research that may have implications for the treatment of executive dysfunction, and to some issues to consider in thinking of how such information could guide future therapies. We start with a brief review of current practice in the rehabilitation of executive dysfunction, as well as a discussion of some difficulties inherent in the concept of executive functioning.

CURRENT PRACTICE IN REHABILITATION

Overview

Executive dysfunction creates a unique challenge for rehabilitation professionals and will often require drawing from a variety of techniques to address specific deficits in daily functioning. In practice, rehabilitation efforts for addressing executive deficits typically include teaching compensatory strategies for completing daily tasks and circumventing problem spots (for a review, see Sohlberg & Mateer, 2001). This may include restructuring environmental demands to eliminate problem-solving requirements (e.g., organizing a client's physical space through labels or reminders;

---

[1]For the purposes of the current discussion, we focus primarily on the domain of executive cognitive functions, which has been most heavily researched to date. Exciting advances are being made in other domains as well, and the interested reader is referred to Cicerone et al. (2006) or Stuss and Levine (2002) for an introduction.

posting operating instructions next to the microwave, laundry machine, or computer) or teaching task-specific routines (e.g., riding the bus, making phone calls, housecleaning). At times, practice and routines may extend to more generalized activities, such as running errands or planning activities. A rehabilitation specialist provides structure in terms of planning, monitoring, supporting, and giving feedback on task completion. With success, such assistance is gradually decreased over time.

Interventions for Specific Skill Sets

Error Monitoring

While treatment of executive dysfunction is often by necessity multifaceted, some rehabilitation approaches focus treatment on improving specific executive skill sets, such as error monitoring, goal management, problem solving, or multitasking. For example, one group of techniques addresses difficulties in self-monitoring by attempting to improve an individual's ability to predict performance. In principle, improving a person's ability to predict his or her behavior and its consequences should allow the individual to identify discrepancies and consider alternative courses of action. Using such concrete tasks as the Tower of London, where individuals move colored beads between different-sized pegs to create specific patterns, researchers are able to provide concrete feedback on discrepancies between prediction of performance and final outcome. As the Tower of London task requires anticipation of errors in order to achieve a successful solution, it provides a useful instrument for monitoring a patient's ability to predict outcomes. Using such tasks, researchers and clinicians have been able to improve the *prediction* of performance; that is, an individual may be more likely to identify a difficult task up front (for a review, see Cicerone, 2002). As noted by Ownsworth, McFarland, and Young (2000), such improvements in self-regulatory strategies can lead to an increased awareness of deficits and a more realistic anticipatory awareness of situations where patients may experience difficulty.

Problem Solving

Whereas anticipating areas of difficulty or deficiency can be an important first step to improving daily functioning, second-line intervention techniques focus more specifically on improving problem-solving abilities through compensatory strategies. The most common approach is training in metacognitive strategies that provide heuristics allowing the client to break more complex tasks into series of rehearsed steps. Perhaps the best-known example of such an approach is goal management training (GMT), developed by Levine et al. (2000).

Based on Duncan's (1986) model of goal neglect, GMT is aimed at teaching clients a framework for problem solving and staying on track. Individuals are taught the five stages of a general-purpose algorithm (see Table 12.1) that can be used in a variety of settings to aid in task completion. Using this type of approach, Levine et al. (2000) have shown improvement in patients' problem solving following a brief 1-hour intervention. In one study (Levine et al., 2000), 30 patients approximately 3–4 years after traumatic brain injury were randomly assigned to brief trials of either GMT or motor skills training (15 in each group). Those individuals who received GMT showed posttraining improvement on paper-and-pencil tasks designed to mimic daily activities that are problematic for individuals with goal neglect (e.g., proofreading, answering questions regarding a hypothetical seating chart, completing a pencil-and-paper grouping task according to specific rules). The control group receiving motor skills training (e.g., mirror tracing, mirror-reversed reading) did not evidence such improvement. In an additional single-case study (Levine et al., 2000), GMT led to observable improvements in meal preparation in a 35-year-old postencephalic patient, suggesting utility in a clinical setting. An interesting case study by Schweizer et al. (2008) applied GMT to a 41-year-old man with executive deficits due to cerebellar damage. Treatment led to improvements on measures of sustained attention planning, and organization that persisted over time and translated into real-life functional gains.

Von Cramon, Matthes-von Cramon, and Mai (1991) implemented a problem-solving training program similarly focused on five domains: (1) problem orientation, (2) problem definition and formulation, (3) generating alternatives, (4) decision making, and (5) solution verification. Treatment was administered to a group of 20 individuals with brain injuries of various etiologies, who were identified as "poor problem solvers" on the basis of psychometric testing and observable behavioral data. Results indicated improvements on tests of categorization and planning for approximately half the participants receiving training. Statistically significant improvements were also seen on intelligence subtasks assessing inductive reasoning and the identification of similarities. Improvements in behavioral ratings of common problem-solving errors were seen in approximately a quarter of

TABLE 12.1. Goal Management Training (GMT) Heuristic

1. *Stop*: "What am I doing?"
2. *Define*: Define the main task.
3. *List*: List the steps needed to complete the task.
4. *Learn*; "Do I know these steps?"
5. *Check*: "Am I doing what I planned to do?"

Note. Based on Levine et al. (2000).

the trained group. However, at least two participants showed worse performance on some measures after training, noting that they felt confused with "all these things to consider" or bored with the tasks. Still, the group receiving problem-solving therapy showed improvements as compared to a memory training group, suggesting that a specific intervention to address problem solving can lead to improvements over and above the benefit of more general treatment factors (e.g., therapist attention, mental effort).

Multitasking

Yet another group of interventions focuses on the common difficulty of multitasking in individuals with executive dysfunction. Different approaches used to address this problem include direct training through completion of dual-task activities, use of periodic auditory alerts to shift focus, and training in cognitive strategies to compensate for areas of difficulty. Direct training using rehearsal of dual-task activities has shown mixed results, including limited generalizability to more real-world settings—a result commonly found across such "restorative" interventions. In a study by Stablum, Umiltà, Mogentale, Carlan, and Guerrini (2000), improvements in dual-task performance were seen with practice over 5 weeks both in a group of individuals with closed head injury and in a separate group with anterior communicating artery aneurysms. Gains were detected on a neuropsychological measure tapping executive abilities and attention (the Paced Auditory Serial Addition Test) and, for the group with aneurysms, a self-report measure of daily functioning (the Cognitive Failures Questionnaire; Broadbent, Cooper, FitzGerald, & Parkes, 1982; Gronwall, 1977). Improvements in performance persisted to some extent at a 12-month follow-up in the aneurysm group. The group with head injuries did not complete testing at 12 months.

Individuals with executive dysfunction often show a certain degree of "stickiness" in their daily lives; that is, switching between tasks, concepts, or activities does not happen spontaneously. To address such problems, periodic auditory alerts can provide helpful reminders to switch or redirect attention. In a study by Manly, Hawkins, Evans, Woldt, and Robertson (2002), 10 individuals with brain injuries benefited from the implementation of periodic auditory alerts when they were completing a task emphasizing frequent switching for successful completion. With alerts, the patient group showed performance equal to that of controls on two primary outcome measures: the number of tasks completed within a given time frame, and the amount of time spent on each task. Switching itself, then, improved with prompting. Interestingly, these results occurred even though the prompts did not lead to an immediate switch between tasks. Instead, with prompting, the time spent on each task more closely resembled that of uninjured control subjects. With the advent of hand-held devices that can provide alerts (e.g., portable timers, paging systems, personal digital assistants), the use of auditory alerts provides a clinical tool for supporting daily functioning.

In contrast to training client to use external devices, Fasotti, Kovacs, Eling, and Brouwer (2000) sought to improve multitasking abilities by training individuals in the use of internal cognitive strategies to deal with the pressures of time management. Training involved the teaching of a four-step cognitive strategy centered on the concept of "Let me give myself enough time." Participants were provided with education on how time pressure can affect performance and on ways for dealing with that pressure, including (1) recognizing time pressure in real-world contexts, (2) preventing time pressure by having a plan, (3) dealing with time pressure by having an "emergency plan," and (4) monitoring performance. Techniques were rehearsed via a series of real-world-style videos involving remembering directions to a hypothetical location or instructions on how to complete an unfamiliar computer task. Significant support was provided by a therapist early in training and was slowly reduced as each individual showed success. To mirror real-life performance more closely, distractors were added over time, including a radio playing in the background. With training, participants were better able to monitor performance in an ongoing manner by reiterating information, asking for clarification, managing distractors, and asking for short pauses. However, a control group who did not receive education on the impact of time pressure and were instead instructed essentially to focus more and not get distracted showed similar (albeit somewhat smaller) improvements. Gains in each group were maintained at a 6-month follow-up.

Explicit Verbal Reasoning

Perhaps a more general approach to addressing executive deficits is through the training of self-instructional strategies that can be applied across a variety of situations. Based on Vgotsky and Luria's early conceptualizations of volitional behavior being modified by inner speech, self-instructional techniques share the common goal of creating an inner dialogue to help guide behavior. Though somewhat similar to the heuristics of metacognitive strategies used for problem solving, explicit verbal reasoning strategies are often more broadly focused on teaching a way of talking to oneself, as opposed to training the use of a specific algorithm.

Foxx, Martella, and Marchand-Martella (1989) developed a training program focused on improving problem-solving skills by encouraging participants to assess socially relevant problem situations by using a set of practical criterion questions ("Who would you talk to?", "What would you say?", "Where would you look for help?"). The goals of such questions were to organize information and help individuals generate the best response to a problem situation. Using such an approach with three individuals with brain injuries, Foxx et al. (1989) were able to show that training led to an improved ability to generate answers to these questions. In addition, anecdotal reports suggested that at least two of the three participants verbally rehearsed the strategy before addressing new problem situations, implying that the questions were internalized over time and used as an effective form of self-talk for problem solving in social settings.

Other techniques involve the verbal modeling of effective problem solving by a therapist, with the premise that an affected individual will gradually internalize such procedures. For instance, Marshall et al. (2004) implemented a training program based on research in the fields of education and educational psychology, involving formalized modeling of effective problem solving and strategy use by a therapist. When this program was applied in a group of 20 individuals at least 20 months following a traumatic brain injury, improvements were seen on a "Twenty questions"-type task (the Rapid Assessment of Problem Solving test) similar to the one used during training. Trained individuals asked more useful questions, adopted new strategies for solving problems that were not presented during training, and showed less random guessing. Training gains were maintained at a 1-month follow-up.

Even more generalized training routines consist of having clients verbalize actions before and during task performance. A typical procedure progresses through three stages: A client verbalizes behavior aloud, then whispers, and then verbalizes silently (inner speech). Cicerone and Giancino (1992) implemented such a training program in a group of six individuals with brain injuries (five with traumatic brain injuries, 1 with falx meningioma) and impairments in planning and self-monitoring. As a result of training, five of the six participants exhibited a reduction in errors; the largest decrease occurred during the first stage of training, suggesting that verbalizing performance aloud can be beneficial in decreasing the rate of errors.

Other Aspects of Current Practice

In practice, rehabilitation of executive dysfunction is by necessity multifaceted. Rath, Simon, Langenbahn, Sherr, and Diller (2003), for example, have added a separate component to their problem-solving program that specifically addresses the motivational and affective components of problem solving and feelings of "emotional overload" commonly faced by individuals with executive dysfunction. Moreover, although we have focused primarily on the rehabilitation of executive cognitive functions, therapeutic attention is also most often paid to physiological factors that affect executive functioning (e.g., nutrition, sleep, activity level, medication) and to commonly co-occurring symptoms, such as impaired self-awareness of deficits.

To date, rehabilitation efforts to address executive deficits have focused on training patients in compensatory strategies based on a small number of theoretical models of cognition. The impact that such strategies may have on neural networks has been largely ignored, probably because such interventions have had a functional focus and because the neural systems involved in regulating behavior are so complex.

PINNING DOWN EXECUTIVE FUNCTIONS

Any intervention that results in new learning will lead to changes in the brain. When considering ways in which research on neuroplasticity can inform rehabilitative efforts for executive functions, we consider such interventions what Cicerone et al. (2006) would term *direct remediation*. Whereas most current practices focus at the level of compensation or training of strategies, direct remediation attempts aim to elicit change at the level of the underlying cognitive process. This is not to say that such interventions are aimed at reinstating previous pathways or abilities, but rather that they have as a goal improving impairment-level outcome measures related to a specific cognitive process.

We have previously suggested (Lillie & Mateer, 2006) that rehabilitation efforts with the goal of altering specific neural networks will benefit from focused work in a narrowly defined area. For executive functions, this can become a daunting task. Unlike sensory or motor functions, for which clear links can be made between specific abilities and cortical areas, executive functions are more diffusely located and less well defined and at times involve complex cortical and subcortical pathways that evolve over the completion of a task (e.g., cerebellar–thalamic–cortical circuit; Ide & Li, 2010). In fact, executive abilities that are most readily apparent in novel, unstructured settings may actually show a reduction in brain activity as a task is learned. Providing repeated practice to target specific brain regions may thus be difficult, to say the least. Further complicating the issue is the fact that poor performance has at times been associated with reduced brain activation (e.g., Cazalis et al., 2006), while at other times disrupted performance has been associated with recruitment of additional brain regions in patients as compared to normal controls (e.g., Christodoulou et al., 2001), or with increased levels of activation (e.g., Scheibel et al., 2003). In addition, similar levels of performance have been found in patient groups and controls, despite differing patterns of cerebral activation (e.g., Cader, Cifelli, Abu-Omar, Palace, & Matthews, 2006; McAllister et al., 1999). Predicting a preferred outcome, then, becomes challenging. Is it desirable to show an increase or reduction in brain activity over time, activity more closely resembling that of normal controls, or some alternative? If performance on outcome measures is consistent with that expected in control subjects, is it problematic that alternative neuronal substrates are used?

Even if specific functional abilities and their neuroanatomical substrates can be identified for various executive functions, the question remains of whether rehabilitation efforts targeting such specific abilities will be effective in eliciting change both in the area of impairment and in other, associated activities. Although incorporating efforts geared toward generalization is a necessary component of any cognitive rehabilitative program (unless task-specific learning is the treatment goal), it is important to identify whether improvements can be expected on similarly structured activities; otherwise, the eventual relevance to daily living is questionable. As Cicerone et al. (2006) have observed, it may be that a holistic or multimodal rehabilitation program, perhaps in combination with specific training elements, will be more effective for treating executive dysfunction and elicit the best outcome. Because executive function deficits are so complex, we anticipate that such focused intervention efforts will ideally take place within the context of a more broadly based rehabilitative plan addressing the myriad of concerns associated with executive dysfunction. Whether such task-specific interventions will be useful components of a larger rehabilitative plan is an empirical question that has yet to be answered.

IMPLICATIONS OF CURRENT RESEARCH ON NEUROPLASTICITY

Potential Mechanisms of Change

Recent research on neuroplasticity suggests that brain structure can be altered via several different mechanisms. Those most relevant to executive functions are briefly described below. For more comprehensive reviews, the reader is referred to other chapters in this text (e.g., Kolb, Cioe, & Williams, Chapter 2; Nudo & Bury, Chapter 4) as well as Bach-y-Rita (2003) and Levin and Grafman (2000).

Multiplexing and Unmasking

Multiplexing in the brain refers to the fact that neurons and fibers participate in multiple functions (Bach-y-Rita, 2003). As opposed to one network for one type of processing, there are redundancies built into the system, so that multiple inputs may access the same cell or network of cells. As summarized by Bach-y-Rita (2003), these multiple inputs may provide a basis for the rerouting of processing pathways and may provide the neural basis for plastic changes with training: If one input is no longer available to the system (e.g., through injury or disease), alternative inputs are "unmasked," allowing for modified access to existing networks. Although unmasking is not likely to explain massive reorganization, some combination of initial unmasking and growth of new connections may underlie plastic changes (Ergenzinger & Pons, 2000).

It is unclear how multiplexing may effect recovery from executive dysfunction. Perhaps initial unmasking primes the system for intervention attempts by revealing alternative inputs. Or perhaps initial reorganization makes intervention attempts more difficult by changing the typical pathways involved in higher-order processing or by reinforcing new and undesirable inputs to higher-level networks. On the more optimistic side, perhaps there is a way for rehabilitation specialists to encourage use of these alternative pathways to circumvent problem spots. Similar to the compensatory training used at the functional level in rehabilitation, supporting the use of alternative pathways for accessing existing networks through training may lead to compensation for injury at the neuronal level. At the bare minimum, these findings suggest a *potential* in the brain for rerouting, implying that even after injury, there may be a possibility of creating new pathways to support functional abilities.

A second finding of this line of research with implications for the treatment of executive dysfunction is that simultaneous reorganization occurs at both cortical and subcortical levels. As described by Xu and Wall (2000) in reference to the reorganization of hand maps in primates, such findings suggest a widespread, central reorganization following injury that is not limited to intracortical change. Understanding how subcortical substrates and mechanisms interact with cortical changes could help further elucidate the types of intervention that may be most successful—or, more practically, may suggest where to monitor for change in intervention studies. For example, executive functions are subserved by a large network of both cortical and subcortical structures. When we are examining change at the highest level of functional ability, it will be important to consider the implications of concurrent changes at lower levels.

Lastly, similar to much of the research on neuroplasticity in general, our understanding of multiplexing and unmasking is grounded in work on the somatosensory system. As discussed later (see "Conceptual Considerations"), the neural networks involved in cognition may respond differently from the motor and sensory systems to injury.

Nonsynaptic Transmission

Historically, our understanding of cortical activity has been based on concepts of synaptic transmission. More recently, however, researchers have been exploring alternative pathways of communication in the brain, including *volume transmission* (VT). VT refers to the diffusion of transmitters, as well as other neuroactive substances, through the volume of extracellular space (Syková, 2005). These substance bind to extrasynaptic (usually high-affinity) binding sites located on neurons, axons, and glial cells. This type of cellular communication has been implicated in such functions as vigilance, sleep, chronic pain, hunger, depression, memory formation, and long-term potentiation and depression. Such communication may play a role in plastic changes within the central nervous system (Syková, 2005).

Nonsynaptic transmission has implications for executive dysfunction, because this form of cellular communication has been implicated in processes requiring continued activity over a period of time, such as setting the overall tone of cortical functioning. As described by Luria (1973, p. 44), "[i]t is only under optimal waking conditions that man can receive and analyse information, that the necessary selective systems of connections can be called to mind, his activity programmed, and the course of his mental processes checked, his mistakes corrected, and his activity kept to the proper course." Without an overall cortical tone that can support higher-order processing, executive cognitive control is impossible. Similarly, when we consider other executive abilities (such as activation-regulating functions), it is clear that nonsynaptic transmission may have an impact on the full spectrum of executive functions.

In memory and learning research, nonsynaptic transmission has been shown to be tightly coupled with synaptic modification, suggesting that such processes may provide a mechanism to facilitate synaptic change (Mozzachiodi & Byrne, 2010). Additionally, synaptic and nonsynaptic changes in different anatomical regions can make distinct contributions to behavioral modification (Mozzachiodi & Byrne, 2010). Understanding the timing, location, and role of such nonsynaptic change in the modification of networks associated with executive abilities would have important implications for rehabilitation.

Pathological processes in the central nervous system, including those that often affect executive functions (e.g., traumatic brain injuries, dementia, stroke), alter the extracellular environment through morphological changes such as swelling, loss of dendritic processes, and demyelination. Such changes can decrease the effectiveness of VT, and hence can impair executive functions relying on such forms of transmission. Because VT has been implicated in processes such as long-term potentiation and depression, as well as in memory formation, dysfunction of this important transmitter pathway may have implications for rehabilitative efforts. If learning opportunities and synaptic change are limited by shifts in VT, intervention attempts may be less successful.

Nonsynaptic transmission also bears consideration in the development of pharmacological interventions for executive functions. Some have suggested that VT may serve as the principal mode of action for psychoactive drugs (Bach-y-Rita, 2003). Anisotropic diffusion, which preferentially channels the movement of substances in the extracellular space in one direction and may be responsible for some degree of specificity in VT, is often disrupted in pathological states (Syková, 2005). This disruption interrupts the normal flow of signal transmission and may contribute to functional deficits (Syková, 1997). As anisotrophy has been detected in tissue of the cerebellum, hippocampus, and along white matter tracts, including the corpus callosum (Syková, 1997), its disruption may affect key structures involved in executive functions and have implications for pharmacological treatments aimed at ameliorating dysfunction.

Plasticity of Limbic versus Eulaminate Cortices

Prefrontal limbic and eulaminate (six-layered) cortices are structurally and functionally distinct, and have their own unique patterns of connectivity with subcortical and cortical areas (Barbas, 2000). Rehabilitation strategies may differ for these two regions, suggesting that distinct approaches may be required to address changes in executive cognitive functions (subserved by eulaminate cortices) as compared to other types of executive functions, such as behavioral self-regulatory functions or activation-regulating functions (which are more closely linked to medial structures). As discussed by Barbas (2000), the patterns of connections of prefrontal limbic and eulaminate cortices have implications for the extent to which these cortices exhibit plasticity after injury, as well as for their relative vulnerability in neurological and psychiatric disease. Limbic cortices in adult monkeys, for example, show more widespread and diverse connections than eulaminate cortices do, and have considerably higher levels of developmentally associated proteins (GAP-43, NOS; Barbas, 2000). It appears, then, that limbic cortices may retain some of the connectional and neurochemical features seen in development to a greater extent than other areas do. This may imply a greater potential for plasticity in these areas, as well as an increased susceptibility to injury or disease.

Understanding the mechanisms underlying this inherent plasticity may suggest intervention strategies that could maximize this potential and, in turn, result in functional improvement following damage (Barbas, 2000). These patterns may also suggest that the cognitive executive functions subserved by eulaminate cortices may be more resistant to change than the behavioral self-regulatory functions or activation-regulating functions subserved by more plastic limbic cortices.

Importantly, the idea that the prefrontal cortex has a limbic component reiterates a common finding that plastic changes in the brain are influenced by behavioral significance (see Nudo & Bury, Chapter 4, this volume). It is important for rehabilitation specialists, then, to use tasks and materials that engage the treated individuals, in order to maximize the underlying potential for change.

Vicariation

Vicariation refers to the ability of one brain region to subsume activities for which it was not originally designed. Although phylogeny predisposes cortical areas to participate in specific abilities (e.g., primary visual cortex with vision, motor cortex with movement, frontal regions for higher-level processing), these predetermined functions are not set in stone and can be altered under certain conditions. The most commonly used example is the activation of primary visual cortex through touch by blind Braille readers (e.g., Sadato, 2005). Without input from the visual system, vicariation allows for adaptation of visual cortex for other functions. To put this another way, without visual input, the cortical area generally predisposed to visual input is overtaken by other functions. Another example would include the recovery of somatosensory functions following stroke where new foci of activation can be detected in the lesioned hemisphere after functional recovery (e.g., Jablonka, Burnat, Witte, & Kossut, 2010), suggesting that new areas have subsumed the ability in the spared cortex. Vicariation sets the stage for plastic changes in the brain, then, by providing a medium in which alterations can occur. Without such flexibility, cortical losses would result in more permanent and debilitating outcomes.

In terms of rehabilitation, vicariation highlights several important features of recovery. First, cortical areas that are not in use for their intended functions may be overtaken in time. This suggests that challenging the system after injury is important in order to preserve abilities (issues of the timing of such challenges are discussed later). It also suggests, though, that the spontaneous recovery process can result in undesirable changes if cortical areas are subsumed by unanticipated processes (e.g., competition between motor and cognitive recovery). Second (and on a more positive note), vicariation suggests that even after injury to specific cortical areas some degree of flexibility is maintained within the system, so that other cortical areas can respond to previously unintentioned inputs. This provides a basis for suggesting that intervention has the potential to lead to desirable changes at the cortical level.

In terms of executive cognitive functions, it is unclear what role vicariation would play in the recovery process. It is unlikely that posterior systems would subserve higher-level abilities, even following injury or disease; however, vicariation may suggest that cortical areas adjacent to key structures linked to executive abilities (e.g., dorsolateral prefrontal cortex, anterior cingulate cortex, orbitofrontal cortex), but not previously predisposed to participate in executive functions, have the potential to subserve new abilities.

Synaptogenesis

Many of the previously discussed processes have implications soon after injury. Long-lasting changes in cortical function following injury or disease require modifications in synaptic connectivity. It has been suggested that functional connections, rather than raw numbers of neurons, determine computational power in the cerebral cortex and distinguish humans from other mammals of comparable size (Turkstra, Holland, & Bays, 2003). The ability to modify these connections allows for learning throughout the lifespan. Both changes in synaptic efficacy and axonal sprouting have been implicated in changes seen in cerebral networks after reorganization of function (Nudo, Barbay, & Kleim, 2000). In terms of executive cognitive abilities, it is possible that rehabilitation efforts can capitalize on the brain's ability to maximize synaptic efficacy and promote axonal sprouting through tailored practice and rehearsal. Other researchers (e.g., Sun & Alkon, 2010; Wurtman, Cansev, Sakamoto, & Ulus, 2009) Have focused on possible pharmacologic agents and nutrition supplements purported to support synaptogenesis which may have future implications for the treatment of executive abilities.

Neurogenesis

One of the more intriguing developments in the field of neuroplasticity is the recent understanding of the potential for neurogenesis within the adult cerebral cortex. Although exciting implications are being studied in terms of stem cell research, and factors that may induce or enhance adult mammalian neurogenesis are being identified and may lead to various types of therapeutic interventions to enhance regeneration (Turkstra et al., 2003), neurogenesis is likely to have limited applications to the rehabilitation of executive dysfunction. Whereas an understanding of the substrates that support growth of new neurons could lead to intervention strategies that support such changes (e.g., pharmacological interventions), there is little direct evidence that neurogenesis plays a significant role in either experience-dependent changes in behavior or behavioral recovery after injury (Turkstra et al., 2003). (For a more complete discussion, see Kolb et al., Chapter 2, this volume.)

Reorganization of Function

Most of the processes identified above result in a potential for reorganization of function in the brain after injury or disease. Such reorganization can occur in different ways (summarized in Grady & Kapur, 1999); it has been identified in various studies as involving activation of perilesional tissue or extension of specialized areas into adjacent tissue, recruitment of homotopic areas of the contralateral hemisphere, or takeover of networks with related functions (for a review, see Muñoz-Cespedes, Rios-Lago, Paul, & Maestu, 2005). At times, tasks have been shown to be completed via altered functional neuroanatomical networks in patient groups as compared to normal controls (e.g., Levine et al., 2002). Although most research on reorganization of function has focused on motor and sensory domains, studies of recovery from aphasia suggest that plastic changes can lead to functional changes in complex cognitive tasks (e.g., language). Changes in reorganization may be long-lasting and depend upon postinjury experience. Some authors now describe reorganization as the principal process responsible for spontaneous recovery of function after acquired brain damage (e.g., Hallett, 2000).

Reorganization occurs in a competitive environment. As summarized by Nudo et al. (2000), spontaneous recovery in the absence of postinfarct training can result in degenerative changes in the physiology of remaining structures. Conversely, training can lead to an expansion in the cortical areas responsible for specific functions. Both of these findings suggest that postinjury rehabilitation efforts are important and that specific training can lead to structural changes in neural systems.

CONCEPTUAL CONSIDERATIONS

If reorganization of function is an active process after injury or during the course of a disease, our challenge as rehabilitation specialists is to determine ways in which this new understanding of brain plasticity can inform treatment regimens to maximize the potential for functional recovery. In the area of executive dysfunction, such work is affected by several conceptual considerations.

The Construct of Executive Functioning

Defining the Problem

As mentioned previously, identifying the construct of executive functioning can at times be difficult. Any effort that hopes to capitalize on plasticity of the recovering brain will benefit from a focused area of interest, in terms of both the specific ability being tested (e.g., planning) and the proposed site of potential change (e.g., middorsolateral frontal cortex). This may be a challenge in the broadly defined domain of executive functioning and will require further refinement of proposed areas of difficulty.

When rehabilitation specialists are focusing on a specific problem area, considering how such abilities map onto neural structures may help identify the types of interventions that may be most beneficial. For example, executive cognitive abilities such as planning, sequencing, or problem solving, which are most closely linked to dorsolateral prefrontal cortex, may be affected by plastic changes related to unmasking, vicariation, or synaptogenesis. It may be possible that challenging a specific neural network, as in some interventions in the sensory–motor domain (e.g., Nudo et al., 2000), will elicit change at the neuronal level. Whether such change can lead to functional improvement remains to be seen, but such alterations have been linked to functional improvements in other domains (Nudo et al., 2000; Pulvermüller et al., 2001), suggesting that the possibility exists. For other executive abilities, such as activation-regulating functions, which have been most closely linked to medial structures, it may be that other plastic changes in the brain, such as alterations in nonsynaptic transmission, may be more relevant, and thus the type of intervention strategy may differ (e.g., pharmacotherapy).

Probing the Problem

A related consideration in the domain of executive functions is developing ways to probe the problem in question. Many of the tests used to assess executive functioning are nonspecific and may not have the sensitivity required to detect change at the level of an identified ability. Working to refine our assessment of executive dysfunction will be an important precursor to developing more specific measures and paradigms for executive abilities. In the meantime, researchers may benefit from focusing on one outcome measure from a more broadly used test (e.g., semantic clustering on the California Verbal Learning Test, perseverative errors on the Wisconsin Card Sorting Test), looking at profiles across different tasks, or tracking specific difficulties in everyday life (e.g., via the Dysexecutive Questionnaire). Although monitoring for change at such a focused level may seem far removed from the day-to-day challenges of individuals with executive deficits, such finite analyses are necessary to determine local effects of training. Strategies geared toward generalization can be implemented once local changes have been detected.

Alternatively, as our interest lies both in functional outcome and in the neural structures underlying such abilities, probing the problem may incorporate some form of imaging to elucidate the type and extent of cerebral damage. One pattern of damage or disease may respond better (or worse) to intervention attempts than another. As executive abilities are diffusely located throughout the cortex and involve a complex interplay of multiple cortical and subcortical regions, identifying the necessary underlying substrates for intervention attempts will be challenging.

Training

The concept of training in the domain of executive functions faces two problems. First, as noted previously, executive abilities are most often required to solve novel or unfamiliar tasks. Repetition of a task, then, may actually lead to a reduction in the need for executive problem solving. How does one provide practice and rehearsal on a task without causing it to become mundane or overlearned? Perhaps one answer lies in the work of Nudo and colleagues (see Nudo et al., 2000, for a summary) suggesting that skill building is more important than basic repetition. It seems that tasks graded in level of difficulty may be most efficient at eliciting change at the neural level. Such hierarchically structured activities are not new in the area of rehabilitation, with Attention Process Training (APT; Sohlberg & Mateer, 1987) perhaps serving as the best example. Working on one specific area of difficulty and slowly increasing complexity may provide a means of consistently challenging executive systems.

Second, as noted by Kilgard and Merzenich (1998), experience is necessary but not sufficient to induce plasticity. Tasks also need to carry some type of behavioral significance. Rehabilitation efforts may be more successful at the neuronal level if the tasks and stimuli used are important or relevant to the individual.

Effectiveness

Defining the effectiveness of any intervention is necessarily complex and multifaceted. In the case of intervention strategies capitalizing on neuroplasticity, effectiveness includes a minimum of two components: (1) change or modification at the neural level and (2) change at the functional level. Although these outcomes are ultimately linked, different studies may focus on one, the other, or both of them, as each can serve as an independent research goal. A concurrent question involves tracking "poorer" recovery patterns, perhaps linked to spontaneous recovery, to determine which types of neuronal change result in worse outcomes. Such information could guide intervention attempts by identifying the types of alterations at the neural level that are less ideal and the environments/conditions that promote undesirable effects.

Tracking change at the functional level is most likely to comprise pre-/posttreatment evaluation of various outcome measures, including neuropsychological test data, functional outcome measures, and/or behavioral questionnaires assessing everyday functioning. Each of these types of evaluations is limited by the same conceptual issues discussed above, including a need to clearly define the area of interest.

The challenges inherent in any assessment of an intervention strategy become all the more pronounced in assessing interventions for executive functioning. For example, researchers will have to determine whether change can be sufficiently captured by a single outcome measure or whether a more multifaceted evaluation, adding to the complexity of statistical analyses, is required. Determining whether there is a cutoff point that will capture improvement or whether an analysis that allows for a continuum of outcomes will be more appropriate may be difficult when complex executive abilities are being assessed. Each of these decisions affects the likelihood of detecting change and determines whether this change will be meaningful at a broader level. In some instances (e.g., preliminary studies), a less conservative approach may be preferred; at other times, a stricter requirement may be desired to detect change at a level that may be evident in daily functioning.

Imaging

Tracking change at the neural level is likely to include some type of imaging data. In the area of executive functioning, such information is particularly important, as in some studies behavioral output has been found to be equivalent whereas the underlying cognitive processes involved before and after intervention may change (e.g., Christodoulou et al., 2001). Some types of executive dysfunction have been linked to less efficient processing strategies than those of normal controls, so that detecting change in the systems used to complete a task will be all the more relevant. Making the study of change even more difficult is the fact that executive abilities involve a diffuse set of networks. Functional imaging techniques benefit from a focused area of interest, and the use of subtraction procedures necessitates structuring cognitive tasks in such a way that only the ability of interest differs from one condition to the next. For complex executive tasks that require the convergence of information across multiple domains of functioning and involve a diffuse network of cortical and subcortical structures, tracking change becomes complicated.

As noted by Ward and Frackowiak (2006), if the relationships between patterns of brain activation and outcome are not clearly understood, interpreting data from functional imaging studies becomes very difficult. In the design of functional imaging studies, such factors as cognitive equivalence of tasks, strategy differences, performance differences, and differences in skill level or difficulty are all fundamentally important (Rickard, 2000; Ward & Frackowiak, 2006), especially when clinical samples are to be compared to normal controls. Even still, interpretations of altered networks can be limited by individual differences, processing differences, bilateral activation in normal controls, and statistical factors, among others (see Rickard, 2000, for a discussion). It has been suggested that converging evidence from multiple measures of neural activity (e.g., functional magnetic resonance imaging, positron emission tomography, electroencephalography, magnetoencephalography) may provide the best support for changes in neural structure. Newer techniques, such as transcranial magnetic stimulation (TMS) and diffusion tensor imaging (DTI), have shown promise in tracking plasticity (Levin, 2003; Hallett, 2007). DTI, which visualizes disruptions in white matter connections, may have particular relevance for tracking executive deficits and changes in underlying networks.

Neuroplasticity

In addition to the challenges posed by the construct of executive functioning itself, several limiting factors suggested by research on neuroplasticity must be mentioned here.

Recruitment of New Areas

First, recruitment of new areas to complete a function is not necessarily desirable. For example, as reviewed in Ward and Frackowiak (2006), some patients with chronic stroke activate additional motor regions when completing a hand grip task, compared to normal controls. Overactivations are often bilateral, suggesting some type of plastic change occurring at the cortical level. Importantly, however, those individuals with overactivations as compared to the control group have *poorer* functional outcomes, suggesting that the recruitment of activity in these regions does not facilitate recovery. Similarly, as noted by Schallert et al. (2000), use can be related to both neuroplasticity and neurodegeneration after focal injury as networks take over adjacent territory. Some plastic changes in the brain may actually make functional recovery more difficult. Such findings suggest that tracking both neurophysiological measures and functional outcome will be necessary to define improvement.

Timing

There is some evidence to suggest that intervention at too early a point in the recovery process can actually lead to poorer outcomes (e.g., Kozlowski, James, & Schallert, 1996) or that the timing of interventions should heed certain critical periods in the recovery process (e.g., Jang, 2009). However, other research suggests that there is great potential for improvement in the first 6 months to 2 years following an injury. The rehabilitation specialist is thus left in the difficult position of determining how to maximize potential of the recovering brain while not implementing challenging treatment regimens too soon after injury. Some have suggested that rehabilitation routines should consist of support during the initial phases of recovery, with more intensive interventions occurring over the longer term. As noted by Muñoz-Cepedes et al. (2005), there is no clear delineation of when recovery is "complete," suggesting that individuals may be able to show some functional improvement even years after injury or disease.

Intensity

Similar to the issue of timing is the suggestion that overuse of a system can actually be detrimental at both a cortical and a functional level. As reviewed by Schallert et al. (2000), a series of studies in rats suggest that forcing overuse of an affected limb after injury leads to retardation of functional improvement and an expansion of the original lesion. But at the same time, repetition is necessary for eliciting change (Kilgard & Merzenich, 1998; Nudo et al., 2000). The rehabilitation specialist, then, is faced with the additional barrier of providing focused, challenging repetition without overtaxing the system by providing training that is too intense. Such issues are also likely to interact with timing, as noted above: It may be possible to provide more intensive treatment later in the recovery process, whereas similar training in early stages of recovery may be ill advised (see Jang, 2009, for an example of the impact of critical periods).

Age

The impact of age on neuroplastic processes is a complicated issue that is better addressed elsewhere (see various chapters in the current volume). Interventions for executive deficits may be similar across the age spectrum, but are likely to vary along important lines such as timing, intensity, and the types of materials used. For example, whereas enriched environments have been shown to be beneficial to adult animals recovering from injury, the same may not hold for injuries to developing nervous systems, where such environments can result in increased dendritic density without accompanying increases in functional connections (Turkstra et al., 2003). Conversely, the expected potential for improvements in children may be greater than that for adults, depending on the age at which injury occurs.

Motor/Sensory–Motor versus Cognitive Domains

To date, with some notable exceptions (e.g., Pulvermüller et al., 2001), studies of neuroplasticity have generally focused on the domain of motor or sensory–motor functioning. It has been suggested that some of the plasticity inherent in this system is due to the high degree of overlap among different systems and the multiple redundancies of information. Similar redundancies may not be recapitulated in cognitive systems, however, and this may restrict the types or degree of possible plastic change. Others, however, have argued that "cortex is cortex" and that there is no reason why the principles of neuroplasticity studied in the motor domain should not translate into domains of cognition. Whether cognitive neural systems respond differently to intervention from motor or sensory–motor systems is an empirical question that remains to be answered.

Injury Characteristics

Several characteristics of the injury itself will have an impact on treatment regimens. For example, there are inherent differences between focal and diffuse damage to the brain. In animal studies, most of the research to date on neuroplasticity has focused on focal damage, although more diffuse injuries have also been studied. It is likely that the potential for change or the types of interventions used for each of these injuries will differ. Diffuse injury is more likely to be associated with white matter damage and widespread changes to brain neurochemistry. Focal damage will be determined in large part by the size of the lesion itself. As noted by Nudo et al. (2000), there are probably limits on vicariation of function. Though the proportion of remaining tissue required to subsume affected abilities is unclear, it is clear that for neuroplastic change to lead to functional improvements following damage or injury, some residual functional network needs to remain. Similarly, as noted by Schallert et al. (2000), not only the size but the location of the lesion within the cortex may play an important role in the types of interventions that may be successful in implementing change.

FUTURE DIRECTIONS

New Treatment Regimens

We see the possibility of new treatment regimens that will maximize the potential of the recovering brain for reorganizing executive functions. At this writing, it is unclear what such interventions will look like, and their development will require the creativity of a variety of rehabilitation specialists. Besides some interventions for working memory and higher-order attentional skills reviewed elsewhere in this volume (see O'Connell & Robertson, Chapter 11), there are currently no published treatments for executive dysfunction guided by our current understanding of research on neuroplasticity. However, the exciting advances being made in other domains suggest that such strategies are possible.

A starting point for developing new strategies, perhaps, is an understanding of the impact of current interventions. One similarity across approaches is the common goal of exerting conscious control over previously automated processes, or, to put it another way, of making common internal processes explicit. Strategies designed to formalize problem solving (e.g., GMT), prediction of one's own performance, or self-talk mirror naturally occurring processes, such as having an organized way of approaching problems, making a prediction of whether a task will be difficult or easy, or conducting an internal dialogue during problem solving, respectively. Such formalized strategies can be thought to combat the seemingly automated, stimulus-driven responses of individuals with executive function deficits. Interestingly, reestablishment of executive control has been linked primarily to activation of the dorsolateral prefrontal cortex (e.g., Kübler, Dixon, & Garavan, 2006), which may be damaged or disconnected from other networks through injury or disease. The findings of efficacy with such interventions thus suggest that the damaged brain maintains some potential for improvement, either by rerouting connections around such problem areas or by using a different neural network to complete such functions. Principles of neuroplasticity would suggest that these interventions capitalize on the brain's underlying potential to reorganize functions through such processes as unmasking, vicariation, or synaptogenesis. But are there still ways to influence such changes more directly?

Perhaps another way of conceptualizing intervention strategies comes from the developmental literature. Some researchers (e.g., Zelazo & Müeller, 2002) have made a distinction between "cool" cognitive aspects of executive function (associated with dorsolateral regions of the prefrontal cortex) and more "hot" affective aspects (associated with ventral and medial regions), and have followed the development of such processes across early childhood. Such distinctions may provide another means of developing tasks intended to focus on one specific aspect of the broader domain of executive abilities. An example of a task tapping "cool" executive abilities would be self-ordered pointing (e.g., Archibald & Kerns, 1999), which requires an individual to point to different items on subsequent pages of a repeated array. Whereas planning and working memory are required for completion, the emotional salience, beyond a certain level of motivation and willingness to please the examiner, is minimal. By contrast, gambling tasks (e.g., Bechara, Tranel, & Damasio, 2000), in which there is an emotional component linked to the use of rewards and consequences, are thought to elicit more "hot" aspects of executive control or to tap decision making about events that have emotionally significant consequences.

Current rehabilitative efforts have primarily focused on what would be considered "cool" executive abilities elicited by more abstract, decontextualized problems. But individuals with executive dysfunction tend to show problems across a variety of domains. Tasks intended to tap more "hot," affective aspects of decision making may provide a means of broadening the framework of intervention strategies or focusing on different aspects of problem solving (e.g., problem solving with and without a salient affective component). In terms of our discussion of neuroplasticity, such "hot" executive functions may provide access to different neural substrates (e.g., ventral and medial regions of the prefrontal cortex), and thus may be a means of integrating the more plastic limbic system into rehabilitative attempts.

Studying Typical Reorganization

Equally important to the development of specific intervention strategies is the study of the typical course of reorganization following injury or disease. By understanding the types of cerebral changes that lead to improved or worsened function, as well as the environmental conditions associated with such changes, we can better predict the types of neural changes and environmental conditions to foster or avoid.

Treatment Variables and Methods

As in other domains (see various chapters in the current volume), elucidating the impact of some of the major variables in treatment will be important to developing new interventions for complex executive abilities. Issues such as desired timing, intensity, and age factors will require exploration so that the functional impact of intervention approaches can be maximized.

Another likely development in the area will be pairing treatment regimens with pharmacological agents (e.g., dopamine, amphetamines, cholinergic agents) or with physiological interventions (e.g., TMS). Although pairing efforts are underway (for a review, see Nadeau & Wu, 2006), the planning of pharmacological treatment appears complex: Agents that have shown to be neuroprotective when administered soon after injury (e.g., *N*-methyl-D-aspartate receptor antagonist MK-801) can be debilitating when administered later (Schallert & Hernandez, 1998), and agents shown to be neuroprotective in animals (e.g., calcium channel antagonists) may be harmful when administered in humans.

Summary

The complexity of executive functioning suggests that interventions in this domain may lag behind those in other areas. A particular limitation remains the lack of specificity in tools designed to assess executive abilities. However, due to executive deficits' high impact on daily functioning and their prevalence across a wide array of injuries, diseases, and disorders, determining ways to improve such abilities will remain a high priority for practicing clinicians. It may be that interventions to improve the general tone of the system (e.g., pharmacological agents to address decreased activation and drive) will precede more specific interventions to address deficits in executive cognitive functions.

CONCLUDING REMARKS

Over the last several years, a key message emerging from research on neuroplasticity is that the lesioned brain and the normal brain are different when it comes to the potential for change (Ward & Frackowiak, 2006). As noted by Barbas (2000) and others, evidence suggests that when the nervous system is damaged by injury or affected by disease, it may revert to a more chaotic pattern of synaptic contacts (perhaps comparable to that seen in development), and may be more able to change structure and function than a typical brain. These factors, combined with the potential for plasticity discussed above, suggest that a more complete understanding of the circumstances facilitating the establishment of appropriate connections may improve intervention attempts by rehabilitation specialists (Barbas, 2000). The combined evidence to date suggests that the brain undergoes many plastic changes following injury or disease in an attempt to repair or compensate for damage. A fuller understanding of these changes may move us toward a new understanding of rehabilitation for brain injury.

Several challenges face the researcher in attempting to translate theory and research on neuroplasticity into treatment regimens for executive dysfunction, including limitations of the broad-based concept of executive functioning, as well as issues related to neuroplasticity itself. Translating findings from the basic research into treatment regimens will necessarily be complex and will require the cooperation of a team of specialists. Nevertheless, with the knowledge that the brain is more plastic than was once believed, the prospect of maximizing this underlying potential is an exciting one.

REFERENCES

Antonucci, A. S., Gansler, D. A., Tan, S., Bhadelia, R., Patz, S., & Fulwiler, C. (2006). Orbitofrontal correlates of aggression and impulsivity in psychiatric patients. *Psychiatry Research, 147*(2–3), 213–220.

Archibald, S. J., & Kerns, K. A. (1999). Identification and description of new tests of executive functioning in children. *Child Neuropsychology, 5*(2), 115–129.

Bach-y-Rita, P. (2003). Theoretical basis for brain plasticity after a TBI. *Brain Injury, 17*(8), 643–651.

Barbas, H. (2000). Neuroanatomic basis for reorganization of function after prefrontal damage in primates. In H. S. Levin & J. Grafman (Eds.), *Cerebral reorganization of function after brain damage* (pp. 84–108). New York: Oxford University Press.

Bechara, A., Tranel, D., & Damasio, H. (2000). Characterization of the decision-making deficit of patients with ventromedial prefrontal cortex lesions. *Brain, 123*(11), 2189–2202.

Boghi, A., Rasetti, R., Avidano, F., Manzone, C., Orsi, L., D'Agata, F., et al. (2006). The effect of gender on planning: An fMRI study using the Tower of London task. *NeuroImage, 33*(3), 999–1010.

Broadbent, D. E., Cooper, P. F., FitzGerald, P., & Parkes, K. R. (1982). The Cognitive Failures Questionnaire (CFQ) and its correlates. *British Journal of Clinical Psychology, 21*(Pt. 1), 1–16.

Cader, S., Cifelli, A., Abu-Omar, Y., Palace, J., & Matthews, P. M. (2006). Reduced brain functional reserve and altered functional connectivity in patients with multiple sclerosis. *Brain, 129*, 527–537.

Cazalis, F., Feydy, A., Valabrègue, R., Pélégrini-Issac, M., Pierot, L., & Azouvi,

P. (2006). fMRI study of problem-solving after severe traumatic brain injury. *Brain Injury, 20*(10), 1019–1028.

Christodoulou, C., DeLuca, J., Ricker, J. H., Madigan, N. K., Bly, B. M., Lange, G., et al. (2001). Functional magnetic resonance imaging of working memory impairment after traumatic brain injury. *Journal of Neurology, Neurosurgery and Psychiatry, 71*, 161–168.

Cicerone, K. D. (2002). The enigma of executive functioning: Theoretical contributions to therapeutic interventions. In P. J. Eslinger (Ed.), *Neuropsychological interventions: Clinical research and practice* (pp. 246–265). New York: Guilford Press.

Cicerone, K. D., & Giancino, J. T. (1992). Remediation of executive function deficits after traumatic brain injury. *NeuroRehabilitation, 2*(3), 12–22.

Cicerone, K. D., Levin, H., Malec, J., Stuss, D., & Whyte, J. (2006). Cognitive rehabilitation interventions for executive function: Moving from bench to bedside in patients with traumatic brain injury. *Journal of Cognitive Neuroscience, 18*(7), 1212–1222.

Dockery, C. A., Hueckel-Weng, R., Birbaumer, N., & Plewnia, C. (2009). Enhancement of planning ability by transcranial direct current stimulation. *Journal of Neuroscience, 29*(22), 7271–7277.

Duncan, J. (1986). Disorganization of behavior after frontal lobe damage. *Cognitive Neuropsychology, 3*, 271–290.

Ergenzinger, E. R., & Pons, T. P. (2000). Growth of new connections and adult reorganizational plasticity in the somatosensory system. In H. S. Levin & J. Grafman (Eds.), *Cerebral reorganization of function after brain damage* (pp. 68–83). New York: Oxford University Press.

Fasotti, L., Kovacs, F., Eling, P. A. T. M., & Brouwer, W. H. (2000). Time pressure management as a compensatory strategy training after closed head injury. *Neuropsychological Rehabilitation, 10*(1), 47–65.

Foxx, R. M., Martella, R. C., & Marchand-Martella, N. E. (1989). The acquisition, maintenance, and generalization of problem-solving skills by closed head-injured adults. *Behavior Therapy, 20*, 61–76.

Grady, C. L., & Kapur, S. (1999). The use of neuroimaging in neurorehabilitative research. In D. T. Stuss, G. Winocur, & I. H. Robertson (Eds.), *Cognitive neurorehabilitation* (pp. 47–58). New York: Cambridge University Press.

Gronwall, D. M. A. (1977). Paced auditory serial-addition task: A measure of recovery from concussion. *Perceptual and Motor Skills, 44*, 367–373.

Gunstad, J., Cohen, R. A., Paul, R. H., Luyster, F. S., & Gordon, E. (2006). Age effects in time estimation: Relationship to frontal brain morphometry. *Journal of Integrative Neuroscience, 5*(1), 75–87.

Hallett, M. (2000). Plasticity. In J. C. Mazziotta, A. W. Toga, & R. Frackowiak (Eds.), *Brain mapping: The disorders* (pp. 569–586). San Diego, CA: Academic Press.

Hallett, M. (2007). Transcranial magnetic stimulation: A primer. *Neuron, 55*, 187–199.

Ide, J. S., & Li, C.-S. R. (2010). A cerebellar thalamic cortical circuit for error-related cognitive control. *NeuroImage, 54*(1), 455–464.

Jablonka, J. A., Burnat, K., Witte, O. W., & Kossut, M. (2010). Remapping of the somatosensory cortex after a photothrombotic stroke: Dynamics of the compensatory reorganization. *Neuroscience, 165*(1), 90–110.

Jang, S. H. (2009). A review of the ipsilateral motor pathway as a recovery mechanism in patients with stroke. *Neurorehabilitation, 24*(4), 315–320.

Kilgard, M. P., & Merzenich, M. M. (1998). Cortical map reorganization enabled by nucleus basalis activity. *Science, 279*(5357), 1714–1718.

Kozlowski, D. A., James, D. C., & Schallert, T. (1996). Use-dependent exaggeration of neuronal injury after unilateral sensorimotor cortex lesions. *Journal of Neuroscience, 16*(15), 4776–4786.

Kübler, A., Dixon, V., & Garavan, H. (2006). Automaticity and reestablishment of executive control: An fMRI study. *Journal of Cognitive Neuroscience, 18*(8), 1331–1342.

Levin, H. S. (2003). Neuroplasticity following non-penetrating traumatic brain injury. *Brain Injury, 17*(8), 665–674.

Levin, H. S., & Grafman, J. (Eds.). (2000). *Cerebral reorganization of function after brain damage.* New York: Oxford University Press.

Levine, B., Cabeza, R., McIntosh, A. R., Black, S. E., Grady, C. L., & Stuss, D. T. (2002). Functional reorganisation of memory after traumatic brain injury: A study with H(2)(15)O positron emission tomography. *Journal of Neurology, Neurosurgery and Psychiatry, 73*(2), 173–181.

Levine, B., Robertson, I. H., Clare, L., Carter, G., Hong, J., Wilson, B. A., et al. (2000). Rehabilitation of executive functioning: An experimental–clinical validation of goal management training. *Journal of the International Neuropsychological Society, 6*, 299–312.

Lillie, R., & Mateer, C. A. (2006). Constraint-based therapies as a proposed model for cognitive rehabilitation. *Journal of Head Trauma Rehabilitation, 21*(2), 119–130.

Luria, A. R. (1973). *The working brain: An introduction to neuropsychology* (B. Haigh, Trans.). New York: Basic Books.

Manly, T., Hawkins, K., Evans, J., Woldt, K., & Robertson, I. H. (2002). Rehabilitation of executive function: Facilitation of effective goal management on complex tasks using periodic auditory alerts. *Neuropsychologia, 40*, 271–281.

Marshall, R. C., Karow, C. M., Morelli, C. A., Iden, K. K., Dixon, J., & Cranfill, T. B. (2004). Effects of interactive strategy modelling training on problem-solving by persons with traumatic brain injury. *Aphasiology, 18*(8), 659–673.

McAllister, T. W., Saykin, A. J., Flashman, L. A., Sparling, M. B., Johnson, S. C., Guerin, S. J., et al. (1999). Brain activation during working memory 1 month after mild traumatic brain injury: A functional MRI study. *Neurology, 53*(6), 1300–1308.

Mozzachiodi, R., & Byrne, J. H. (2010). More than synaptic plasticity: Role of nonsynaptic plasticity in learning and memory. *Trends in Neurosciences, 33*(1), 17–26.

Muñoz-Cespedes, J. M., Rios-Lago, M., Paul, N., & Maestu, F. (2005). Functional neuroimaging studies of cognitive recovery after acquired brain damage in adults. *Neuropsychology Review, 15*(4), 169–183.

Nadeau, S. E., & Wu, S. S. (2006). CIMT as a behavioral engine in research on physiological adjuvants to neurorehabilitation: The challenge of merging animal and human research. *NeuroRehabilitation, 21*, 107–130.

Nudo, R. J., Barbay, S., & Kleim, J. A. (2000). Role of neuroplasticity in functional recovery after stroke. In H. S. Levin & J. Grafman (Eds.), *Cerebral reorganization of function after brain damage* (pp. 168–197). New York: Oxford University Press.

Ownsworth, T. L., McFarland, K., & Young, R. M. (2000). Development and standardization of the Self-Regulation Skills Interview (SRSI): A new clinical assessment tool for acquired brain injury. *Clinical Neuropsychologist, 14*(1), 76–92.

Pulvermüller, F., Neininger, B., Elbert, T., Mohr, B., Rockstroh, B., Koebbel, P., et al. (2001). Constraint-induced therapy of chronic aphasia following stroke. *Stroke, 32*, 1621–1626.

Rath, J. F., Simon, D., Langenbahn, D. M., Sherr, R. L., & Diller, L. (2003). Group treatment of problem-solving deficits in outpatients with traumatic brain injury: A randomized outcome study. *Neuropsychological Rehabilitation, 13*(4), 461–488.

Rickard, T. C. (2000). Methodological issues in functional magnetic resonance imaging studies of plasticity following brain injury. In H. S. Levin & J. Grafman (Eds.), *Cerebral reorganization of function after brain damage* (pp. 304–317). New York: Oxford University Press.

Sadato, N. (2005). How the blind "see" Braille: Lessons from functional magnetic resonance imaging. *Neuroscientist, 11*(6), 577–582.

Schallert, T., Bland, S. T., Leasure, J. L., Tillerson, J., Gonzales, R., Williams, L., et al. (2000). Motor rehabilitation, use-related neural events, and reorganization of the brain after injury. In H. S. Levin & J. Grafman (Eds.), *Cerebral reorganization of function after brain damage* (pp. 145–167). New York: Oxford University Press.

Schallert, T., & Hernandez, T.D. (1998). GABAergic drugs and neuroplasticity after brain injury: Impact of functional recovery. In L. Goldstein (Ed.), *Restorative neurology: Advances in the pharmacotherapy of recovery after stroke* (pp. 91–120). Armonk, NY: Futura Press.

Scheibel, R. S., Pearson, D. A., Faria, L. P., Kotrla, K. J., Aylward, E., Bachevalier, J., et al. (2003). An fMRI study of executive functioning after severe diffuse TBI. *Brain Injury, 17*(11), 919–930.

Schweizer, T. A., Levine, B., Rewilak, D., O'Connor, C., Turner, G., Alexander, M. P., et al. (2008). *Neurorehabilitation and Neural Repair, 22*(1), 72–77.

Shafritz, K. M., Kartheiser, P., & Belger, A. (2005). Dissociation of neural systems mediating shifts in behavioral response and cognitive set. *NeuroImage, 25*(2), 600–606.

Sohlberg, M. M., & Mateer, C. A. (1987). Effectiveness of an attention-training program. *Journal of Clinical and Experimental Neuropsychology, 9*(2), 117–130.

Sohlberg, M. M., & Mateer, C. A. (2001). Management of dysexecutive symptoms. In M. M. Sohlberg & C. A. Mateer (Eds.), *Cognitive rehabilitation: An integrative neuropsychological approach* (pp. 230–268). New York: Guilford Press.

Stablum, F., Umiltà, C., Mogentale, C., Carlan, M., & Guerrini, C. (2000). Rehabilitation of executive deficits in closed head injury and anterior communicating artery aneurysm patients. *Psychological Research, 63*, 265–278.

Stuss, D., & Levine, B. (2002). Adult clinical neuropsychology: Lessons from studies of the frontal lobes. *Annual Review of Psychology, 53*, 401–433.

Sun, M. K., & Alkon, D. L. (2010). Pharmacology of protein kinase C activators: Cognition-enhancing and antidementic therapeutics. *Pharmacology and Therapeutics, 127*(1), 66–77.

Syková, E. (1997). The extracellular space in the CNS: Its regulation, volume and geometry in normal and pathological neuronal function. *Neuroscientist, 3*, 28–41.

Syková, E. (2005). Glia and volume transmission during physiological and pathological states. *Journal of Neural Transmission, 112*, 137–147.

Turkstra, L. S., Holland, A. L., & Bays, G. A. (2003). The neuroscience of recovery and rehabilitation: What have we learned from animal research? *Archives of Physical Medicine and Rehabilitation, 84*, 604–612.

von Cramon, D. Y., Matthes-von Cramon, G., & Mai, N. (1991). Problem-solving deficits in brain-injured patients: A therapeutic approach. *Neuropsychological Rehabilitation, 1*(1), 45–64.

Ward, N. S., & Frackowiak, R. S. J. (2006). The functional anatomy of cerebral reorganisation after focal brain injury. *Journal of Physiology—Paris, 99*, 425–436.

Wurtman, R. J., Cansev, M., Sakamoto, T., & Ulus, I. H. (2009). Use of phosphatide precursors to promote synaptogeneis. *Annual Review of Nutrition, 29*, 59–87.

Xu, J., & Wall, J. T. (2000). Rapid reorganization of subcortical and cortical maps in adult primates. In H. S. Levin & J. Grafman (Eds.), *Cerebral reorganization of function after brain damage* (pp. 130–144). New York: Oxford University Press.

Zelazo, P. D., & Müeller, U. (2002). Executive function in typical and atypical development. In U. Goswami (Ed.), *Handbook of childhood cognitive development* (pp. 445–469). Oxford: Blackwell.

CHAPTER 13

What Rehabilitation Clinicians Can Do to Facilitate Experience-Dependent Learning

McKAY MOORE SOHLBERG
LAURIE EHLHARDT POWELL

The accumulating evidence supporting experience-dependent learning offers much hope to those with cognitive impairments due to acquired brain injury. However, as discussed throughout this text, the recovery landscape is complex. The various neural mechanisms believed to underlie experience-dependent learning, including unmasking of existing circuits, modification of synaptic connectivity and interhemispheric competition (Gonzalez Rothi, 2001), do not account for the whole recovery story. Task requirements and context also greatly influence function. For example, Stuss (2006) reviews lesion studies suggesting that when task demands are manipulated, there is fluid recruitment of different processes throughout the brain as required by the current task. Similarly, plasticity appears to operate differently, depending upon the specific neural network; experience-induced functional changes after stroke are thought to occur most rapidly in the motor, language, and visual systems (Calvert et. al., 2000; Thulborn, Carpenter, & Just, 1999). There are increasing studies using a variety of neurophysiological markers showing remediation-involved changes in cortical connectivity (e.g., Keller & Just, 2009; Kim et al., 2009). However, the differential responsiveness of various brain networks to targeted input is only beginning to be systematically studied, and conflicting evidence abounds. The goal of this chapter is to examine the impact of a specific domain of structured experience on postinjury learning and recovery: the domain of instructional practices (Owen, Hampshire, Grahn, Stenton, Dajany, et al., 2010).

Our challenge as rehabilitation specialists is to optimize experience-dependent learning and, by extension, neuronal plasticity for the most advantageous functional gain. Neuronal plasticity is the mechanism underlying all learning and represents an "obligatory consequence of all neural activity (even mental practice), and environmental pressures, functional significance and experience are critical factors" (Pascual-Leone, Amedi, Fregni, & Merabet, 2005, p. 395). As clinicians, we seek to organize the factors related to the learning experiences that can promote this plasticity. The field of instruction provides clinicians with a construct and set of practices that can facilitate experience-dependent learning.

REHABILITATION TREATMENT APPROACHES AND THE ROLE OF INPUT

The field of cognitive–linguistic rehabilitation has traditionally classified treatment approaches into two groups: interventions that target change at the level of impairment (i.e., *restorative approaches*) and those that target change at the level of activity or behavior (i.e., *behavioral approaches*) (Ben-Yishay & Diller, 1993; World Health Organization, 2001). An example of a cognitive intervention that targets impairment is direct attention training (Sohlberg et al., 2003), whereas training the use of external memory aids (Sohlberg et al., 2007) is an example of an intervention that targets activity or behavior. Impairment-based interventions are generally believed to be associated with neural restitution/reconnection, whereas behavior-based therapies are thought to be associated with neural reorganization/redistribution and use of adjacent and remote neuronal circuits (Gonzalez Rothi, 2001; Laatsch, Thulborn, Krisky, Shobat, & Sweeney, 2004). Figure 13.1 provides a schematic view of this classification.

The basic distinction between impairment-oriented and behavior- or activity-oriented therapies has theoretical and practical merits. For example, treatment outcomes for impairment-based therapies include changes on corresponding neuropsychological or standardized tests, as well as functional gains in the activities that are dependent upon the impaired cognitive–linguistic processes. Indicators of improvement based on activity-based training are changes in the behaviors or activities trained. There is, however, an important bridge between these approaches: Both require some type of structured environmental experience. Whether therapy consists of repetitively stimulating an impaired cognitive process or training the steps to a functional activity, neuronal plasticity occurs in response to structured input.

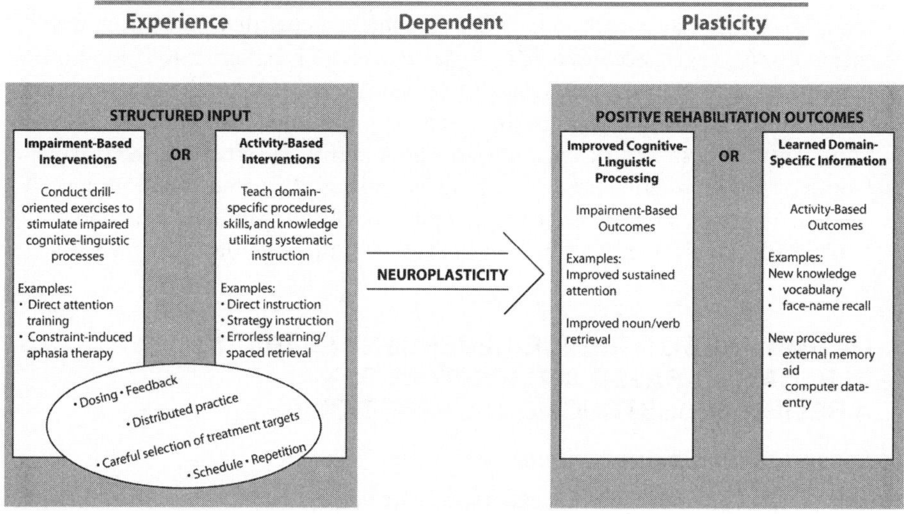

FIGURE 13.1. Schematic depicting structured input associated with rehabilitation outcomes.

The common clinical challenge is how best to structure the input to restore the impaired process and/or achieve the desired behavioral change. This is the task required of rehabilitation professionals and our focus in the remainder of this chapter. Much of this book reviews current evidence that might explain the *underlying mechanisms* (e.g., neuronal plasticity) responsible for positive outcomes following rehabilitation. In this chapter, the goal is to examine evidence supporting the role of *external input*—specifically, instruction—in cognitive–linguistic rehabilitation.

Instructional techniques have not been linked to plasticity per se; however with the advent of diagnostic technologies as discussed throughout this text, this link may soon be established. Currently, we can use the behavioral outcome evidence available in the instructional literature from the fields of both special education and neuropsychology to predict how best to facilitate plasticity and experience-dependent learning. The next section begins with an overview of research evidence from the special education literature—the area that laid the foundation for developing and evaluating effective instructional practices when individuals have damaged learning systems. This literature is highly relevant to working with people who have acquired cognitive–linguistic impairments.

Before we move on to discuss instructional practices, a caveat is in order. Rehabilitation practitioners increasingly recognize the complexity of factors that influence recovery. For example, the importance of context (i.e., environmental variables) and of collaborating with natural supports (e.g., family members, staff) in order to achieve generalization of rehabilitation goals is well accepted (Braga, da Paz, & Ylvisaker, 2005). Certain deficits are more appropriately addressed by altering the environment than by conducting person-oriented interventions (Sohlberg & Mateer, 2001). Similarly, the primacy of emotion and personality variables in recovering from cognitive impairments is acknowledged and factored into the development of many current treatment regimens (High, Sander, Struchen, & Hart, 2005; Ylvisaker, McPherson, Kayes, & Pellett, 2008).

OPTIMIZING EXPERIENCE-DEPENDENT LEARNING IN BEHAVIOR-BASED INTERVENTIONS: A REVIEW OF INSTRUCTIONAL PRACTICES

Lessons from Special Education[1]

The instructional model that has been subjected to the most experimental scrutiny is *direct instruction* (DI), pioneered by Engelmann and Carnine (1991). DI is a comprehensive, explicit instructional method shown to be effective in teaching a wide range of material (e.g., academic and social skills) across different populations with learning challenges, particularly individuals with learning disabilities (Becker, 1978; Engelmann & Carnine, 1991; Stein, Carnine, & Dixon, 1998). DI requires systematic design and delivery of instruction in order to facilitate efficient skill acquisition and generalization. The key techniques associated with the DI design–delivery process include (1) analyzing and sequencing instructional content (i.e., task analysis); (2) training a broad range of examples; (3) using simple, consistent instructional wording; (4) establishing high mastery criteria; (5) providing models and carefully faded prompts; (6) providing high amounts of correct massed practice followed by distributed practice; and (7) sufficient cumulative review (Engelmann & Carnine, 1991; Marchand-Martella, Slocum, & Martella, 2004; Stein et al., 1998).

Glang, Singer, Cooley, and Tish (1992) conducted one of the first studies evaluating DI techniques for treating students with compromised learning due to acquired brain injury. Treatment targets included reasoning skills, math facts and story problems, reading skills, and a self-management strategy. The DI training procedures were customized for each student, depending on his or her particular neuropsychological profile and behavioral/academic needs. The multiple-baseline research design used to evaluate the effects of DI provided experimental support for using this method in the treatment of acquired brain injury.

---

[1]Portions of this instructional literature review were summarized from Ehlhardt et al. (2008).

Strategy-based instruction is another instructional model that has been experimentally evaluated within special education (Englert, Raphael, Anderson, Anthony, & Stevens, 1991; Graham, MacArthur, & Schwartz, 1995; Idol, 1987). This model emphasizes teaching learners to monitor their own thinking, and it may be integrated with the previously described DI approach. Different terms are sometimes used to describe strategy-based instruction, including *procedural facilitators, scaffolded instruction*, and *cognitive strategies* (Baker, Gersten, & Scanlon, 2002; Englert et al., 1991; Harris & Pressley, 1991; Hughes, Ruhl, Schumaker, & Deshler, 2002; Palinscar & Brown, 1984; Stein et al., 1998). Core instructional techniques may include the use of advanced organizers; teacher questions and/or prompts to encourage student self-assessment; strategies for summarizing and elaborating content; and simple outlines of important themes/structures (Baker et al., 2002; Swanson, 2001).

Several meta-analyses have attempted to determine the most effective instructional practices and components within the special education literature (Kavale & Forness, 2000; Mastropieri, Scruggs, Bakken, & Whedon, 1996; Swanson, 1999, 2001; Swanson, Carson, & Sachse-Lee, 1996; Swanson & Hoskyn, 1998). Swanson and colleagues (Swanson, 1999, 2001; Swanson & Hoskyn, 1998) conducted one of the first meta-analyses examining the outcomes of special education instructional practices used to teach a range of academic subjects to children and adults with identified learning disabilities. Following an extensive search yielding over 900 data-based articles, 180 studies were selected that met the inclusion criteria (e.g., presence of a comparison/control group, sufficient data to calculate effect sizes). These studies were categorized into one of four groups, based on the instructional techniques that were utilized. The results indicated that a combined model (the use of DI and strategy-based instruction techniques in concert) produced the largest effect size, followed by strategy-based instruction alone, DI alone, and non-direct/non-strategy-based instruction.

In summary, a rich experimental literature within the field of special education supports the use of explicit instructional techniques as effective teaching methods for individuals with learning disabilities. These techniques include content analysis and sequencing; teacher modeling; high rates of correct, massed practice and distributed practice; and use of advanced organizers. Table 13.1 provides a summary of the experimentally supported instructional techniques.

Lessons from Neuropsychology

A number of instructional practices from the special education literature have been adapted and evaluated within the field of neuropsychology. For example, teacher modeling, an effective instructional technique

TABLE 13.1. Summary of Experimentally Supported Instructional Components and Activities

Design of instruction

- Analyze content to identify "big ideas," concepts, rules, and generalizable strategies.
- Determine specific skills/information, including prerequisites.
- Sequence skills/information from simple to more complex.
- Develop task analyses (i.e., break skills/content down into small, manageable chunks).
- Develop and sequence a broad range of training examples to facilitate generalization.
- Develop simple, consistent instructional wording and scripts to reduce confusion and focus the learner on relevant content.

Delivery of instruction

- Clearly state learning objectives.
- Establish high mastery criteria.
- Provide models and carefully fade prompts and cues to facilitate errorless acquisition.
- "Precorrect" by instructing prerequisite skills/information first or isolating difficult components for extra practice.
- Provide consistent feedback (e.g., immediately model the correct response after the client makes a mistake).
- Provide high amounts of correct, massed practice followed by distributed practice.
- Provide sufficient, cumulative review (i.e., integrate new with old material).
- Individualize instruction, including instructional pacing.
- Conduct ongoing assessment to gauge skill retention.

intended to reduce the risk of errors during the acquisition phase of learning (Marchand-Martella et al., 2004), has been extensively studied under the label of *errorless learning* in the neuropsychology field (e.g., Evans et al., 2000; Hunkin, Squires, Aldrich, & Parkin, 1998a; Tailby & Haslam, 2003; Wilson, Baddeley, Evans, & Shiel, 1994). Several error-control rehabilitation techniques have been studied in individuals with acquired brain injury. Spaced retrieval is a form of distributed practice that facilitates the successful recall of information over expended time intervals. Method of vanishing cues (MVC) (Glisky et al., 1986b) is an error control technique in which the client is given progressively stronger or weaker cues following recall attempts of the targeted information (e.g., Brush & Camp, 1998; Cherry, Simmons, & Camp, 1999; Clare et al., 2000; Clare, Roth, Wilson, Carter, & Hodges, 2002; Melton & Bourgeois, 2005).

We (the current authors) participated in the Evidence-Based Practice subcommittee of the Academy of Neurologic Communication Disorders and Sciences, charged with reviewing the literature to develop evidence-based clinical practice guidelines (including instructional techniques) for a range of neurogenic communication disorders (Ehlardt et al., 2008). An extensive search and review of the instructional literature from 1986 to

2006 was conducted; various combinations of terms were used to search several databases, including Academic Search Premier, MEDLINE, Education Research Complete, ERIC, PsycINFO, and Psychology and Behavioral Sciences Collection. The search yielded over 850 records and was combined with hand searches of extant references (e.g., studies cited within an article). Fifty-one relevant studies were selected, ranging from single-case designs to randomized controlled trials. Cross-population evidence was included, permitting the study of instructional practices used across populations with functionally equivalent cognitive–linguistic symptoms (e.g., impairments in new learning common to individuals with TBI, schizophrenia, and dementia). Studies of errorless learning and related techniques constituted the majority of the instructional research studies found in the neuropsychological rehabilitation literature.

Errorless learning is a training technique theoretically and empirically grounded in the concept that learning occurring in the absence of errors is stronger and more durable than learning by trial and error (Baddeley & Wilson, 1994; Sidman & Stoddard, 1967; Wilson et al., 1994). Elimination of errors is achieved by (1) providing sufficient models *before* a client is asked to perform the target task or retrieve the target information; (2) encouraging the client to avoid guessing, and immediately correcting errors; (3) carefully fading prompts; (4) breaking down the targeted task into small components when training multistep procedures/skills; and (5) providing practice so that treatment targets are overlearned through repeated successes and a rich schedule of positive reinforcement (Baddeley & Wilson, 1994; Kern et al., 2005; Marchand-Martella et al., 2004; Sohlberg & Turkstra, in press; Wilson et al., 1994). Errorless learning is contrasted with errorful learning (i.e., trial-and-error learning, discovery learning, standard anticipation), in which the client is encouraged to guess the targeted response before being provided with the information (Baddeley & Wilson, 1994; Evans et al., 2000; Sohlberg & Turkstra, in press; Wilson et al., 1994). The benefits of errorless learning are typically reported in individuals with relatively spared procedural memory (memory without recalling the experience of learning) and severe declarative memory loss (memory involving conscious recollection).[2] The benefits are less clear for people with early stage dementia or mild cognitive impairment of the amnestic type (Bier et al., 2008; Dunn & Clare, 2007; Simond et al., 2009).

Results from additional studies qualify these findings by indicating that the benefits of errorless learning may depend on a number of vari-

[2]The memory systems (e.g., nondeclarative vs. declarative) associated with improvements under errorless learning conditions are a subject of debate. Experimental evidence and reviews centered on this topic may be found in several sources (e.g., Evans et al., 2000; Hunkin, Squires, Parkin, & Tidy, 1998b; Riley et al., 2004; Tailby & Haslam, 2003; Wilson et al., 1994), but are not specifically addressed in this chapter.

ables. For example, the degree of memory impairment has been shown to be a factor; individuals with more severe memory impairments may show more robust improvements in learning with errorless methods than those with lesser impairments may (Evans et al., 2000; Riley, Sotiriou, & Jaspal, 2004). The type of training task and recall conditions may also affect outcomes (Evans et al., 2000; Riley et al., 2004; Thoene & Glisky, 1995). For example, Thoene and Glisky (1995) showed that explicit, mnemonic techniques were more effective than implicit (i.e., procedural memory) techniques for teaching arbitrary face–name associations, whereas implicit techniques may prove more beneficial with perceptual–orthographic information (e.g., stem completion tasks).

Consistent with the special education instructional literature, several techniques have been shown to increase the effects of errorless learning and improve instructional outcomes in the adult neurogenic population:

1. *High amounts of correct practice.* Frequent, correct practice has been shown to facilitate learning and retention, particularly when combined with distributed practice (e.g., Ehlhardt, Sohlberg, Glang, & Albin, 2005; Glisky, Schacter, & Tulving, 1986a; Hunkin et al., 1998b; Sohlberg & Turkstra, in press).

2. *Distributed practice/spaced retrieval.* The benefits of distributed practice, specifically spaced retrieval (i.e., expanded rehearsal), have been well documented. Spaced retrieval provides individuals with severe memory loss practice at successfully recalling information over expanded time intervals, which is thought to enhance the "durability of learning" (e.g., Brush & Camp, 1998; Cherry et al., 1999; Clare et al., 2000, 2002; Sohlberg & Turkstra, in press; Turkstra & Bourgeois, 2005).

3. *Forward–backward chaining.* Chaining techniques are frequently used to teach multistep tasks to individuals with severe learning disabilities (Spooner & Spooner, 1984). That is, each new step is individually taught and mastered, then sequentially linked to the preceding step. The method of vanishing cues (MVC), which provides a client with progressively weaker prompts following successful recall of targeted information, is a form of backward chaining developed for people with memory impairments (e.g., Glisky, 1995; Glisky & Delaney, 1996; Hunkin & Parkin, 1995; Komatsu, Mimura, Kato, Wakamatsu, & Kashima, 2000; Riley et al., 2004).

4. *Varied training examples.* Carefully planned, multiple training examples are critical to preventing "stimulus-bound" learning and to facilitating generalization (e.g., Ehlhardt et al., 2005; Glisky & Schacter, 1989; Stark, Stark, & Gordon, 2005).

5. *Effortful processing and self-generation.* Increasing the amount of effort expended by the learner has been shown to enhance the effects

of errorless learning techniques (Dunn & Clare, 2007). Techniques for increasing effort while minimizing errors include giving carefully planned descriptions of the target item before the participant generates an answer (Tailby & Haslam, 2003), or asking evaluative questions before providing the correct answer to the participant (Kalla, Downes, & van den Broek, 2001; Tailby & Haslam, 2003).

The literature supports the benefits of errorless over errorful learning, as well as the other instructional techniques summarized above, for teaching a wide range of activities (information *and* behavior) to individuals with severe memory impairment due to a variety of etiologies (e.g., TBI, dementia, schizophrenia). Examples of how these instructional techniques can be applied to specific learning domains are reviewed below.

Instructional Practices Applied to Teaching Information

The most frequently studied information-learning targets in the experimental instructional literature are word recall, face–name recall, and vocabulary acquisition, with the latter two domains having the most functional relevance.

Face–Name Recall

Clare et al. (2000) evaluated errorless learning techniques to reduce the frequency of "everyday memory problems," including face–name recall and the reduction of repetitive questioning, for six individuals with Alzheimer's dementia. Treatment components included verbal elaboration, the MVC, and expanded rehearsal. Five of the six participants demonstrated significant improvements in recalling targeted information and strategies immediately after treatment and, in some cases, up to 6 months later. These results were later replicated in a controlled experiment involving 12 individuals with early-stage Alzheimer's disease who were retaught face–name associations (Clare et al., 2002). Several other studies have also successfully employed errorless techniques to train face–name recall (e.g., Kalla et al., 2001; Parkin, Hunkin, & Squires, 1998). Not all studies, however, have shown consistent findings. Dunn and Clare (2007), did not find superior effects of error reduction during face–name learning trials in patients with early dementia. There are gaps in our knowledge of what population and task factors benefit from EL.

Vocabulary

Successful participation in many social and vocational activities depends on the ability to recall relevant vocabulary. Glisky et al. (1986a) pioneered the use of the MVC to teach computer-related vocabulary to individuals with severe memory impairments due to acquired brain injury. They demonstrated that the MVC was superior to standard anticipation (i.e., trial-and-error) in training the recall of computer terms matched to definitions; computers were used to deliver the training stimuli and prompts. Under the MVC conditions, the definition for a term would appear on the computer screen (e.g., "programs the computer carries out"), followed by the first letter of the matching term (e.g., "S" for "software"). If the participant was unable to guess the term from the initial letter cue, then subsequent letters were provided until the term was correctly recalled. On subsequent trials, the word fragment appeared smaller by one letter than what the participant had required in the previous trial. The authors reported that although learning was slow and strongly cue-dependent on the initial letter, all participants learned a substantial amount of vocabulary, much of which was retained after 6 weeks; some transfer of knowledge was also observed. These authors went on to conduct a series of studies reevaluating the use of the MVC to train computer-related terms, coupled with systematic, intensive instruction targeting the application of those terms within the contexts of functional tasks (e.g., simple–complex data entry procedures). Aspects of this instruction included high amounts of practice, varied examples, and transfer of training to vocational settings (Glisky, 1995; Glisky et al., 1986a; Glisky & Schacter, 1987, 1988, 1989; Glisky, Schacter, & Tulving, 1986b).

Instructional Practices Applied to Teaching Procedures and Skills

Use of Compensatory Aids

Training patients to use compensatory strategies (e.g., note taking) or external aids (e.g., memory books, personal digital assistants) is the most common rehabilitation technique for managing memory impairments (Sohlberg, 2005). Every study analyzed in a practice guidelines review evaluating the efficacy of using external aids for the management of memory disorders reported positive outcomes and described improved functioning on memory-related activities in association with the implementation of external aids (Sohlberg et. al., 2007). A number of the studies have emphasized the importance of individualizing the training and selection of aids (e.g., Donaghy & Williams, 1998; Svoboda & Richards, 2009) and report that it is useful to provide direct, systematic instruction when teaching a person with cognitive impairment to use an external memory aid (e.g., Fluharty & Priddy, 1993; Hart, Hawkey, & Whyte, 2002; Kim, Burke, Dowds, Boone, & Park, 2000; Ownsworth & McFarland, 1999; Quemada et al., 2003; Schmitter-Edgecombe, Fahy, Whelan, & Long, 1995; Squires, Hunkin, &

Parkin, 1996; van den Broek, Downes, Johnson, Dayus, & Hilton, 2000; Wright et al., 2001; Zencius, Wesolowski, & Burke, 1990). Instructional techniques included use of task analyses with the specific steps for using an aid, as well as sufficient practice and cumulative review, and practice with application in real-world contexts (Sohlberg et al., 2007; Svoboda & Richards, 2009).

Computer-Related Tasks

Hunkin et al. (1998a) used an errorless learning instructional package emphasizing frequent practice to train a 33-year-old male with severe memory impairment due to viral encephalitis in selected word-processing tasks (e.g., opening and editing a file). Following repeated errorless recognition exercises with the targeted tasks, timed practice exercises were repeated nine times during each session until firm performance was achieved; repetitions were subsequently reduced to three and then one per session, depending on the task. The participant learned the targeted word-processing tasks so successfully that he no longer required any prompts. Frequent practice both within and across sessions probably contributed to the participant's improved performance. Todd and Barrow (2008) conducted a study of skill acquisition for touch typing with patients who had memory impairments. Their results showed the benefit of distributed or spaced practice in learning this task.

We (Ehlhardt et al., 2005) developed an instructional package (TEACH-M) based on the experimental instructional literature and evaluated its effectiveness for teaching four individuals with severe memory and executive functions to use a multistep email procedure. The TEACH-M procedures are summarized in Table 13.2. Results of a multiple-baseline-across-participants study revealed positive findings. All four participants learned the seven-step email procedure, reaching the criterion for mastery (100% accuracy for three consecutive sessions) within 7–15 training sessions. Three participants retained the email procedure after a 30-day break, and all participants generalized their skills to an altered (i.e., untrained) interface.

Social Problem-Solving Skills

Research on errorless learning techniques has predominantly focused on teaching relatively simple information (e.g., face–name recall) or tasks reliant on motor procedures (e.g., mouse movements to perform computer tasks). Less understood is the application of these techniques to more complex cognitive strategies. Kern et al. (2005) evaluated the application of errorless learning principles to training in social problem-solving skills among individuals diagnosed with schizophrenia or schizoaffective disorders—

TABLE 13.2. TEACH-M Components

Component	Description
Task analysis	Know the instructional content. Break it up into small steps. Chain steps together.
Errorless learning	Keep errors to a minimum during the acquisition phase. Model target step(s) before the client attempts a new skill or step. Carefully fade support. If an error occurs, demonstrate the correct skill or step immediately and ask the client to do it again. Use simple, consistent instructional wording.
Assessment	Initial: Assess skills before initiating treatment for the first time.
	Ongoing: Probe performance at the beginning of each teaching session or before introducing a new step.
Cumulative review	Regularly integrate and review new skills with previously learned skills.
High rates of correct practice	Practice the skill several times. Distributed practice encourages this.
Metacognition	The prediction–reflection technique, or another appropriate strategy that encourages self-reflection, can be used to encourage active processing of the material.

conditions frequently associated with impairments in new learning/memory and executive functions. Sixty participants were randomly assigned to either the experimental treatment or a control condition (i.e., "symptom management"). The experimental group participated in a social problem-solving training module with three interrelated content components: (1) *receiving skills* (identification of problematic social interactions through videotaped examples); (2) *processing skills* (identification of one of three basic solutions to the targeted social problem); and (3) *sending skills* (practice applying the solutions in role play). With each component, the instructor identified/modeled the specific information and skills appropriate to each video sample, and provided carefully faded cues to facilitate errorless learning. The control group participants received similar content, but with a strong problem-solving component targeting identification of problems associated with their own illness and formulation of interpersonal solutions to their problems. Results showed a significant experimental training group effect favoring errorless learning, with retention of some skills at a 3-month follow-up. It is important to remember that training social *skills* does not necessarily translate to improved social *life*, and intervention in this area must be highly contextualized and target participation-based outcomes (Sohlberg & Turkstra, in press).

Summary

The instructional literature clearly demonstrates that *structuring the manner in which target information or behavior is introduced and reviewed can facilitate learning.* By implication, carefully planning how to train and instruct people with damaged learning systems allows clinicians to optimize experience-dependent learning.

OPTIMIZING EXPERIENCE-DEPENDENT LEARNING IN IMPAIRMENT-BASED TREATMENTS

The goal of impairment-based treatment is to restore impaired cognitive–linguistic processes, rather than to directly train the skills or behaviors (i.e., activities) dependent on these processes. This is distinct from the behavioral interventions discussed in the preceding section, which target the teaching of information or procedures. Instruction is not typically associated with impairment-based interventions. Yet the treatment efficacy research in both domains reveals the importance of *structured, systematic input* to facilitate optimal rehabilitation outcomes. In this section, we review impairment-based interventions with an eye for what the literature suggests are key principles for delivering and reviewing treatment stimuli.

The cognitive–linguistic areas that have been most studied with respect to impairment-based interventions are attention and language. Impairment-based techniques to restore memory function have not been successful; to date, little to no experimental evidence supports the use of drill-oriented exercises to increase underlying memory function (e.g., Glisky et al., 1986a; Sohlberg & Mateer, 2001). The only exceptions are preliminary reports suggesting that drill-oriented prospective memory training may be effective in increasing the amount of time an individual can hold on to and remember to carry out an action (Raskin & Sohlberg, 1996, 2009). Memory has been more commonly addressed via behavioral and compensatory methods reliant on instructional practices, as discussed in the preceding section.

Systematic Input and the Treatment of Attention Impairments

Attention training is based on the premise that particular aspects of attention can be activated and improved through a stimulus–drill approach. The repeated stimulation of attentional systems via systematically graded attention exercises is hypothesized to facilitate changes in attentional functioning, leading to changes in behavior dependent on these skills (Cicerone, 2002; Sohlberg & Mateer, 2001). Most attention training programs assume that aspects of cognition can be isolated and discretely targeted with training exercises. The aspects of attention that are addressed vary widely among interventions and frequently depend upon a theoretical model of attention. Regardless of their operational framework, however, such interventions appear to include functions related to sustaining attention over time (vigilance), capacity for information, shifting attention, speed of processing, and screening out distractions. Some attention efficacy studies evaluate attention interventions that focus on particular attention components, such as reaction time and sustained attention for visual information (e.g., Ponsford & Kinsella, 1992; Serino et al., 2006). Other efficacy studies use attention training programs that include hierarchical tasks to address a continuum of attention components, from basic sustained attention to more complex executive control (e.g., Duval, Coyette, & Seron, 2008; Park, Proulx, & Towers, 1999; Sohlberg, McLaughlin, Pavese, Heidrich, & Posner, 2000).

The practice guidelines for direct attention training (Sohlberg et al., 2003) are based on experimental evidence supporting improvement in attention-based skills with direct training; however, the studies that have reported improvements are open to differing interpretations. Some reports suggest that exercises may promote the acquisition of specific skills and that outcomes may be task-specific (Park & Ingles, 2001). The Sohlberg et al. (2003) literature review suggested that the studies reporting more robust changes following direct attention training (e.g., Cicerone, 2002; Sohlberg et al., 2000) shared the following features: (1) individualized attention exercises; (2) more intensive frequency of treatment; and (3) outcome measures that included a range of different tests sensitive to attention and working memory, and that included activity-based measures using client self-report data. In addition, examination of the older literature in conjunction with the current literature suggested that including strategy or metacognitive training as part of direct attention training increases treatment effectiveness (Duval et al., 2008; Galbiati et al., 2009).

The evidence in the impairment-based attention intervention literature thus shares several features with that in the instructional literature regarding how to structure input, including the notion of systematic, hierarchically graded, sufficiently frequent practice combined with strategy training.

Systematic Input and the Treatment of Language Impairments

Gonzalez Rothi (2006) suggests that interventions aimed at maximizing neuroplastic changes to encourage language recovery after stroke must respect established treatment principles in dosing schedule, experience, practicality of treatment activities, and use/role of feedback. As reviewed by Leon, Maher, and Gonzalez Rothi (Chapter 10, this volume), applications of these treatment principles promote language recovery. Again, close parallels can be drawn between this literature and the instructional literature. Common treatment principles include *sufficient* and *intensive practice.* In the case of aphasia intervention, it is critical to have hundreds of trials—more treatment is better (Odell, Bair, Flynn, Osborne, & Chial, 1997). Intensive therapeutic regimens (e.g., treatment 2–3 hours per day, 7 days a week vs. 1 hour per day, 5 days weekly) have also been associated with favorable treatment outcomes (e.g., Basso & Caporali, 2001). Recently, the research on constraint-induced aphasia therapy has shown the benefits of intensive practice schedules in combination with individualized, incremental shaping of treatment stimuli in the context of practical communication tasks, while avoiding (i.e., "constraining") the use of compensatory behaviors (Maher et al., 2006; Meinzer, Djundja, Barthel, Elbert, & Rockstroh, 2005; Pulvermüller et al., 2001). Other research calls for practice schedules to include mass practice followed by *distributed practice* (e.g., Basso. Capitani, & Vignolo, 1979). Spaced retrieval, a form of distributed practice previously described, has recently been applied to the treatment of anomia (i.e., word retrieval impairments) (Fridriksson, Holland, Beeson, & Morrow, 2005).

Other researchers have also incorporated errorless learning techniques into treatment regimens targeting word retrieval deficits due to aphasia. Raymer and Kohen (2006) combined errorless learning with self-generation of responses to facilitate noun and verb retrieval, using sentence-based treatment stimuli. Participant 1 presented with moderately severe fluent aphasia, while Participant 2 presented with nonfluent aphasia and apraxia of speech. Treatment included presentation of target nouns and verbs across two separate training phases (noun vs. verb therapy) in sentence contexts, according to the following sequence: (1) The clinician modeled the target sentence; (2) the participant read the sentence aloud, receiving prompts to pronounce each word correctly; (3) the clinician next covered the target noun or verb and then the full sentence, followed by the participant's generating the full sentence, including the target word; and (4) treatment targets were practiced in the context of a barrier activity. Steps 1 and 2 represented the errorless learning component of the treatment regimen, while Steps 3 and 4 represented the self-generation component. The self-generation component was included on the basis of research demonstrating that recall is facilitated when individuals are required to self-generate responses (Tailby & Haslam, 2003). A single-participant, time series design was used to evaluate treatment effects. The participant with nonfluent aphasia demonstrated large treatment effect sizes in single-word picture naming for nouns and verbs, as well as generalized improvements in numbers of grammatical sentences and content words following noun therapy. The participant with fluent aphasia improved minimally across tasks.

To summarize, errorless learning techniques, adherence to systematic practice regimens (e.g., intensive, distributed practice), and effortful processing techniques (e.g., self-generation of responses) have been effectively incorporated into treatment regimens targeting language impairments.

CONCLUSIONS

This chapter has focused on evidence from the fields of special education and neuropsychology supporting instructional practices that facilitate experience-dependent learning and, presumably, neuroplasticity through systematic input. This literature suggests that the methods involved in selecting instructional targets and in presenting and reinforcing target material determine learners' outcomes. DI combined with strategy-based instruction has been shown to be a more effective approach than either method alone in teaching children and adults with learning disabilities. Systematic delivery of stimuli, using principles analogous to those discussed in the instructional literature, has also been shown to be important for impairment-based therapies targeting the improvement of attention and language.

Unfortunately, careful adherence to task analyses, practice regimens, and delineation of relevant strategy instruction is not a mainstream practice. Although clinicians typically do not view themselves as the designers and deliverers of curricula, that ultimately must assume these roles in order to implement the treatment principles discussed in this chapter. In addition to the experimental instructional literature, there is evidence suggesting that when rehabilitation therapists are trained to use systematic instructional techniques, patients' outcomes improve (Ducharme & Spencer, 2001; Mozzoni & Bailey, 1996). We conclude this chapter with a call to review the instructional design and delivery principles listed in Tables 13.1 and 13.2. Finally, Figure 13.2 offers a checklist to help clinicians monitor and organize their use of techniques that optimize learning. Increasing our understanding of the neurobiology of recovery may further refine our instructional and training practices. As research reveals the brain mechanisms stimulated by specific types of input, we clinicians can make optimal decisions about dosing, practice schedules, feedback, prompting, and a myriad of other variables related to how we structure input in order for our patients to achieve optimal and efficient rehabilitation outcomes.

REFERENCES

Baddeley, A., & Wilson, B. (1994). When implicit learning fails: Amnesia and the problem of error elimination. *Neuropsychologia, 32*, 53–68.

Baker, S., Gersten, R., & Scanlon, D. (2002). Procedural facilitators and cognitive strategies: Tools for unraveling the mysteries of comprehension and the writing process, and for providing meaningful access to the general curriculum. *Learning Disabilities Practice, 17*(1), 65–77.

Basso, A., Capitani, E., & Vignolo, L. (1979). Influence of rehabilitation of language skills in aphasic patients: A controlled study. *Archives of Neurology, 36*, 190–196.

Basso, A., & Caporali, A. (2001). Aphasia therapy or the importance of being earnest. *Aphasiology, 15*(4), 307–332.

Before the session:

- ☐ Did I determine prerequisite skills/information?
- ☐ Did I sequence the treatment stimuli/targets from simple to more complex and include contextual factors?
- ☐ Did I develop a task analysis, if appropriate?
- ☐ Did I select a broad range of training examples?
- ☐ Did I plan for generalization?

During the session:

- ☐ Did I check for retention of previously trained skills/information before introducing new material?
- ☐ Did I keep my directions clear and simple, and avoid excessive talking during the session?
- ☐ Did I provide models and carefully fade prompts and cues, as appropriate?
- ☐ Did I provide consistent feedback?
- ☐ Did I provide high amounts of correct practice?
- ☐ Did I distribute the practice?
- ☐ Did I take data?
- ☐ Did I incorporate natural supports in order to encourage generalization?

FIGURE 13.2. Structuring input for impairment and activity-based treatment programs: A clinician's checklist.

Becker, W. C. (1978). The national evaluation of Follow Through: Behavioral-theory-based programs come out on top. *Education and Urban Society, 10*(4), 431–458.

Ben-Yishay, Y., & Diller, L. (1993). Cognitive remediation in traumatic brain injury: Update and issues. *Archives of Physical Medicine and Rehabilitation, 74*, 204–213.

Bier, N., Van der Linden, M., Gagnon, L., Desrosiers, J., Adam, S., et al. (20080. Face–name association learning in early Alzheimer's disease: A comparison of learning methods and their underlying mechanisms. *Neuropsychological Rehabilitation, 18*(3), 343–371.

Braga, L. W., da Paz, A. C., & Ylvisaker, M. (2005). Direct clinician delivered versus indirect family supported rehabilitation of children with traumatic brain injury: A randomized controlled trial. *Brain Injury, 19*(10), 819–831.

Brush, J., & Camp, C. (1998). Using spaced retrieval as an intervention during speech–language therapy. *Clinical Gerontologist, 19*(1), 51–64.

Calvert, G., Brammer, M., Morris, R. G., Williams, S. C., King, N., & Matthews, P. M. (2000). Using fMRI to study recovery from acquired dysphasia. *Brain and Language, 71, 391–399.*

Cherry, K. E., Simmons, S. S., & Camp, C. J. (1999). Spaced retrieval enhances memory in older adults with probable Alzheimer's disease. *Journal of Clinical Geropsychology, 5*(3), 159–175.

Cicerone, K. (2002). Remediation of working memory in mild traumatic brain injury. *Brain Injury, 16*(3), 185–195.

Clare, L., Roth, I., Wilson, B., Carter, G., & Hodges, J. (2002). Relearning face–name associations in early Alzheimer's disease. *Neuropsychology, 16*(4), 538–547.

Clare, L., Wilson, B. A., Carter, G., Breen, K., Gosses, A., & Hodges, J. R. (2000). Intervening with everyday memory problems in dementia of the Alzheimer type: An errorless learning approach. *Journal of Clinical and Experimental Neuropsychology, 22*(1), 132–146.

Donaghy, S., & Williams, W. (1998). A new protocol for training severely impaired patients in the usage of memory journals. *Brain Injury, 12*(12), 1061–1070.

Ducharme, J. M., & Spencer, T. F. (2001). Training brain injury rehabilitation therapists to use generalized teaching skills. *Brain Injury, 15*(4), 333–347.

Dunn, J., & Clare, L. (2007). Learning face–name associations in early-stage dementia: Comparing the effects of errorless learning and effortful processing. *Neuropsychological Rehabilitation, 17*(6), 735–754.

Duval, J., Coyette, F., & Seron, X. (20080. Rehabilitation of the central executive component of working memory: A re-organizational approach applied to a single case. *Neuropsychological Rehabilitation, 18*(4), 430–460.

Ehlhardt, L., Sohlberg, M. M., Kennedy, M., Coelho, C., Ylvisaker, M., Turkstra, L., et al. (2008). Evidence-based practice guidelines for instructing individuals with acquired memory impairments: What have we learned in the past 20 years? *Neuropsychological Rehabilitation, 18*(3), 300–342.

Ehlhardt, L., Sohlberg, M. M., Glang, A., & Albin, R. (2005). TEACH-M: A pilot study evaluating an instructional sequence for persons with impaired memory and executive functions. *Brain Injury, 19*(8), 569–583.

Engelmann, S. E., & Carnine, D. W. (1991). *Theory of instruction.* Eugene, OR: Association for Direct Instruction.

Englert, C. S., Raphael, T. E., Anderson, L. M., Anthony, H. M., & Stevens, D. D. (1991). Making writing strategies and self-talk visible: Cognitive strategy instruction in regular and special education classrooms. *American Educational Research Journal, 28*, 337–372.

Evans, J. J., Wilson, B. A., Schuri, U., Andrade, J., Baddeley, A., Bruna, O., et al. (2000). A comparison of "errorless" and "trial and error" learning methods for teaching individuals with acquired memory deficits. *Neuropsychological Rehabilitation, 10*(1), 67–101.

Fluharty, G., & Priddy, D. (1993). Methods of increasing client acceptance of a memory book. *Brain Injury, 7*(1), 85–88.

Fridriksson, J., Holland, A., Beeson, P., & Morrow, L. (2005). Spaced retrieval of anomia. *Aphasiology, 19*(2), 99–109.

Galbiati, S., Recla, M., Pastore, V., Liscio, M., Bardoni, A., et al. (2009). Attention remediation of following traumatic brain injury in childhood and adolescence. *Neuropsychology, 23*(1), 40–49.

Glang, A., Singer, G., Cooley, E., & Tish, N. (1992). Tailoring direct instruction techniques for use with elementary students with brain injury. *Journal of Head Trauma Rehabilitation, 7*(4), 93–108.

Glisky, E. L. (1995). Acquisition and transfer of word processing skills by an amnesic patient. *Neuropsychological Rehabilitation, 5*(4), 299–318.

Glisky, E. L., & Delaney, E. L. (1996). Implicit memory and new semantic learning in posttraumatic amnesia. *Journal of Head Trauma Rehabilitation, 11(2), 31–42.*

Glisky, E. L., & Schacter, D. L. (1987). Acquisition of domain-specific knowledge in organic amnesia: Training for computer-related work. *Neuropsychologia, 25*(6), 893–906.

Glisky, E. L., & Schacter, D. L. (1988). Long-term retention of computer learning by patients with memory disorders. *Neuropsychologia, 26*(1), 173–178.

Glisky, E. L., & Schacter, D. L. (1989). Extending the limits of complex learning in organic amnesia: Computer training in a vocational domain. *Neuropsychologia, 27(1), 107–120.*

Glisky, E. L., Schacter, D. L., & Tulving, E. (1986a). Learning and retention of computer-related vocabulary in memory-impaired patients: Method of vanishing cues. *Journal of Clinical and Experimental Neuropsychology, 8*(3), 292–312.

Glisky, E. L., Schacter, D. L., & Tulving, E. (1986b). Computer learning by memory-impaired patients: Acquisition and retention of complex knowledge. *Neuropsychologia, 24*(3), 313–328.

Gonzalez Rothi, L. J. (2001). Neurophysiologic basis of rehabilitation. *Journal of Medical Speech–Language Pathology, 9*(2), 117–127.

Gonzalez Rothi, L. J. (2006, March). *The power of experience dependent relearning after brain injury: Hope offered to TBI rehabilitation by human rehabilitation studies in other pathophysiologic models.* Paper presented at the Federale Interagency Conference on TBI, Bethesda, MD.

Graham, S., MacArthur, C., & Schwartz, S. (1995). Effects of goal setting and procedural facilitation on the revising behavior and writing performance of students with writing and learning problems. *Journal of Educational Psychology, 87*(2), 230–240.

Harris, K., & Pressley, M. (1991). The nature of cognitive strategy instruction: Interactive strategy instruction. *Exceptional Children, 57,* 392–404.

Hart, T., Hawkey, K., & Whyte, J. (2002). Use of a portable voice organizer to remember therapy goals in traumatic brain injury rehabilitation: A within-subjects trial. *Journal of Head Trauma Rehabilitation, 17*(6), 556–570.

High, W., Sander, A. M., Struchen, M. A., & Hart, K. A.(2005). *Rehabilitation for traumatic brain injury.* New York: Oxford University Press.

Hughes, C., Ruhl, K., Schumaker, J., & Deshler, D. (2002). Effects of instruction in an assignment completion strategy on the homework performance of students with learning disabilities in general education classes. *Learning Disabilities Research and Practice, 17*(1), 1–18.

Hunkin, N. A., & Parkin, A. J. (1995). The method of vanishing cues: An evaluation of its effectiveness in teaching memory impaired individuals. *Neuropsychologia, 33*(10), 1255–1279.

Hunkin, N. M., Squires, E. J., Aldrich, F. K., & Parkin, A. J. (1998a). Errorless learning and the acquisition of word processing skills. *Neuropsychological Rehabilitation, 8*(4), 433–449.

Hunkin, N. M., Squires, E. J., Parkin, A. J., & Tidy, J. A. (1998b). Are the benefits of errorless learning dependent upon implicit memory? *Neuropsychologia, 36*(1), 25–26.

Idol, L. (1987). Group story mapping: A comprehension strategy for both skilled and unskilled readers. *Journal of Learning Disabilities, 20*, 196–205.

Kalla, T., Downes, J. J., & van den Broek, M. (2001). The pre-exposure technique: Enhancing the effects of errorless learning in the acquisition of face–name associations. *Neuropsychological Rehabilitation, 11*(1), 1–16.

Kavale, K. A., & Forness, S. R. (2000). Policy decisions in special education: The role of meta-analysis. In R. Gersten, E. P. Schiller, & S. Vaughn (Eds.), *Contemporary special education research* (pp. 281–326). Mahwah, NJ: Erlbaum.

Keller, T. A., & Just, M. A. (2009). Altering cortical connectivity: Remediation-induced changes in the white matter of poor readers. *Neuron, 64*(5), 624–631.

Kern, R. S., Green, M. F., Mitchell, S., Kopelowicz, A., Mintz, J., & Liberman, R. P. (2005). Extensions of errorless learning for social problem-solving deficits in schizophrenia. *American Journal of Psychiatry, 162*(3), 513–519.

Kim, H. J., Burke, D. T., Dowds, M. M., Boone, K., & Park, G. J. (2000). Electronic memory aids for outpatient brain injury: Follow-up findings. *Brain Injury, 14*(2), 187–196.

Komatsu, S., Mimura, M., Kato, M., Wakamatsu, N., & Kashima, H. (2000). Errorless and effortful processes involved in the learning of face–name associations by patients with alcoholic Korsakoff's syndrome. *Neuropsychological Rehabilitation, 10*(2), 113–132.

Laatsch, L. K., Thulborn, K. R., Krisky, C. M., Shobat, D. M., & Sweeney, J. A. (2004). Investigating the neurobiological basis of cognitive rehabilitation therapy with fMRI. *Brain Injury, 18*(10), 957–974.

Maher, L., Schmadeke, S., Pingel, K., Haley, J. A., Ciampitti, M., Ochipa, C., et al. (2006, November). *A RCT of constraint induced language therapy for aphasia.* Paper presented at the convention of the American Speech–Language–Hearing Association, Miami, FL.

Marchand-Martella, N. E., Slocum, T. A., & Martella, R. C. (Eds.). (2004). *Introduction to direct instruction.* Boston: Pearson/Allyn & Bacon.

Mastropieri, M. A., Scruggs, T. E., Bakken, J. P., & Whedon, C. (1996). Reading comprehension: A synthesis of research in learning disabilities. In T. E. Scruggs & M. A. Mastropieri (Eds.), *Advances in learning and behavioral disabilities* (Vol. 10, pp. 277–303). Greenwich, CT: JAI Press.

Meinzer, M., Djundja, D., Barthel, G., Elbert, T., & Rockstroh, B. (2005). Long-term stability of improved language functions in chronic aphasia after constraint-induced therapy. *Stroke, 36*, 1462–1466.

Melton, A. K., & Bourgeois, M. S. (2005). Training compensatory memory strategies via the telephone for persons with TBI. *Aphasiology, 19*(3–5), 353–364.

Mozzoni, M. P., & Bailey, J. S. (1996). Improving training methods in brain injury rehabilitation. *Journal of Head Trauma Rehabilitation, 11*(1), 1–17.

Odell, K. H., Bair, S., Flynn, M., Workinger, M., Osborne, D., & Chial, M. (1997). Retrospective study of treatment outcome for individuals with aphasia. *Aphasiology, 11*(4–5), 415–432.

Owen, A. M., Hampshire, A., Grahn, J., Stenton, R., Dajani, S., et al. (2010).

Putting brain training to the test. *Nature: International Weekly Journal of Science, 465*, 775–778.

Ownsworth, T. L., & McFarland, K. (1999). Memory remediation in long-term acquired brain injury: Two approaches in diary training. *Brain Injury, 13*(8), 605–626.

Palinscar, A. S., & Brown, A. L. (1984). Reciprocal teaching of comprehension-fostering and comprehension-monitoring activities. *Cognition and Instruction, 1*(2), 117–175.

Park, N. W., & Ingles, J. L. (2001). Effectiveness of attention rehabilitation after an acquired brain injury: A meta-analysis. *Neuropsychology, 15*(22), 199–210.

Park, N. W., Proulx, G. B., & Towers, W. M. (1999). Evaluation of the Attention Process Training Programme. *Neuropsychological Rehabilitation, 1*, 241–257.

Parkin, A. J., Hunkin, N. M., & Squires, E. J. (1998). Unlearning John Major: The use of errorless learning in the reacquisition of proper names following herpes simplex encephalitis. *Cognitive Neuropsychology, 15(4), 361–375,*

Pascual-Leone, A., Amedi, A., Fregni, F., & Merabet, L. B. (2005).The plastic human brain cortex. *Annual Review of Neuroscience, 28*, 377–401.

Ponsford, J. L., & Kinsella, G. (1992). Attention deficits following closed head injury. *Journal of Clinical and Experimental Neuropsychology, 14*, 822–838.

Pulvermüller, F., Neininger, B., Elbert, T., Mohr, B., Rockstroh, B., Koebbel, P., et al. (2001). Constraint-induced therapy of chronic aphasia after stroke. *Stroke, 32*, 1621–1626.

Quemada, J. I., Munoz Cespedes, J. M., Ezkerra, J., Ballesteros, J., Ibarra, N., & Urruticoechea, I. (2003). Outcome of memory rehabilitation in traumatic brain injury assessed by neuropsychological tests and questionnaires. *Journal of Head Trauma Rehabilitation, 18*(6), 532–540.

Raskin, S., & Sohlberg, M. (1996). An investigation of prospective memory training in two individuals with traumatic brain injury. *Journal of Head Trauma Rehabilitation, 11*, 32–51.

Raskin, S., & Sohlberg, M. M. (2009). Prospective memory intervention: A review and evaluation of a restrictive intervention. *Brain Impairment, 10*(1), 311–320.

Raymer, A., & Kohen, F. (2006). Word-retrieval treatment in aphasia: Effects of sentence context. *Journal of Rehabilitation Research and Development, 43(3), 367–378.*

Riley, G. A., Sotiriou, D., & Jaspal, S. (2004). Which is more effective in promoting implicit and explicit memory: The method of vanishing cues or errorless learning without fading? *Neuropsychological Rehabilitation, 14*(3), 257–283.

Schmitter-Edgecombe, M., Fahy, J. F., Whelan, J. P., & Long, C. J. (1995). Memory remediation after severe closed head injury: Notebook training versus supportive therapy. *Journal of Clinical and Consulting Psychology, 63*(3), 484–489.

Serino, A., Ciaramelli, E., Di Santantonio, A., Malagu, S., Servadei, F., et al. (2006). Central executive system impairment in traumatic brain injury. *Brain Injury, 20*(1), 23–32.

Sidman, M., & Stoddard, L. T. (1967). The effectiveness of fading in programming simultaneous form discrimination for retarded children. *Journal of the Experimental Analysis of Behavior, 10*, 3–15.

Sohlberg, M. M. (2005). External aids: Expanding our understanding of the most widely used memory rehabilitation technique. In W. High, A. M. Sander, M. A. Struchen, & K. A. Hart (Eds.), *Rehabilitation for traumatic brain injury* *pp. 47–70). New York: Oxford University Press.

Sohlberg, M. M., Avery, J., Kennedy, M., Ylvisaker, M., Coelho, C., Turkstra, L., et al. (2003). Practice guidelines for direct attention training. *Journal of Medical Speech–Language Pathology, 11*(3), xix–xxxix.

Sohlberg, M. M., Ehlhardt, L., Kennedy, M. (2005). Instructional techniques in cognitive rehabilitation: A preliminary report. *Seminars in Speech and Language, 26*(4), 268–279.

Sohlberg, M. M., Kennedy, M., Avery, J. M., Coelho, C., Turkstra, L. S., Ylvisaker, M., et al. (2007). Practice guidelines for external aids for memory rehabilitation. *Journal of Medical Speech–Language Pathology, 15*(1), xv–xvii.

Sohlberg, M. M., & Mateer, C. (2001). *Cognitive rehabilitation: An integrative neuropsychological approach.* New York: Guilford Press.

Sohlberg, M. M., McLaughlin, K., Pavese, A., Heidrich, A., & Posner, M. (2000). Evaluation of Attention Process Training in persons with acquired brain injury. *Journal of Clinical and Experimental Neuropsychology, 22*(5), 656–676.

Sohlberg, M. M., & Turkstra, L. S. (in press). *Optimizing cognitive rehabilitation: Effective instructional methods.* New York: Guilford Press.

Spooner, F., & Spooner, D. (1984). A review of chaining techniques: Implications for future research and practice. *Education and Training of the Mentally Retarded, 19*, 114–124.

Squires, E., Hunkin, N. M., & Parkin, A. J. (1996). Memory notebook training in a case of severe amnesia: Generalizing from paired associate learning to real life. *Neuropsychological Rehabilitation, 6*(1), 55–65.

Stark, C., Stark, S., & Gordon, B. (2005). New semantic learning and generalization in a patient with amnesia. *Neuropsychology, 19*(2), 139–151.

Stein, M. S., Carnine, D., & Dixon, R. (1998). Direct instruction: Integrating curriculum design and effective teaching practice. *Intervention in School and Clinic, 33*(4), 227–234.

Stuss, D. (2006). Frontal lobes and attention: Processes and networks, fractionation and integration. *Journal of the International Neuropsychological Society, 12*(2), 261–271.

Svoboda, E., & Richards, B. (2009). Compensating for anterograde amnesia: A new training method that capitalized on emerging smartphone technologies. *Journal of the International Neuropsychological Society, 15*, 629–638.

Swanson, H. L. (1999). Instructional components that predict treatment outcomes for students with learning disabilities: Support for the combined strategy and direct instruction model. *Learning Disabilities Research and Practice, 14*(3), 129–140.

Swanson, H. L. (2001). Searching for the best model for instructing students with learning disabilities. *Focus on Exceptional Children, 34*(2), 2–15.

Swanson, H. L., Carson, C., & Sachse-Lee, C. M. (1996). A selective synthesis of intervention research for students with learning disabilities. *School Psychology Review, 25*, 370–391.

Swanson, H. L., & Hoskyn, M. (1998). A synthesis of experimental intervention literature for students with learning disabilities: A meta-analysis of treatment outcomes. *Review of Educational Research, 68*, 277–322.

Tailby, R., & Haslam, C. (2003). An investigation of errorless learning in memory-impaired patients: Improving the technique and clarifying the theory. *Neuropsychologia, 41*, 1230–1240.

Thoene, A. I. T., & Glisky, E. (1995). Learning name–face associations in memory impaired patients: A comparison of procedures. *Journal of the International Neuropsychological Society, 1*, 29–38.

Thulborn, K., Carpenter, P., & Just, M. (1999). Plasticity of language-related brain function during recovery from stroke. *Stroke, 30*, 749–754.

Todd, M., & Barrow, C. (2008). Touch type: The acquisition of a useful complex perceptual–motor skill. *Neuropsychological Rehabilitation, 18*(4), 486–606.

Turkstra, L. S., & Bourgeois, M. S. (2005). Intervention for a modern day HM: Errorless learning of practical goals. *Journal of Medical Speech–Language Pathology, 13*(3), 205–212.

van den Broek, M. D., Downes, J., Johnson, Z., Dayus, B., & Hilton, Z. (2000). Evaluation of an electronic memory aid in the neuropsychological rehabilitation of prospective memory deficits. *Brain Injury, 14*(5), 455–462.

Wilson, B. A., Baddeley, A., Evans, J., & Shiel, A. (1994). Errorless learning in the rehabilitation of memory impaired people. *Neuropsychological Rehabilitation, 4*(3), 307–326.

World Health Organization. (2001). *International classification of functioning, disability and health.* Geneva: Author.

Wright, P., Rogers, N., Hall, C., Wilson, B., Evans, J., Emslie, H., et al. (2001). Comparison of pocket-computer memory aids for people with brain injury. *Brain Injury, 15*(9), 787–800.

Ylvisaker, M., McPherson, K., Kayes, N., & Pellett, E. (2008). Metaphoric identity mapping: Facilitating goal-setting and engagement in rehabilitation after traumatic brain injury. *Neuropsychological Rehabilitation, 18*(5–6), 713–741.

Zencius, A., Wesolowski, M. D., & Burke, W. H. (1990). A comparison of four memory strategies with traumatically brain-injured clients. *Brain Injury, 4*(1), 33–38.

CHAPTER 14

Pharmacological Therapies, Rehabilitation, and Neuroplasticity

JOHN C. FREELAND

The majority of pharmacological interventions currently used in rehabilitation are arguably not driven by theories of recovery after brain injury as much as by symptomatic relief. This is perhaps equally true of many pharmacological interventions for other disorders, such as depression and schizophrenia, which have lacked cohesive theoretical rationales fully supported by empirical research. Researchers in the burgeoning area of neuroplasticity are revamping the models of neurological recovery, as well as models of psychiatric disorders such as depression and addiction. Already the great strides in the basic neuroscience of synaptic plasticity and neurogenesis have left large gaps in knowledge for the clinical sciences to explore. Due to these strides, pharmacotherapy is gaining a stronger theoretical basis for future clinical utility.

This chapter surveys the current research that ties pharmacological agents to neuroplasticity, with particular emphasis on the treatment/rehabilitation of neurologically impaired patients to improve cognitive or motor functions. It includes a discussion of the use of pharmacotherapy in conjunction with behavioral and cognitive therapies. Current clinical studies that relate to neuroplasticity are perhaps best described as preliminary, and any comprehensive review must include basic laboratory research with animals in order to paint a complete picture. Looking at any area of pharmacology, neurological recovery, and neuroplasticity will leave the reader examining a field of research with numerous gaps, over which theoretical leaps are required to arrive at any possible clinical utility. Moreover, although this area is one of promise, it also contains cautionary tales of drugs that actually impede recovery but continue to be routinely used in clinical practice.

Pharmacological therapies can be studied in relation to rehabilitation on a number of different dimensions or continua. The degree to which findings can be generalized to clinical practice is often related to the type of study. To help organize the myriad research results in this area, these continua are outlined:

1. The first dimension is that of size (micro to macro levels). This dimension begins at the molecular level of action—for instance, the reduction in calcium influx in response to a drug's impact on an *N*-methyl-D-aspartate (NMDA) receptor. The following is a general breakdown of this dimension, which spans the pharmacology/neuroplasticity literature: molecular, synaptic, neuronal, specific neuronal populations, brain regions, molecular behaviors, and complex behaviors. Other chapters of this volume provide a major detailed background and basis for understanding the research at the synaptic to neural population levels.

2. The second dimension is that of time frames. These can range from milliseconds in the case of many *in vitro* studies to months in clinical outcome studies.

3. The third dimension ranges from *in vitro/in vivo* studies of cell populations in cell preparations to studies of effects within living organisms.

4. Animal versus human is an obvious distinction related to generalization of findings. Within human studies, the specificity of the diagnosis is critical for the generalizability of findings.

5. The next dimension consists of physiological markers versus behavioral markers. In pharmacology and rehabilitation studies, dependent variables range from assays of proteins all the way to composite measurements of cognitive function in persons with dementia. The degree of direct tie-in to the neuroplasticity varies accordingly with the dependent variable measured.

6. Types of pharmacological agents can range from molecules infused into cellular preparations, to experimental agents, to licensed medications.

7. Neuroplasticity paradigms can relate to synaptic plasticity, axonal changes, genetic changes, neurogenesis, or larger morphological changes of neuronal populations.

8. Finally, correlation to neuroplasticity varies greatly. In many behavioral animal studies and most human studies, involvement of specific mechanisms of neuroplasticity is generally inferred rather than directly measured.

In many instances, putting pharmacological studies into the context of synaptic or morphological neuroplasticity requires examining a number of studies together in order to form conceptual linkages among studies. For instance, consider neuroplasticity as related to the effects of amphetamines on recovery after stroke. The following chain of evidence might be formed: Studies back to Bliss and Lomo (1973) support the contention that increased dendritic density appears to modify neuronal activity; other studies have shown an association of brain-derived neurotrophic factor (BDNF) with increases in dendrites (Lu & Chow, 1999); studies have demonstrated that glutamate up-regulates BDNF (Nestler et al., 2002); still other research supports the impact of norepinephrine (NE) on glutamate and the concomitant impact of amphetamine on BDNF (Scheiderer, Dobrunz, & McMahon, 2004). The precise linkage between amphetamine treatment and neuroplasticity at the dendritic or synaptic level is circuitous, but follows a reasonable chain of logic. The network of evidence is even more oblique when rehabilitation is considered as a type of enriched environment or when physiotherapy after stroke is examined as an independent variable analogous to forepaw exercise in a rodent (Walker-Batson et al., 2001). As more sophisticated techniques are being developed, studies are beginning to bridge some of these conceptual gaps; for example, the advent of bromodeoxyuridine (BrdU) has enabled researchers to tie behavioral memory measures to hippocampal neurogenesis.

In the sections that follow, studies of pharmacological agents are discussed, and linkages to relevant background research are explored in relation to these. This discussion begins with relevant animal research with licensed and potential pharmacological agents. Next, human studies related to recovery of motor and cognitive function are reviewed. A final caveat: Although I am aware that synaptic receptor functions may not be the most recent or most conceptually logical manner of organizing aspects of neuroplasticity, the remainder of this chapter is arranged according to these functions. Unfortunately, medications are anything but pure with respect to their effects on neurotransmitter systems, and therefore no classification using neurotransmitter receptor functions can ever be fully satisfactory. The reader is also cautioned that this review is far from exhaustive because of space limitations and should be considered merely a survey of the area.

ACETYLCHOLINE

Acetylcholine (ACh) was the first neurotransmitter to be identified, and the nicotinic and muscarinic receptor types are still those established by 19th-century research. It is perhaps the most studied neurotransmitter system related to cognition. Numerous animal studies have directly tied neuroplasticity to ACh-related processes. Again, only a brief survey of this research is provided here.

Nicotine is an ACh receptor agonist, but is also known to have an agonistic effect on dopamine. Brown and Kolb (2001) found that rats injected with nicotine that were exposed to an enriched locomotor environment showed increases in dendritic spine length and dendritic spine density, relative to saline-injected controls. This was noted in the nucleus accumbens and medial frontal cortex, but not the parietal cortex. In an associated behavioral study, Brown, Gonzalez, Whishaw, and Kolb (2001) also found that nicotine given before and after a medial frontal brain lesion to rats improved the rats' Morris water maze performance. In fact, the nicotine-treated rats with lesions performed as well as the sham-lesioned rats without nicotine. Verbois, Scheff, and Pauly (2003) evaluated whether chronic nicotine infusion could attenuate deficits induced by traumatic brain injury (TBI) in alpha-7-cholinergic expression. After being cortically contused and then chronically dosed with nicotine, rats demonstrated a reversal of nicotinic receptor density loss in the hippocampus. In a more recent study using both *in vitro* and *in vivo* studies with two cholinesterase inhibitors, Jin, Xie, Mao, and Greenberg (2006) used the BrdU labeling technique to identify newborn neurons. These drugs resulted in substantial increases in neuroproliferation as measured by BrdU. Conner, Chiba, and Tuszynski (2005) reported finding that rats with damage to the cholinergic system demonstrated substantially less neuronal plasticity after focal cortical lesions. Their study of the reorganization of the motor cortex at the cell population level showed a very different response to motor training after cortical lesions if the cholinergic system was selectively damaged. The cholinergic-specific injury was produced with an immunotoxin that selectively damaged the cholinergic neurons of the basal forebrain systems, and this substantially interfered with the reorganization of the motor cortex after cortical lesion.

In a study designed as an analogue to current dosing practices in dementia, Barnes et al. (2000) used the cholinesterase inhibitors donepezil and galantamine in a study with older rats. They measured maze learning, hippocampal long-term potentiation (LTP) induction, and nicotinic receptor density and affinity. The drug treatment significantly extended LTP decay times. Not only did the ACh inhibitors elevate the number of nicotinic receptors within the hippocampus and neocortex, but LTP decay was significantly positively correlated with nicotinic receptor binding in the hippocampus.

Murphy, Foley, O'Connell, and Regan (2006) gave chronic doses of the ACh inhibitor tacrine (as well as deprenyl and nefiracetam, discussed later) to rats exposed to several learning paradigms. The drug-treated rats were then compared to those raised in complex environments and social colonies. The primary histological dependent measure was an immunological marker of polysialic acid (PSA) associated with the neural cell adhesion molecule (NCAM), now strongly tied to the synaptic reorganization in the hippocampus that is associated with new learning. Rats treated with these clinical medications, which produce putative cognitive enhancement, showed increases in NCAM-PSA similar to those found in rats raised in an enriched environment. In fact, combining the drugs with an enriched environment did not further elevate the NCAM-PSA. Murphy et al. concluded that the synaptic modifications are the most likely explanation for the putative cognition-enhancing properties of these medications.

The most widely used and clinically tested class of medications for cognitive impairment is undoubtedly the cholinesterase inhibitors. The target disorders of most intense interest have been the dementias, especially Alzheimer's disease (AD). The progression of this literature is long, and a full discussion of it would be beyond the space limitations of this chapter. Instead, I only focus here on recent reviews of randomized controlled trials (RCTs). Kaduszkiewicz, Zimmermann, Beck-Bornholdt, and van den Bussche (2005) reviewed 22 RCTs that found positive effects for the ACh agonists but noted that the effect sizes were minimal. In the United Kingdom similar conclusions have led the National Centre for Clinical Excellence to declare this pharmacological treatment to be cost-effective only for moderate or severe AD. Others have asserted that response to cholinesterase inhibitors may be sufficient in selected patients to warrant their usage (Overshott & Burns, 2005). Although this research has provided no panacea, it has produced methodologies for assessing the next generation of medications in dementia. The clinical trials with ACh drugs raise a question drawn from the study by Murphy et al. (2006): If the patients selected for clinical trials already come from such "enriched environments" (i.e., rehabilitation units) that the neuroplastic changes that the ACh drugs might have otherwise produced have already occurred, is the use of the drugs justifiable? In other studies, the selection of different outcome variables (such as activities of daily living or behavioral difficulties) may explain the general enthusiasm for ACh medications among those who care for persons with dementia (Erkinjuntti et al., 2002).

Clinical research on ACh medications has also involved areas outside of the dementias. Pashek and Bachman (2003) reported significant gains in language, cognition, and motor speech abilities following administration of donepezil to a single participant with stable nonfluent aphasia. In a study of patients with postacute TBI, Zhang, Plotkin, Wang, Sandel, and Lee (2004) examined the effects of donepezil on short-term memory and sustained attention, using a 24-week double-blind crossover RCT. They found that donepezil increased neuropsychological test scores for both short-term memory and sustained attention.

Finally, researchers have often questioned whether the clear-cut distinction usually made between vascular dementia and AD actually reflects common clinical presentation. In a recent placebo-controlled study of a combination of vascular dementia and AD, galantamine was found to produce not only cognitive change, but also robust changes in activities of daily living and behavioral symptoms (Erkinjuntti et al., 2002).

NOREPINEPHRINE

NE has long been associated with attention, but there is also a wealth of research tying it to impulsivity, sympathetic nervous system activity, mood disorders, and drug abuse/addiction. The volume of NE-related studies in rodents precludes a thorough review here. A theoretical overview was published by Goldstein (2000). This area of research began with a landmark study by Feeney, Gonzalez, and Law (1982), who studied the effects of amphetamine, haloperidol, and physical restraint on recovery from unilateral sensory–motor cortex ablation. They measured narrow-beam walking and reported that a single postinjury dose of amphetamine accelerated recovery, whereas haloperidol retarded recovery. Widely cited, this 1982 article supported amphetamine as a putative agent in recovery, and large clinical trials of amphetamine treatment for stroke have been published as recently as 2006. Boyeson and Feeney (1990) noted that intraventricular administration of NE facilitated motor recovery in lesioned rats. Again, they assessed the effect on motor recovery by using the beam-walking task. NE was found to be the critical neurotransmitter in facilitating motor recovery.

The nature of the NE/amphetamine ameliorative effect was initially postulated to be related to diathesis, but evidence from researchers such as Dahl and Sarvey (1989) supports stronger links to neuroplasticity. The NE neurons of the locus coeruleus project to the hippocampus, providing the noradrenergic innervations necessary for hippocampus-dependent learning and memory. Dahl and Sarvey reported induction of LTP in hippocampal *in vitro* preparations in response to a noradrenergic agonist. Goldstein and Bullman (1997) completed a study that tied the NE/amphetamine research on beam walking in rodents to later constraint-induced therapy in humans. They tested whether the critical effect of NE on motor behavior was produced by administration of NE contralateral to the lesion or ipsilateral to the lesion, and found that the NE effect on recovery appeared to be a function of its effect on contralateral sensory–motor cortex. Stroemer, Kent, and Hulsebosch (1998) studied the effects of D-amphetamine on behavioral performance and neurogenesis in lesioned rats. At intervals, a proportion of rats were sacrificed, and immunoreactants (GAP-43 and synaptophysin) were examined. The amphetamine-treated group showed signs of increased neurogenesis in forelimb, hindlimb, and parietal regions ipsilateral to the infarction, compared to the sham-treated control group. There were also signs of greater synaptogenesis between 14 and 60 days after infarction in ipsilateral and contralateral cortices, compared to the non-amphetamine-treated control group. These data demonstrated that the occurrence of neuritic growth followed by synaptogenesis in the neocortex occurred in a pattern that corresponded both spatially and temporally with the behavioral recovery that D-amphetamine accelerated.

In their *in vitro* study of rats' hippocampal brain sections (see above), Dahl and Sarvey (1989) found that NE induced not only LTP, but long-term depression (LTD) in the hippocampal dentate gyrus. Scheiderer et al. (2004) supported the role of NE independent of glutamate in inducing LTD in the hippocampus. In a study of D-deprenyl on cognitive function following TBI, rats received fluid percussion TBI bilaterally to the entorhinal cortex (Zhu, Hamm, Reeves, Povlishock, & Phillips, 2000). Significant cognitive improvement was recorded in the rats treated with D-deprenyl. From a histological point of view, the noradrenergic fiber integrity was most clearly associated with enhanced neurogenesis of the hippocampus.

Clinical studies related to NE and recovery began to appear after the landmark study by Feeney et al. (1982). The most commonly tested pharmacological interventions in recovery from neurological injury in rehabilitation have been NE agonists such as amphetamine and methylphenidate. Stroke is the diagnosis with the greatest number of clinical studies related to NE enhancement. In the earliest of these studies, Crisostomo, Duncan, Propst, Dawson, and Davis (1988) assigned four of eight patients within 10 days of an ischemic stroke to a single dose of amphetamine combined with physical therapy. The amphetamine showed an ameliorative effect on motor performance the following day. Since the Crisostomo et al. study, there have been at least seven placebo-controlled trials of amphetamine for stroke. The initial trials in the mid-1990s were relatively small (Reding, Solomon, & Borucki, 1995; Walker-Batson, Smith, Curtis, Unwin, & Greenlee, 1995). The Walker-Batson et al. study, with five treated patients, supported the earlier findings of Crisostomo et al. However, larger studies (Gladstone et al., 2006; Sonde, Nordstrom, Nilsson, Lokk, & Viitanen, 2001; Treig, Werner, Sachse, & Hesse, 2003) have failed to support the use of amphetamine for recovery of motor function after stroke. Questions remain related to these results, such as the linkage with physiotherapy, dosing regimen, and time since stroke onset. To contextualize these findings, Kidwell, Liebeskind, Starkman, and Saver (2001) reviewed 178 controlled trials of treatments for ischemic stroke in the 20th century, of which only 3 met conventional criteria for positive results. A very thorough review of NE and stroke up to 2003 can be found in the Cochrane Collaboration Database (Martinsson, Wahlgreen, & Hardemark, 2003).

In contrast to the conflicting findings for amphetamine's effects on motor function, one double-blind placebo-controlled study of its effects on aphasic symptoms has shown generally more positive findings. Researchers from several different centers (Walker-Batson et al., 2001) studied 21 patients with ischemic stroke who were randomly assigned to receive amphetamine or a placebo. The dosing regimen was similar to that used in the earlier motor function study by Walker-Batson et al. (1995). The findings at 1 week after the dosing trial and at a 6-month follow-up included better scores on the Porch Index of Communicative Ability. Although the follow-up results failed to reach significance when corrected for multiple comparisons, the findings supported ameliorative effects of amphetamine in the cognitive–language domain.

Methylphenidate, another putative NE agonist, has been examined in clinical trials for its effect on recovery from neurological injury. A research group from the University of Texas Medical Center studied 23 patients with complicated mild to severe TBI in a double-blind placebo-controlled trial of methylphenidate (Perna, 2006; Plenger et al., 1996). The Disability Rating Scale scores were higher for the methylphenidate-treated group at 30 days but not at 90 days. The group receiving methylphenidate also showed an advantage at 30 days in the domains of attention/concentration and motor memory; again, however, these differences were not apparent at 90 days. Attrition appears to have been a factor in the follow-up, as the 90-day findings approached significance. More recently, Whyte et al. (2004) have reported a double-blind crossover RCT of methylphenidate in 34 clients with postacute brain injuries. Each participant received a daily dose or placebo on alternating weeks for 6 weeks. Whyte et al. reported a significant effect on processing speed (in both laboratory tasks and caregiver ratings) during the methylphenidate treatment. There were no crossover effects for distractibility or sustained attention.

Another NE agonist, atomoxetine, was recently examined along with venlafaxine in a training target zone study using a transcranial magnetic stimulation paradigm (Foster, Good, Fowlkes, & Sawaki, 2006). The atomoxetine-treated group showed an increase of movements in the training target zone, a finding associated with neuroplastic changes on the motor strip. A new paradigm using transcranial magnetic stimulation to elicit corticomotor neuronal excitability has links to neuroplasticity. Early work in this area suggests that the NE agonists reboxetine and yohimbine may enhance cortical excitability (Plewnia, Bartels, Cohen, & Gerloff, 2001; Plewnia et al., 2002). This noninvasive procedure has potential as a technique for early human preclinical trials.

GAMMA-AMINOBUTYRIC ACID

Gamma-aminobutyric acid (GABA) is widely distributed throughout the brain and is considered the ubiquitous inhibitory neurotransmitter. In the cortex and hippocampus, most GABA activity is in interneurons. Glutamate and GABA, as the primary excitatory and inhibitory inputs, are thought to work together to achieve a coordinated balance in the nervous system (Foster & Kemp, 2006). Benzodiazepines (BZDs) are the most widely used GABA-associated drugs that have putative agonistic properties. When initially introduced, BZDs were thought to be virtually devoid of negative effects, but they are now known to carry risks of dependence, withdrawal, and negative side effects related to cognition. They are particularly associated with deficits in visual–spatial ability, speed of processing, and verbal learning. Although BZDs are widely used to ensure amnesia during anesthesia, Perna (2006) has remarked that BZDs administered chronically after a lesion can slow brain recovery.

GABA has been tied for some time to the neurochemical cascades that follow brain injury. Albensi and Janigro (2003) studied the effects of brain trauma on LTP and LTD responses in hippocampal regions. Their results are similar to those of other studies that point to glutamate and GABA mechanisms as the links between brain injury and changes in LTP. Other research points to a possible inoculatory effect of BZDs in neural trauma. One study examined the effects of diazepam on survival and cognitive performance in rats after TBI (O'Dell, Gibson, Wilson, DeFord, & Hamm, 2000). Rats treated prior to TBI with diazepam had significantly lower mortality than saline-treated rats, and surviving animals had significantly shorter latencies to complete the Morris water maze test 11–15 days after injury. Chronic administration of BZDs has very different effects. Van Sickle, Cox, Schak, Greenfield, and Tietz (2002) found that chronic BZD administration leads to a substantial reduction in NMDA receptor currents in the hippocampus. Gomez-Pinilla, Dao, Choi, and Ryba (2000) investigated whether the GABA system can influence the expression of basic fibroblast growth factor (FGF-2) in the hippocampus, striatum, and caudal cerebral cortical region. The GABA agonist diazepam was injected into adult rats, and results of nuclease protection assays showed significant increases in FGF-2 messenger RNA (mRNA) in the hippocampus and striatum, but not in the caudal cerebral cortical region. Their research supports the contention that diazepam up-regulates FGF-2 expression in select areas of the brain, suggesting that GABA may promote neuroplasticity.

In an investigation of the effects of the short-acting BZD derivative midazolam on stroke patients, eight patients underwent baseline testing for motor function, aphasia, and neglect, after which midazolam was administered (Lazar et al., 2002). Patients were tested during the 2-hour period following administration, and again 2 hours after the drug effects had passed. All patients showed a return of the stroke sequelae that had previously resolved, and each returned to baseline 2 hours after midazolam administration. In a review and meta-analysis of the cognitive effects of withdrawal from long-term BZD use, Barker, Greenwood, Jackson, and Crowe (2004) concluded that cognitive impairment related to BZDs does show some remission after withdrawal but full restoration of function does not occur.

Maubach (2006) reported that in contrast to the amnesic effect of the BZD agonists that potentiates GABA(a) receptor function, newer GABA(a) antagonists have been shown to improve performance in animal models of memory formation. Unfortunately, these compounds have been anxiogenic and proconvulsant, and hence are not suitable for clinical use. More recently, GABA($alpha^5$) selective antagonists have been developed that enhance learning and memory in animal models, but are devoid of the adverse effects.

DOPAMINE

An important neurotransmitter in the development of psychopharmacology, dopamine is important in motor disorders involving the basal ganglia, such as Parkinson's disease. Dopamine imbalances in the frontal lobes are believed to cause deficits in attention, memory, and problem solving. The nucleus accumbens and striatum dopamine receptors are associated with pleasure, addiction, and reinforcement. The primary antipsychotic drugs are targeted at dopamine, especially the older class. The newer atypical antipsychotics have strong antagonistic action with serotonin, as well as substantial cholinergic and adrenergic effects. Antipsychotics have long been associated with structural alterations in the caudate nucleus and in dendrites in the prefrontal cortex—changes that suggest drug-induced plasticity. These striatal changes are generally assumed to relate to side effects more than therapeutic effects. Other neuropathological findings related to schizophrenia and antipsychotics remain somewhat clouded by disease-versus-treatment confounds (Harrison, 1999). In studying one of the last cohorts of patients with schizophrenia who were not treated with antipsychotics, Jellinger and Riederer (1977) found signs of generalized gliosis in the caudate nuclei in 46% of the drug-treated group, but only 4% in the drug-naive group. Unlike drugs affecting most other neurotransmitter systems, both dopamine agonists and dopamine antagonists are commonly associated with neurological recovery. On the whole, dopamine antagonists have generally been used in rehabilitation settings to control agitated and aggressive behaviors; this is done despite the lack of any double-blind placebo-controlled trials with these compounds (Fleminger, Greenwood, & Oliver, 2003). Most of the studies using dopamine agonists have been employed to test the hypothesis of improved cognitive function.

Feeney et al. (1982)'s landmark research investigated both amphetamine and haloperidol in rats following cerebral infarction. As noted earlier, a single dose of haloperidol retarded recovery from infarction as measured by balance beam walking. Interestingly, Boyeson and Feeney (1990) noted 8 years later that intraventricular administration of dopamine did not affect recovery, leading them to posit that the deleterious effects of haloperidol may be mediated through the adrenergic system.

More recent studies have focused on histological changes associated with neuroplastic changes, and most have focused on the newer antipsychotics, which antagonize both dopamine and serotonin. Zhao, Puurunen, Schallert, Sivenius, and Jolkkonen (2005) evaluated the effect of risperidone and fluoxetine on histological and functional outcome after experimental stroke in aged rats. Their study showed that risperidone acutely impaired behavioral performance, but did not affect histological or functional outcome in aged rats subjected to cortical photothrombosis. Pillai, Terry, and Mahadik (2006) investigated the effects of first- and second-generation antipsychotics on nerve growth factor (NGF) and BDNF with long-term usage. Compared to control animals, all treated animals showed a reduction in these neuroplasticity-related cytokines, but the data suggest that the newer drugs have less deleterious effects than the older medications. Lipska, Khaing, Weickert, and Weinberger (2001) studied the effects of antipsychotic drugs (haloperidol and clozapine) on unlesioned rats and rats with neonatal ventral hippocampal lesions, an animal model for schizophrenia. They found the antipsychotics reduced BDNF mRNA in the hippocampus. In lesioned rats, the drugs also tended to reduce BDNF mRNA in the prefrontal cortex.

Other behaviorally oriented research with animals has explored the newer antipsychotics. Investigating the effects of risperidone and olanzepine on adult rats, Wilson, Gibson, and Hamm (2003) found that chronic administration of haloperidol, but not olanzapine, impaired cognitive performance after TBI in rats. Green, Patil, Marsden, Bennett, and Wigmore (2006) tested memory by using object discrimination. The results showed that both drugs significantly improved object discrimination performance after 21 days. In addition, olanzapine significantly increased cell proliferation in the subventricular zone and prefrontal cortex, but not the dentate gyrus. Nitsche et al. (2006) investigated the effect of dopaminergic mechanisms on NMDA-receptor-dependent neuroplasticity; their findings suggest that D2 receptors play a major supporting role in inducing neuroplasticity in the motor cortex. In a study of an atypical antipsychotic, quetiapine (and the antidepressant venlafaxine), Xu et al. (2006) subjected rats to chronic restraint stress and then measured hippocampal cell proliferation and BDNF expression. Their findings demonstrated that the decreased hippocampal cell proliferation and BDNF expression otherwise caused by the restraint-induced stress were prevented by quetiapine administration (and by venlafaxine). Bai, Zhang, and Li (2004) found that chronic dosing of clozapine and olanzapine up-regulated BCL-2 mRNA, strongly associated with neuroplasticity, in rats' frontal cortex and hippocampus.

Wakade, Mahadik, Waller, and Chiu (2002) studied neurogenesis in the adult rat brain in response to risperidone and olanzapine. When compared to controls and animals treated with haloperidol, the animals treated with atypical neuroleptics showed a twofold to threefold increase in newly divided cells in the subventricular zones.

A study of five dopamine agonists—bromocriptine, cabergoline, dihydroergocryptine, pergolide, and ropinirole—with ischemically injured rats (Micale et al., 2006) found several palliative effects. When rats that were exposed to hypobaric hypoxia were first pretreated with one of the dopamine agonists, they showed faster recovery from amnesia. Animals were taught an avoidance procedure prior to occlusive ischemia of the carotid artery, and later were exposed to dopaminergic agonists for 7 days. The number of successful avoidance trials was higher in treated rats than in controls and was related to the dose of the dopamine agonist. As noted in the discussion of ACh, Murphy et al. (2006) gave chronic doses of deprenyl, a drug known to raise dopamine level (as well as levels of ACh and NE), to rats exposed to several learning paradigms. The drug-treated rats were then compared to those raised in complex environments and social colonies. Murphy et al. concluded that deprenyl produced putative neuroplastic effects, based on increases of NCAM-PSA that were similar to those for rats raised in an enriched environment. In another study of D-deprenyl's effects on cognitive function following TBI, rats received fluid percussion TBI bilaterally to the entorhinal cortex (Zhu et al., 2000). Significant cognitive improvement was recorded in rats treated with D-deprenyl. The researchers concluded that, histologically, the noradrenergic fiber integrity was most closely associated with enhanced neurogenesis of the hippocampus.

Most controlled human studies of dopamine have used dopamine agonists as the independent measure. The dependent measures range from emergence from coma to executive functions. The majority of dopamine antagonist studies in TBI or stroke have used dependent behavioral measures such as agitation or aggression. In clinical studies that report cognitive gains, one could question whether these are direct cognitive effects or consequences of better behavioral control.

Hughes, Colantonio, Santaguida, and Paton (2005) administered amantadine as a means of increasing consciousness after prolonged traumatic coma. In a sample of 123 adults with severe TBI, 46.4% of cases treated with amantadine emerged from coma, compared to 37.9% of controls; this was not a significant difference. In an outcome study (Meythaler, Brunner, Johnson, & Novack, 2002), 35 patients with TBI related to transportation accidents participated in a double-blind crossover RCT investigating the clinical efficacy of amantadine. The results included improvements on the Mini-Mental State Exam, the Disability Rating Scale, the Glasgow Coma Scale, and the Functional Independent Measure in the group that received amantadine during the first 6 weeks of recovery. The contrast group, which received the active drug during the second 6 weeks, showed improvements on the Mini-Mental State Exam and the Disability Rating Scale. Kraus et al. (2005) investigated the effects of amantadine on chronic TBI. In an open-label study, 22 subjects received 400 mg of amantadine daily for 12 weeks. The patients showed significant improvements on neuropsychological tests of executive functioning. Positron emission tomography (PET) data suggested a significant increase in left prefrontal cortex glucose metabolism, which was significantly correlated with the executive domain scores.

In an interesting single-case study of a patient with encephalopathy secondary to drug overdose, Arciniegas, Frey, Anderson, Brousseau, and Harris (2004) and colleagues found substantial improvements in motivation, attention, memory, and executive function coinciding with the introduction of amantadine. When the patient later elected to reduce his dose of amantadine, symptoms returned, and then improved upon the patient's recommencing the original dose. Another single-case study reported by French researchers (Ben Smail, Samuel, Rouy-Thenaisy, Regnault, & Azouvi, 2005) found that bromocriptine improved memory, attention, and speed of processing in a patient with parkinsonian symptoms secondary to brain trauma.

SEROTONIN

The bulk of basic research on serotonin is rooted in the fundamental psychiatric research into mood disorders. Some of the landmark literature in the past decade has related to the impact of stress upon hippocampal neurogenesis. Malberg (2004) has reviewed the effect of antidepressants on aspects of neuroplasticity. In another review, Silva (2004) concluded that a growing body of evidence supports the critical role of decreased neuroplasticity in the etiology of mood disorders. When serotonin is considered in relationship to widely used medications in rehabilitation, the atypical antipsychotics are characterized by some as having greater antagonism of serotonin than of dopamine, but these medications have been included in the discussion of dopamine above. In relation to rehabilitation and recovery from neurological injury, Mitchell and Neumaier (2005) have reviewed articles that tie the 5-HT6 serotonin receptors to higher cognitive processes such as memory. In a review of BDNF and serotonin, Mattson, Maudsley, and Martin (2004) have emphasized the up-regulation of BDNF by serotonin and the effect of BDNF on enhancing the growth and survival of serotonergic neurons.

Nibuya, Morinobu, and Duman (1995) investigated the influence of antidepressant drug treatment on expression of BDNF and its receptor trkB. Male rats were administered once-daily electroconvulsive shock (which increases BDNF mRNA twofold) and either vehicle, tranylcypromine, imipramine, desipramine, sertraline, or mianserin (haloperidol, morphine, and cocaine were also used). Chronic, but not acute, treatment with several antidepressants (tranylcypromine, sertraline, desipramine, or mianserin) significantly increased trkB mRNA in hippocampus. Chronic administration of nonantidepressant psychotropic drugs (morphine, cocaine, or haloperidol) did not increase levels of BDNF mRNA in the hippocampus in response to restraint stress. Another study of BDNF expression treated rats with imipramine or tranylcypromine for 20 days (Russo-Neustadt, Beard, & Cotman, 1999). The combination of physical activity and antidepressant treatment for the 20-day period led to a significant potentiation of BDNF mRNA levels within the dentate gyrus. These results suggest that physical exercise may be a potential enhancer of treatment response to antidepressants.

Antidepressant effects upon hippocampal neurogenesis in the adult rat were explored in a study by Malberg, Eisch, Nestler, and Duman (2000), which used BrdU as a marker for dividing cells. The experiments conducted showed that chronic antidepressant treatment significantly increased the number of BrdU-labeled cells in the dentate gyrus and hilus of the hippocampus. The investigators administered several different classes of antidepressants, all of which were found to increase BrdU-labeled cells. Windle and Corbett (2005) investigated fluoxetine and recovery of motor function after focal ischemia in rats. More specifically, they examined whether chronic administration of fluoxetine combined with physical practice affected recovery of function on three separate tests (forelimb reaching, forelimb preference, and limb coordination) after focal ischemia in rats. Fluoxetine combined with rehabilitation therapy did not alter the degree or rate of recovery of function in treated compared to nontreated rats.

As noted in the discussion of dopamine, Zhu et al. (2000) found that D-deprenyl improved cognitive function and enhanced neuroplasticity after TBI in rats. The synaptic plasticity in the hippocampus appeared most closely related to the noradrenergic fiber integrity. Alboni, Benatti, Capone, Corsini, Caggia, et al. (2010), found changes in BDNF in the frontal cortex and hippocampus in response to escitalopram, dependent on the time course of administration. Their findings corresponded with the recovery patterns in clinical use of SSRIs.

A great deal of research in the area of depression has focused on the effects of stress upon neurogenesis. Duman, Nakagawa, and Malberg (2001) found that antidepressant treatment up-regulated the cyclic adenosine monophosphate and neurotrophin signaling pathways involved in plasticity. The authors concluded that depression may be associated with a disruption of mechanisms governing cell survival and plasticity in the brain. In a more recent study that explored not only neurogenesis but an important new area of newborn neuron survival, Banasr, Soumier, Hery, Mocaer, and Daszuta (2006) explored a new antidepressant, agomelatine. Chronic (3-week), but not acute (4-hour) or subchronic (1-week), administration of agomelatine increased cell proliferation and neurogenesis in the ventral dentate gyrus. Extending treatment over several weeks, however, increased survival of newly formed neurons in the entire dentate gyrus area.

Dam, Tonin, Sale, and Pizzolato (1996) studied the effects of fluoxetine and maprotiline (an NE reuptake blocker) on recovery in patients with poststroke hemiplegia. A total of 52 subjects were assigned to receive one of the medications or a placebo while undergoing 3 months of physiotherapy. The greatest improvements in activities of daily living were observed in the fluoxetine group, and the smallest in the maprotiline group. Fluoxetine yielded a significantly larger number of patients with good recovery than did either maprotiline or placebo. These effects were not related to the medication's efficacy for treating depressive symptoms. In a double-blind placebo-controlled trial of the antidepressant trazadone, 27 inpatients in a rehabilitation program received either placebo or trazodone 44 days after stroke (Reding et al., 1986). Patients with either a clinical diagnosis of depression or abnormal Zung Depression Scale scores showed a consistent trend toward greater improvement in activities of daily living with trazadone than with placebo. More recently, patients in early stages of recovery from severe TBI were given a trial of sertraline (Meythaler, Depalma, Devivo, Guin-Renfroe, & Novack, 2001). No improvement with this selective serotonin reuptake inhibitor was found.

GLUTAMATE

Glutamate is the excitatory neurotransmitter most closely tied to NMDA, alpha-amino-3-hydroxy-5-methyl-4-isoxazole propionic acid (AMPA), and kainite, all of which are linked to LTP and LTD (Johnson & Kotermanski, 2006). Although currently only 3 common drugs are generally associated with glutamate (ketamine, memantine, and modafinil), there are 12 drugs in at least Phase I trials at this writing. Lynch (2006) has coined the term *AMPAkine* to refer to the small molecules that positively modulate AMPA-type glutamate receptors, and thereby enhance fast excitatory neurotransmission throughout the brain.

Memantine is an antagonist of glutamate through the NMDA receptors. Unlike other NMDA antagonists (e.g., ketamine), which produce pernicious side effects, memantine does not produce such effects because it is a noncompetitive receptor antagonist (Parsons, Danysz, & Quack, 1999). Although *in vitro* evidence of dopamine enhancement exists, *in vivo* studies support the contention that memantine works predominantly through its effect upon glutamate (Schwenkreis et al., 1999). Shearman et al. (2006) found an increase in extracellular ACh by memantine in the nucleus accumbens and the ventral tegmental regions. Despite a flurry of research related to memantine, large clinical trials have demonstrated less than robust treatment effects. Dansyz and Parsons (2003) tested the contention whether glutamate-mediated neurotoxicity in AD was caused by NMDA receptors' being stimulated in a tonic rather than a phasic manner. They found that over activation of the NMDA receptors could be countered by memantine. This led to concomitant changes in LTP in the hippocampus. Krystal, Tolin, Sanacora, Castner, Williams, et al. (2009), have proposed treatments tailored to NMDA receptor plasticity in anxiety disorders in a recent paper proposing that neuroplasticity targets would improve the efficacy of many aspects of pharmacotherapy.

In a study of memantine (and another NMDA antagonist, MK-801), lesioned rats were tested in a radial maze test (Zajaczkowski, Quack, & Danysz, 1996). Memantine had no effect on normal rats, but in lesioned rats memantine reversed the lesion-induced deficits in memory. In a study using transgenic mice designed to model AD (Minkeviciene, Banerjee, & Tanila, 2004), researchers found that memantine improved spatial learning in the Morris water maze, but had no effect on locomotor activity or aggressive behavior.

A recent Cochrane review (McShane, Areosa Sastre, & Minakaran, 2006), found that two out of three studies conducted for at least 6 months showed only small beneficial cognitive effects of memantine in moderate to severe AD, whereas effects on mild to moderate AD were even more marginal. The review did find that patients taking memantine were slightly less likely to develop agitation. Koch, Szecsey, and Haen (2004) have recommended that the target indications for memantine ought to be enhancing drive, producing an antispastic effect, and increasing vigilance.

A study using transcranial magnetic stimulation as the primary dependent variable investigated the effect of memantine on motor excitability in humans (Schwenkreis et al., 1999). When memantine was used for 8 days, it was noted to enhance intracortical inhibition and reduce intracortical facilitation in comparison to placebo. Although the direct connection to neuroplasticity of this technique is still being researched, it holds promise as a new noninvasive means of measuring some drug effects. Nitsche, Kuo, Karrasch, Wachter, Leibentanz, et al. (2009), found similar findings in a singled-blinded, placebo-controlled, randomized crossover study using citalopram.

RACETAMS

Piracetam, a derivative compound of GABA, was originally described as a *nootropic* (i.e., cognition-enhancing) member of the racetam family. There are at least 10 compounds in this category, and these have received considerable attention since the 1960s. (The term *nootropics* has now been expanded to include most of the medications discussed in this chapter.) Explanations for racetams' possible mechanisms of action have focused on the membrane hypothesis, with both neuronal and vascular mechanisms considered to explain the drugs' putative effects. The neuronal effects discussed include effects on neurotransmission, neuroprotective effects, and effects on neuroplasticity. Clinical research with these drugs is wide-ranging, including cognitive disorders, vertigo, myoclonus, dyslexia, and sickle cell anemia (Winblad, 2005).

As noted in the discussion of ACh and dopamine, Murphy et al. (2006) gave chronic doses of nefiracetam, another member of the racetam family, to rats exposed to several learning paradigms. The drug-treated rats were then compared to those raised in complex environments and social colonies. Their primary histological dependent measure was the immunological marker NCAM-PSA, now strongly tied to synaptic reorganization in the hippocampus. The rats treated with nefiracetam showed increases of NCAM-PSA similar to those of rats raised in an enriched environment. In fact, combining the drugs with an enriched environment did not further elevate the NCAM-PSA. Murphy et al. concluded that the synaptic modification is the most likely explanation for the putative cognition-enhancing properties of these medications.

Using a prospective, double-blind, placebo-controlled design Kessler, Thiel, Karbe, and Heiss (2000) investigated whether piracetam would improve language recovery in poststroke aphasia. Neuropsychological tests and activation PET measurements of cerebral blood flow were completed with 24 patients. After 6 weeks of speech treatment, the piracetam-treated group improved on six language measures, whereas the placebo-treated group only improved on three measures. PET scanning showed more regions of activation for the piracetam-treated group. In a Cochrane review, Flicker and Grimley Evans (2004) concluded that piracetam did not produce significant improvements in cognition over those of placebo treatment.

OTHER MEDICATIONS

In a study of lithium and its impact on neurogenesis (Chen, Rajkowska, Du, Seraji-Bozorgzad, & Manji, 2000), adult mice were treated chronically with lithium while being injected with the BrdU-labeling agent. Immunohistochemical analysis undertaken 1 day after the last injection showed that lithium produced a significant (25%) increase in the BrdU-labeled cells in the dentate gyrus, in comparison to placebo.

In one of the first studies of sleep disorders after neurological injury, Kemp, Biswas, Neumann, and Coughlan (2004) investigated the efficacy of melatonin in treating post-TBI sleep disturbance. A double-blind crossover RCT was conducted to compare melatonin and amitriptyline in a small sample of patients presenting with chronic sleep disturbance after TBI. No differences were found in sleep latency or quality for either drug compared to baseline; however, the melatonin users reported improved daytime alertness compared to baseline, and amitriptyline users reported increased sleep duration compared to baseline. Mirakur, Moorhead, Stanfield, McKirdy, Sussman, et al. (2009), reported that in 18 patients with bipolar disorder, a decline in gyrification over 4 years was associated with BDNF valine[66] methionine variant. These patients were taking various medications for their disorders over the study period, so pharmacological implications were obscure but the atropic changes which occurred over the course of the disease in comparison to controls has implication for understanding neuroplastic factors in affective disorders.

PRESCRIBING PATTERNS

Our current knowledge related to medications and neuroplasticity after neurological injury represents the metaphorical two-edged sword. On the one hand, a great deal of potential benefit may unfold as our knowledge base improves; on the other hand, indications of the deleterious effects of same drugs (e.g., first-generation antipsychotics) appear adequate for practitioners to avoid their use in all but the most desperate circumstances. Goldstein (1995) investigated the prescribing patterns for hospitalized patients with the diagnosis of TBI. In a study of 85 patients, 48% were prescribed neuroleptics/dopamine antagonists and 40% BZDs. In comparison, only 24% were given anticonvulsants, of which most were older, more sedating anticonvulsants (phenytonin or phenobarbitone). Despite the growing evidence available even in 1995, the doctors prescribing for these patients did not appear to have attended to published findings related to recovery. This is a cautionary tale that should be regarded with care.

CONCLUSIONS

The current overall state of research into clinical medications to enhance recovery from neurological injury has been a story of numerous, small, incremental results without the hoped-for great strides forward. No class of medication has been widely accepted as invariably effective at an indisputable level of improvement in cognitive function for any neurological disorder. Cholinergic medications are the most widely researched group of medications, but their overall levels of effectiveness remain topics of continued debate. Despite the early enthusiasm for NE agonists caused by laboratory research, this class of drugs has been anything but a panacea in recovery from stroke or brain injury. Early hope for the racetams has diminished after large, well-controlled trials failed to meet earlier expectations. The glutamate-related medications, which arguably have the strongest link to adult neuroplasticity, have failed to produce unequivocally robust treatment effects in the population with dementia.

Research into the neuroplasticity aspects of current clinical medications has been more encouraging than clinical effectiveness studies have been. Perhaps current laboratory findings at the level of neuropeptides, the synaptic level, or the neuronal level are exquisitely sensitive, as they often correlate with relatively small clinical findings. A less sanguine view is that current methods have yet to tap into critical aspects of neuroplasticity that will lead to breakthroughs in aiding the recovery from neurological injury.

After many decades of the belief that the adult mammalian brain essentially did not regenerate after injury, new molecular and cellular bases for regenerative responses are beginning to change the fundamental tenets of recovery (see Kolb, Cioe, & Williams, Chapter 2, this volume). Technological advances are leading researchers to ask questions that were almost unthinkable even a decade or so ago. Many polypeptides that regulate the induction and inhibition of regeneration have been uncovered. What are clearly missing at this juncture are pharmacological compounds that can accomplish the following: deliver specific neurotrophic factors, guide axon regrowth, inhibit gliotic scarring, mediate the survival of newborn neurons, switch apoptosis on or off, or mediate the impact of the immune system on damaged cells. Perhaps in the future, texts will be divided into these more logical divisions related to neuroplasticity as the science moves away from older paradigms.

In the search for means of limiting the impact of neurological injury, most research has focused on morphological changes or on neurochemical abnormalities. Until recently, most diagnoses of disorders in the nervous system have almost entirely focused on morphological changes. Although this morphological emphasis is understandable, it has led down many blind alleys. Studies of the best-known area of adult neurogenesis, the hippocampus, have primarily taken a morphological approach until recently. More recent studies are beginning to explore the role and function of newborn cells. This deeper knowledge of the function of neuroplastic processes is critical if research is to move more adeptly from the lab to the clinic (Eisch, 2002).

Research on recovery from neurological injury is fraught with promising hypotheses from animal studies that eventually have not come to fruition in clinical trials. This is certainly the case with NE and ACh medications. One possible explanation for this disconnection between the animal and the clinical literature could lie in a familiar culprit in behavioral science—difference among species. Rakic (2002) has recently reviewed many of the differences among mammalian species and within primates with regard to adult neurogenesis. Morphological differences between rodents and primates can be substantial, and the timing of neurogenic periods can also be considerably different, even with regard to defining adulthood. These substantial differences may in part explain the frequent failure of laboratory work to generalize to later clinical trials. Readers should also bear in mind that many of the larger current clinical trials are testing hypotheses raised in the 1980s, when the multiple molecular systems involving receptor subtypes, second-messenger systems, and gene expression were little more than weakly supported speculations.

Another relatively simple explanation of why so much animal research has not resulted in clinically effective treatment might lie in the Murphy et al. (2006) study. Interestingly, they found that anticholinesterase inhibitors increased evidence of neuroplasticity, but did not have an additive effect beyond that achieved with an enriched environment. Conceptualizing rehabilitation for humans with neurological injury as analogous to an enriched environment for rodents raises the question: Is the potential neuroplasticity in clinical settings already achieved by rehabilitation, and hence does further medication add only marginal benefit?

Enthusiasm for new models of brain repair should not overshadow the potential "down sides" to this area. In his recent text on neuroplasticity, Möller (2006) outlines a number of neurological signs and symptoms that are caused or exacerbated by neuroplasticity. Certainly several iatrogenic disorders in psychiatry, such as tardive dyskinesia, are already tied to neuroplastic changes.

Much of the research on neuroplasticity has been in exploring the family of polypeptides known as neurotrophins, such as NGF or BDNF. These factors not only are important in the survival of neurons, but aid in differentiation of neurons and the development of axonal connections. New drugs that directly turn the neurotrophins on and off may represent the next big stage in pharmacological development. Apoptosis is another area that is becoming better understood in the development of several neurodegenerative diseases. A number of possible intervention points with apoptosis-related neurotrophins hold promise for pharmacological development (Yuan & Yankner, 2000). The AMPA-enhancing compounds that were named AMPAkines by Lynch (2006) represent a rich area for future development. Insulin receptors are also another interesting targets, as they have recently been tied to animal learning. Angiotensin receptors are other modulators not primarily associated with the central nervous system, but there is some evidence for their involvement with learning and memory (Amadio, Govoni, Alkon, & Pascale, 2004). Cataloguing the potential new developments in medications that may capitalize on neuroplastic changes is a task that appears to be growing exponentially.

Like psychiatry and other fields of human behavior, rehabilitation is undergoing a revolution in its basic theoretical underpinnings. Considering the impact of medications upon neuroplasticity is fundamental to any up-to-date clinical practice, despite the relative inconclusiveness current in the field. The clinical scientist who takes on learning this 21st-century neuroscience has several daunting challenges: a whole alphabet soup of new agents; a more dynamic process of neurological repair than was once thought; a reevaluation of the role of glia cells; and an ever larger role for genetics. Besides these substantial intellectual challenges, the clinical researcher must regularly question the antiquated models of recovery that were so widely accepted only a decade or so ago. The future of rehabilitation appears linked to the burgeoning field of neuroplasticity. Ideally, further work in this area will lead to the long-awaited development of robust therapeutics that will fundamentally alter the nature of recovery from neurological injury.

REFERENCES

Albensi, B. C., & Janigro, D. (2003). Traumatic brain injury and its effects on synaptic plasticity. *Brain Injury, 17*(8), 653–663.

Alboni, S., Benatti, O., Capone, G., Corsini, D., Caggia, F., Tascedda, F., et al. (2010). Time-dependent effects of escitalopram on brain derived neurotrophic factor (BNDF) and neuroplasticity related targets in the central nervous systems of rats. *European Journal of Pharmacology, 643*, 180–187.

Amadio, M., Govoni, S., Alkon, D. L., & Pascale, A. (2004). Emerging targets for the pharmacology of learning and memory. *Pharmacological Research, 50*(2), 111–122.

Arciniegas, D. B., Frey, K. L., Anderson, C. A., Brousseau, K. M., & Harris, S. N. (2004). Amantadine for neurobehavioural deficits following delayed post-hypoxic encephalopathy. *Brain Injury, 18*(12), 1309–1318.

Bai, O., Zhang, H. H., & Li, X. M. (2004). Antipsychotic drugs clozapine and olanzapine upregulate BCL-2 mRNA and protein in rat frontal cortex and hippocampus. *Brain Research, 1010*(1–2), 81–86.

Banasr, M., Soumier, A., Hery, M., Mocaer, E., & Daszuta, A. (2006). Agomelatine, a new antidepressant, induces regional changes in hippocampal neurogenesis. *Biological Psychiatry, 59*(11), 1087–1096.

Barker, M. J., Greenwood, K. M., Jackson, M., & Crowe, S. F. (2004). Persistence of cognitive effects after withdrawal from long-term benzodiazepine use: A meta-analysis. *Archives of Clinical Neuropsychology, 19*(3), 437–454.

Barnes, C. A., Meltzer, J., Houston, F., Orr, G., McGann, K., & Wenk, G. L. (2000). Chronic treatment of old rats with donepezil or galantamine: Effects on memory, hippocampal plasticity and nicotinic receptors. *Neuroscience, 99*(1), 17–23.

Ben Smail, D., Samuel, C., Rouy-Thenaisy, K., Regnault, J., & Azouvi, P. (2005). Bromocriptine in traumatic brain injury. *Brain Injury, 20*(1), 111–115.

Bliss, T. V. P., & Lomo, T. (1973). Long-lasting potentiation of synaptic transmission in dentate area of anesthetized rabbit following stimulation of perforant path. *Journal of Physiology, 232*(2), 331–356.

Boyeson, M. G., & Feeney, D. M. (1990). Intraventricular norepinephrine facilitates motor recovery following sensorimotor cortex injury. *Pharmacology, Biochemistry, and Behavior, 35*(3), 497–501.

Brown, R. W., Gonzalez, C. L., Whishaw, I. Q., & Kolb, B. (2001). Nicotine improvement of Morris water task performance after fibra–formix lesion is blocked by mecamylamine. *Behavioural Brain Research, 119*(2), 185–192.

Brown, R. W., & Kolb, B. (2001). Nicotine sensitization increases dendritic length and spine density in nucleus accumbens and cingulate cortex. *Brain Research, 899*(1–2), 94–100.

Chen, G., Rajkowska, G., Du, F., Seraji-Bozorgzad, N., & Manji, H. K. (2000). Enhancement of hippocampal neurogenesis by lithium. *Journal of Neurochemistry, 75*(4), 1729–1734.

Conner, J. M., Chiba, A. A., & Tuszynski, M. H. (2005). The basal forebrain cholinergic system is essential for cortical plasticity and functional recovery following brain injury. *Neuron, 46*(2), 173–179.

Crisostomo, E. A., Duncan, P. W., Propst, M., Dawson, D. V., & Davis, J. N. (1988). Evidence that amphetamine with physical therapy promotes recovery of motor function in stroke patients. *Annals of Neurology, 23*(1), 94–97.

Dahl, D., & Sarvey, J. M. (1989). Norepinephrine induces pathway-specific long-lasting potentiation and depression in the hippocampal dentate gyrus. *Proceedings of the National Academy of Sciences USA, 86*(12), 4776–4780.

Dam, M., Tonin, P., Sale, E., & Pizzolato, G. (1996). Effects of fluoxetine and maprotiline on functional recovery in poststroke hemiplegic patients undergoing rehabilitation therapy: Response. *Stroke, 27*(11), 2145–2146.

Danysz, W., & Parsons, C. G. (2003). The NMDA receptor antagonist memantine as a symptomatological and neuroprotective treatment for Alzheimer's disease: Preclinical evidence. *International Journal of Geriatric Psychiatry, 18*, S23–S32.

Duman, R. S., Nakagawa, S., & Malberg, J. (2001). Regulation of adult neurogenesis by antidepressant treatment. *Neuropsychopharmacology, 25*(6), 836–844.

Eisch, A. J. (2002). Adult neurogenesis: Implications for psychiatry. In M. A. Hofman, G. J. Boer, A. J. G. D. Holtmaat, E. J. W. Van Someren, J. Verhaagen, & D. F. Swaab (Eds.), *Progress in brain research: Vol. 138. Plasticity in the adult brain: From genes to neurotherapy* (pp. 315–342). Amsterdam: Elsevier.

Erkinjuntti, T., Kurz, A., Gauthier, S., Bullock, R., Lilienfeld, S., & Damaraju, C. V. (2002). Efficacy of galantamine in probable vascular dementia and Alzheimer's disease combined with cerebrovascular disease: A randomised trial. *Lancet, 359*(9314), 1283–1290.

Feeney, D. M., Gonzalez, A., & Law, W. A. (1982). Amphetamine, haloperidol, and experience interact to affect rate of recovery after motor cortex injury. *Science, 217*(4562), 855–857.

Fleminger, S., Greenwood, R. J., & Oliver, D. L. (2003). Pharmacological management for agitation and aggression in people with acquired brain injury. *Cochrane Database of Systematic Reviews, Issue 1, Art. No. CD003299.*

Flicker, L., & Grimley Evans, J. (2004). Piracetam for dementia or cognitive impairment: Reviews. *Cochrane Database of Systematic Reviews*, Issue 1, Art. No. CD001011.

Foster, A. C., & Kemp, J. A. (2006). Glutamate- and GABA-based CNS therapeutics. *Current Opinion in Pharmacology, 6*(1), 7–17.

Foster, D. J., Good, D. C., Fowlkes, A., & Sawaki, L. (2006). Atomoxetine enhances a short-term model of plasticity in humans. *Archives of Physical Medicine and Rehabilitation, 87*(2), 216–221.

Gladstone, D. J., Danells, C. J., Armesto, A., McIlroy, W. E., Staines, W. R., Graham, S. J., et al. (2006). Physiotherapy coupled with dextroamphetamine for rehabilitation after hemiparetic stroke: A randomized, double-blind, placebo-controlled trial. *Stroke, 37*(1), 179–185.

Goldstein, L. B. (1995). Prescribing of potentially harmful drugs to patients admitted to hospital after head-injury. *Journal of Neurology, Neurosurgery and Psychiatry, 58*(6), 753–755.

Goldstein, L. B. (2000). Effects of amphetamines and small related molecules on recovery after stroke in animals and man. *Neuropharmacology, 39*(5), 852–859.

Goldstein, L. B., & Bullman, S. (1997). Effects of dorsal noradrenergic bundle lesions on recovery after sensorimotor cortex injury. *Pharmacology, Biochemistry, and Behavior, 58*(4), 1151–1157.

Gomez-Pinilla, F., Dao, L., Choi, J., & Ryba, E. A. (2000). Diazepam induces FGF-2 mRNA in the hippocampus and striatum. *Brain Research Bulletin, 53*(3), 283–289.

Green, W., Patil, P., Marsden, C. A., Bennett, G. W., & Wigmore, P. M. (2006). Treatment with olanzapine increases cell proliferation in the subventricular zone and prefrontal cortex. *Brain Research, 1070*(1), 242–245.

Harrison, P. J. (1999). The neuropathological effects of antipsychotic drugs. *Schizophrenia Research, 40*(2), 87–99.

Hughes, S., Colantonio, A., Santaguida, P. L., & Paton, T. (2005). Amantadine to enhance readiness for rehabilitation following severe traumatic brain injury. *Brain Injury, 19*(14), 1197–1206.

Jellinger, K., & Riederer, P. (1977). Brain monoamines in metabolic (endotoxic) coma: Preliminary biochemical study in human postmortem material. *Journal of Neural Transmission, 41*(4), 275–286.

Jin, K., Xie, L., Mao, X. O., & Greenberg, D. A. (2006). Alzheimer's disease drugs promote neurogenesis. *Brain Research, 1085*, 183–188.

Johnson, J. W., & Kotermanski, S. E. (2006). Mechanism of action of memantine. *Current Opinion in Pharmacology, 6*(1), 61–67.

Kaduszkiewicz, H., Zimmermann, T., Beck-Bornholdt, H. P., & van den Bussche, H. (2005). Cholinesterase inhibitors for patients with Alzheimer's disease: Systematic review of randomised clinical trials. *British Medical Journal, 331*(7512), 321–323.

Kemp, S., Biswas, R., Neumann, V., & Coughlan, A. (2004). The value of melatonin for sleep disorders occurring post-head injury: A pilot RCT. *Brain Injury, 18*(9), 911–919.

Kessler, J., Thiel, A., Karbe, H., & Heiss, W. D. (2000). Piracetam improves activated blood flow and facilitates rehabilitation of poststroke aphasic patients. *Stroke, 31*(9), 2112–2116.

Kidwell, C. S., Liebeskind, D. S., Starkman, S., & Saver, J. L. (2001). Trends in acute ischemic stroke trials through the 20th century. *Stroke, 32*(6), 1349–1359.

Koch, H. J., Szecsey, A., & Haen, E. (2004). NMDA-antagonism (memantine): An alternative pharmacological therapeutic principle in Alzheimer's and vascular dementia. *Current Pharmaceutical Design, 10*(3), 253–259.

Kraus, M. F., Smith, G. S., Butters, M., Donnell, A. J., Dixon, E., Yilong, C., et al. (2005). Effects of the dopaminergic agent and NMDA receptor antagonist amantadine on cognitive function, cerebral glucose metabolism and D2 receptor availability in chronic traumatic brain injury: A study using positron emission tomography (PET). *Brain Injury, 19*(7), 471–479.

Krystal, J. H., Tolin, D. F., Sanacora, G., Castner, S. A., Williams, G. V., Aikins, D. E., et al. (2009). Neuroplasticity as a target for the pharmacotherapy for anxiety disorders, mood disorders, and schizophrenia. *Drug Discovery Today, 14*(13/14), 690–697.

Lazar, R. M., Fitzsimmons, B. F., Marshall, R. S., Berman, M. F., Bustillo, M. A., Young, W. L., et al. (2002). Reemergence of stroke deficits with midazolam challenge. *Stroke, 33*(1), 283–285.

Lipska, B. K., Khaing, Z. Z., Weickert, C. S., & Weinberger, D. R. (2001). BDNF mRNA expression in rat hippocampus and prefrontal cortex: Effects of neonatal ventral hippocampal damage and antipsychotic drugs. *European Journal of Neuroscience, 14*(1), 135–144.

Lu, B., & Chow, A. (1999). Neurotrophins and hippocampal synaptic transmission and plasticity. *Journal of Neuroscience Research, 58*(1), 76–87.

Lynch, G. (2006). Glutamate-based therapeutic approaches: AMPAkines. *Current Opinion in Pharmacology, 6*(1), 82–88.

Malberg, J. E. (2004). Implications of adult hippocampal neurogenesis in antidepressant action. *Journal of Psychiatry and Neuroscience, 29*(3), 196–205.

Malberg, J. E., Eisch, A. J., Nestler, E. J., & Duman, R. S. (2000). Chronic antidepressant treatment increases neurogenesis in adult rat hippocampus. *Journal of Neuroscience, 20*(24), 9104–9110.

Martinsson, I., Wahlgreen, N., & Hardemark, H.-G. (2003). Amphetamines for improving recovery after stroke: Review. *Cochrane Database of Systematic Reviews*, Issue 3, Art. No. CD002090.

Mattson, M. P., Maudsley, S., & Martin, B. (2004). BDNF and 5-HT: A dynamic duo in age-related neuronal plasticity and neurodegenerative disorders. *Trends in Neurosciences, 27*(10), 589–594.

Maubach, K. A. (2006). The GABA(a) receptor as a potential target for the treatment of cognitive dysfunction. *Drugs of the Future, 31*(2), 151–162.

McShane, R., Areosa Sastre, A., & Minakaran, N. (2006). Memantine for dementia. *Cochrane Database of Systematic Reviews*, Issue 2, Art. No. CD003154.

Meythaler, J. M., Brunner, R. C., Johnson, A., & Novack, T. A. (2002). Amantadine to improve neurorecovery in traumatic brain injury-associated diffuse axonal injury: A pilot double-blind randomized trial. *Journal of Head Trauma Rehabilitation, 17*(4), 300–313.

Meythaler, J. M., Depalma, L., Devivo, M. J., Guin-Renfroe, S., & Novack, T. A. (2001). Sertraline to improve arousal and alertness in severe traumatic brain injury secondary to motor vehicle crashes. *Brain Injury, 15*(4), 321–331.

Micale, V., Incognito, T., Ignoto, A., Rampello, L., Sparta, M., & Drago, F. (2006). Dopaminergic drugs may counteract behavioral and biochemical changes induced by models of brain injury. *European Neuropsychopharmacology, 16*(3), 195–203.

Minkeviciene, R., Banerjee, P., & Tanila, H. (2004). Memantine improves spatial learning in a transgenic mouse model of Alzheimer's disease. *Journal of Pharmacology and Experimental Therapeutics, 311*(2), 677–682.

Mirakur, A., Moorhead, T. W. J., Stanfield, A. C., McKirdy, J., Sussman, J. E. D., Hall, J., et al. (2009). *Biological Psychiatry, 66*, 293–297.

Mitchell, E. S., & Neumaier, J. F. (2005). 5-HT6 receptors: A novel target for cognitive enhancement. *Pharmacology and Therapeutics, 108*(3), 320–333.

Moller, A. (2006). *Neural plasticity and disorders of the nervous system.* Cambridge, UK: Cambridge University Press.

Murphy, K. J., Foley, A. G., O'Connell, A. W., & Regan, C. M. (2006). Chronic exposure of rats to cognition enhancing drugs produces a neuroplastic response identical to that obtained by complex environment rearing. *Neuropsychopharmacology, 31*(1), 90–100.

Nestler, E. J., Barrot, M., DiLeone, R. J., Eisch, A. J., Gold, S. J., & Monteggia, L. M. (2002). Neurobiology of depression. *Neuron, 34*(1), 13–25.

Nibuya, M., Morinobu, S., & Duman, R. S. (1995). Regulation of BDNF and TRKB messenger-RNA in rat-brain by chronic electroconvulsive seizure and antidepressant drug treatments. *Journal of Neuroscience, 15*(11), 7539–7547.

Nitsche, M. A., Kuo, M.-F., Karrasch, R., Wächter, B., Leibetanz, D., & Paulus, W. (2009). Serotonin affects transcranial direct current-induced neuroplasticity in humans. *Biological Psychiatry, 66*, 503–508.

Nitsche, M. A., Lampe, C., Antal, A., Liebetanz, D., Lang, N., Tergau, F., et al. (2006). Dopaminergic modulation of long-lasting direct current-induced cortical excitability changes in the human motor cortex. *European Journal of Neuroscience, 23*(6), 1651–1657.

O'Dell, D. M., Gibson, C. J., Wilson, M. S., DeFord, S. M., & Hamm, R. J. (2000). Positive and negative modulation of the GABA(a) receptor and outcome after traumatic brain injury in rats. *Brain Research, 861*(2), 325–332.

Overshott, R., & Burns, A. (2005). Treatment of dementia. *Journal of Neurology, Neurosurgery and Psychiatry, 76*, V53–V59.

Parsons, C. G., Danysz, W., & Quack, G. (1999). Memantine is a clinically well tolerated *N*-methyl-D-aspartate (NMDA) receptor antagonist: A review of preclinical data. *Neuropharmacology, 38*(6), 735–767.

Pashek, G. V., & Bachman, D. L. (2003). Cognitive, linguistic, and motor speech effects of donepezil hydrochloride in a patient with stroke-related aphasia and apraxia of speech. *Brain and Language, 87*(1), 179–180.

Perna, R. (2006). Brain injury: Benzodiazepines, antipsychotics, and functional recovery. *Journal of Head Trauma Rehabilitation, 21*(1), 82–84.

Pillai, A., Terry, A. V., & Mahadik, S. P. (2006). Differential effects of long-term treatment with typical and atypical antipsychotics on NGF and BDNF levels in rat striatum and hippocampus. *Schizophrenia Research, 82*(1), 95–106.

Plenger, P. M., Dixon, C. E., Castillo, R. M., Frankowski, R. F., Yablon, S. A., & Levin, H. S. (1996). Subacute methylphenidate treatment for moderate to moderately severe traumatic brain injury: A preliminary double-blind placebo-controlled study. *Archives of Physical Medicine and Rehabilitation, 77*(6), 536–540.

Plewnia, C., Bartels, M., Cohen, L., & Gerloff, C. (2001). Noradrenergic modulation of human cortex excitability by the presynaptic alpha(2)-antagonist yohimbine. *Neuroscience Letters, 307*(1), 41–44.

Plewnia, C., Hoppe, J., Hiemke, C., Bartels, M., Cohen, L. G., & Gerloff, C. (2002). Enhancement of human cortico-motoneuronal excitability by the selective norepinephrine reuptake inhibitor reboxetine. *Neuroscience Letters, 330*(3), 231–234.

Rakic, P. (2002). Neurogenesis in adult primates. In M. A. Hofman, G. J. Boer, A. J. G. D. Holtmaat, E. J. W. Van Someren, J. Verhaagen, & D. F. Swaab (Eds.), *Progress in brain research: Vol. 138. Plasticity in the adult brain: From genes to neurotherapy* (pp. 3–16). Amsterdam: Elsevier.

Reding, M. J., Orto, L. A., Winter, S. W., Fortuna, I. M., Diponte, P., & McDowell, F. H. (1986). Antidepressant therapy after stroke: A double-blind trial. *Archives of Neurology, 43*(8), 763–765.

Reding, M. J., Solomon, B., & Borucki, S. (1995). Effect of dextroamphetamine on motor recovery after stroke. *Neurology, 45*(4), A222.

Russo-Neustadt, A., Beard, R. C., & Cotman, C. W. (1999). Exercise, antidepressant medications, and enhanced brain derived neurotrophic factor expression. *Neuropsychopharmacology, 21*(5), 679–682.

Scheiderer, C. L., Dobrunz, L. E., & McMahon, L. L. (2004). Novel form of long-term synaptic depression in rat hippocampus induced by activation of alpha 1 adrenergic receptors. *Journal of Neurophysiology, 91*(2), 1071–1077.

Schwenkreis, P., Witscher, K., Janssen, F., Addo, A., Dertwinkel, R., Zenz, M., et al. (1999). Influence of the *N*-methyl-D-aspartate antagonist memantine on human motor cortex excitabirity. *Neuroscience Letters, 270*(3), 137–140.

Shearman, E., Rossi, S., Szasz, B., Juranyi, Z., Fallon, S., Pomara, N., et al. (2006). Changes in cerebral neurotransmitters and metabolites induced by acute donepezil and memantine administrations: A microdialysis study. *Brain Research Bulletin, 69*(2), 204–213.

Silva, J. A. C. (2004). From restoration of neuroplasticity to the treatment of depression: Clinical experience. *European Neuropsychopharmacology, 14*, S511–S521.

Sonde, L., Nordstrom, M., Nilsson, C. G., Lokk, J., & Viitanen, M. (2001). A double-blind placebo-controlled study of the effects of amphetamine and physiotherapy after stroke. *Cerebrovascular Diseases, 12*(3), 253–257.

Stroemer, R. P., Kent, T. A., & Hulsebosch, C. E. (1998). Enhanced neocortical neural sprouting, synaptogenesis, and behavioral recovery with D-amphetamine therapy after neocortical infarction in rats. *Stroke, 29*(11), 2381–2393.

Treig, T., Werner, C., Sachse, M., & Hesse, S. (2003). No benefit from D-amphetamine when added to physiotherapy after stroke: A randomized, placebo-controlled study. *Clinical Rehabilitation, 17*(6), 590–599.

Van Sickle, B. J., Cox, A. S., Schak, K., Greenfield, L. J., & Tietz, E. I. (2002). Chronic benzodiazepine administration alters hippocampal CA1 neuron excitability: NMDA receptor function and expression. *Neuropharmacology, 43*(4), 595–606.

Verbois, S. L., Scheff, S. W., & Pauly, J. R. (2003). Chronic nicotine treatment attenuates alpha 7 nicotinic receptor deficits following traumatic brain injury. *Neuropharmacology, 44*(2), 224–233.

Wakade, C. G., Mahadik, S. P., Waller, J. L., & Chiu, F. C. (2002). Atypical neuroleptics stimulate neurogenesis in adult rat brain. *Journal of Neuroscience Research, 69*(1), 72–79.

Walker-Batson, D., Curtis, S., Natarajan, R., Ford, J., Dronkers, N., Salmeron, E., et al. (2001). A double-blind, placebo-controlled study of the use of amphetamine in the treatment of aphasia. *Stroke, 32*(9), 2093–2097.

Walker-Batson, D., Smith, P., Curtis, S., Unwin, H., & Greenlee, R. (1995). Amphetamine paired with physical therapy accelerates motor recovery after stroke: Further evidence. *Stroke, 26*(12), 2254–2259.

Whyte, J., Hart, T., Vaccaro, M., Grieb-Neff, P., Risser, A., Polansky, M., et al. (2004). Effects of methylphenidate on attention deficits after traumatic brain injury: A multidimensional randomized controlled trial. *American Journal of Physical Medicine and Rehabilitation, 83*(6), 401–420.

Wilson, M. S., Gibson, C. J., & Hamm, R. J. (2003). Haloperidol, but not olanzapine, impairs cognitive performance after traumatic brain injury in rats. *American Journal of Physical Medicine and Rehabilitation, 82*(11), 871–879.

Winblad, B. (2005). Piracetam: A review of pharmacological properties and clinical uses. *CNS Drug Reviews, 11*(2), 169–182.

Windle, V., & Corbett, D. (2005). Fluoxetine and recovery of motor function after focal ischemia in rats. *Brain Research, 1044*(1), 25–32.

Xu, H. Y., Chen, Z., He, J., Haimanot, S., Li, X. K., Dyck, L., et al. (2006). Synergetic effects of quetiapine and venlafaxine in preventing the chronic restraint stress-induced decrease in cell proliferation and BDNF expression in rat hippocampus. *Hippocampus, 16*(6), 551–559.

Yuan, J. Y., & Yankner, B. A. (2000). Apoptosis in the nervous system. *Nature, 407*(6805), 802–809.

Zajaczkowski, W., Quack, G., & Danysz, W. (1996). Infusion of (+)-MK-801 and memantine: Contrasting effects on radial maze learning in rats with entorhinal cortex lesion. *European Journal of Pharmacology, 296*(3), 239–246.

Zhang, L., Plotkin, R. C., Wang, G., Sandel, M. E., & Lee, S. (2004). Cholinergic augmentation with donepezil enhances recovery in short-term memory and sustained attention after traumatic brain injury. *Archives of Physical Medicine and Rehabilitation, 85*(7), 1050–1055.

Zhao, C. S., Puurunen, K., Schallert, T., Sivenius, J., & Jolkkonen, J. (2005). Behavioral and histological effects of chronic antipsychotic and antidepressant drug treatment in aged rats with focal ischemic brain injury. *Behavioural Brain Research, 158*(2), 211–220.

Zhu, J., Hamm, R. J., Reeves, T. M., Povlishock, J. T., & Phillips, L. L. (2000). Postinjury administration of D-deprenyl improves cognitive function and enhances neuroplasticity after traumatic brain injury. *Experimental Neurology, 166*(1), 136–152.

Index

The letter *f* following a page number indicates figure; the letter *t* indicates table.

B

D

E

N

Q

R

S

W